Documenting Occupational Therapy Practice

SECOND EDITION

Karen M. Sames, MBA, OTR/L, FAOTA

*Associate Professor of Occupational Science
and Occupational Therapy
St. Catherine University
St. Paul, Minnesota*

Pearson

Boston   Columbus   Indianapolis   New York   San Francisco   Upper Saddle River
Amsterdam   Cape Town   Dubai   London   Madrid   Milan   Munich   Paris   Montreal   Toronto
Delhi   Mexico City   Sao Paulo   Sydney   Hong Kong   Seoul   Singapore   Taipei   Tokyo

Library of Congress Cataloging-in-Publication Data

Sames, Karen M.
  Documenting occupational therapy practice / Karen M. Sames. — 2nd ed.
     p. ; cm.
  Includes bibliographical references and index.
  ISBN 0-13-199948-6
  1. Occupational therapy—Practice. 2. Medical records. 3. Medical protocols. I. Title.
  [DNLM: 1. Occupational Therapy—organization & administration. 2. Medical Records—standards.
WB 555 S187d 2010]

  RM735.4.S264 2010
  615.8'515—dc22

                                                                    2009023194

Publisher: Julie Alexander
Publisher's Assistant: Regina Bruno
Editor-in-Chief: Mark Cohen
Development Editor: Melissa Kerian
Assistant Editor: Nicole Ragonese
Director of Marketing: Karen Allman
Executive Marketing Manager: Katrin Beacom
Marketing Specialist: Michael Sirinides
Senior Marketing Assistant: Judy Noh
Production Manager: Fran Russello

Cover Art Director: Jayne Conte
Cover Designer: Bruce Kenselaar
Cover Art: Agb\Shutterstock; Photo courtesy of
   Karen M. Sames; Courtesy of www.istockphoto.com
Full-Service Project Management: Swapnil K. Vaidya
Composition: GGS Higher Education Resources,
   A division of PreMedia Global, Inc.
Printer/Binder: Edwards Brothers, Inc.
Cover Printer: Lehigh-Phoenix Color Corp.
Text Font: 10/12, Melior

Credits and acknowledgments borrowed from other sources and reproduced, with permission, in this textbook appear on appropriate page within text.

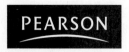

www.pearsonhighered.com

10 9 8 7 6 5 4 3 2 1
ISBN 10:   0-13-199948-6
ISBN 13: 978-0-13-199948-0

CONTENTS

▼ SECTION II ▼
ETHICAL AND LEGAL CONSIDERATIONS   53

▼ SECTION IV ▼

SCHOOL SYSTEM DOCUMENTATION   175

PREFACE

For many years, I wished for a book that could be used by students to learn about documentation and at the same time be used by clinicians to improve the quality of documentation in the field. Eventually, I realized that I could, and should, write that book. As a college professor, I spend a great deal of time reading written work produced by occupational therapy students. As a peer reviewer, I read client charts that insurance companies were unsure about—charts that were so poorly written that the insurers could not decide whether the services were medically necessary and appropriate.

For these reasons, I decided to begin the long and challenging task of writing this book. It took over 3 years from the time I started talking about writing it to the actual printing of the first edition of the book. It took another 3 years to revise it for the second edition. Federal rules and professional standards changed while I was writing this book, forcing me to revise and add topics as the book evolved.

During the process of writing this book, I learned even more about writing. I learned that I write better in the morning than in the afternoon. I learned that I have difficulty knowing when to use the word "that" (refers to a specific object) as opposed to the word "which" (not specific to an object). I learned about comma and semicolon placement in sentences. Just because I pause when I speak the sentence out loud does not mean that rules of proper punctuation call for a comma. I learned the difference between a hyphen, an em dash, and an en dash. Finally, I learned to say "on the basis of," instead of "based on."

My hope for this book is that it gets used; that it is not simply put up on a shelf. I want it to be written in, to have pages flagged, and to have the spine well broken from repeated use. Normally, I would be appalled at the vision of food-stained, rumpled pages in a book. But I think this book is different. If it retains its original pristine condition, then it hasn't served its reader well.

ACKNOWLEDGMENTS

This book would not have been possible without the help and support of several people. First, I want to thank the editorial staff at Pearson Health Science, especially Melissa Kerian and Mark Cohen, for their persistence and willingness to let me write this book in my own voice. I owe many thanks to Swapnil K. Vaidya and his team at GGS Higher Education Resources, a division of PreMedia Global, Inc., for their work in copyediting the text. The drafts of this book were sent by Pearson Health Science to many unnamed reviewers who were occupational therapy and occupational therapy assistant practitioners and educators. Because each reviewer read the draft from a different perspective, some of the feedback conflicted from one reviewer to the next. I did my best to accommodate as much of the feedback I was given as possible, but ultimately my revisions were based on what I thought was important. I'd like to acknowledge all the reviewers for this book whose feedback was critical in my revision. I appreciate the time it took each of them to read and comment on the text, their candor in criticizing it, and the overwhelming encouragement they provided.

I was fortunate to participate in several writers' retreats while working on the revision of this book. I want to thank the leaders of the retreats, Cecelia Conchar Farr, JoAnn Cavalero, and Gabrielle Civil for providing such a supportive environment in which to write. In addition, the other women at the retreat helped provide the right balance of privacy, encouragement, humor, and food to keep me writing. The retreat was sponsored by St. Catherine University (formerly The College of St. Catherine), championed by Dean Susan Cochrane, and sustained by the generous gifts of the Denny family.

I would also like to thank the faculty and staff of the Department of Occupational Science and Occupational Therapy of St. Catherine University for their continuous support during the course of my writing. I am so fortunate to work in an environment where people encourage each other and help each other out. In particular, I want to thank Linda Buxell, Nancy Flinn, MaryLou Henderson, Kathleen Matuska, Brenda Frie, and Paula Rabaey for being sounding boards when I needed them and for the ideas they shared with me about writing in general, and writing this book in particular. I want to thank Barb Gilbertson for serving as a hand model for the cover of this book.

Finally, I want to thank my family. My husband Wayne, son Ethan (the English major), and younger daughter Emily provided quiet support. My older daughter Amanda provided very vocal criticism with just the right touch of humor to keep me going.

Karen M. Sames

REVIEWERS

SECOND EDITION

Diane Anderson, MPH, OTR/L
Chair, Occupational Therapy
College of St. Scholastica
Duluth, Minnesota

Gail Bass, Ph.D., OTR/L
Assistant Professor, Occupational Therapy
University of North Dakota
Grand Forks, North Dakota

Rachelle Dorne, Ed.D., OTR/L
Associate Professor, Occupational Therapy
Nova Southeastern University
Ft. Lauderdale-Davie, Florida

Catherine Emery, MS, OTR/L
Assistant Professor, Occupational Therapy
Alvernia College
Reading, Pennsylvania

Tamera K. Humbert, D.Ed., OTR/L
Associate Professor, Occupational Therapy
Elizabethtown College
Elizabethtown, Pennsylvania

Nancy A Lowenstein, MS, OTR/L, BCPR
Clinical Associate Professor, Occupational
    Therapy
Boston University
Boston, Massachusettts

Lori Reynolds, MOT, OTR/L
Assistant Professor/Fieldwork Coordinator,
    Occupational Therapy
Spalding University
Louisville, Kentucky

Katie L. Serfas, OTD, OTR/L
Clinical Assistant Professor, Occupational
    Therapy and Occupational Science
University of Missouri-Columbia
Columbia, Missouri

Michelle M. Sheperd, MEd, OTR
Program Director, Occupational Therapy
Brown Mackie College
South Bend, Indiana

Janeene Sibla, OTD, MS, OTR/L
Director/Associate Professor Occupational
    Therapy
University of Mary
Bismarck, North Dakota

Barbara J. Williams, OT, OTR
Director/Assistant Professor, Occupational
    Therapy Program
University of Southern Indiana
Evansville, Indiana

FIRST EDITION

Alma R. Abdel-Moty, MS, OTR
Clinical Assistant Professor, Occupational
    Therapy Program
Florida International University
Miami, Florida

Gail S. Bass, OTR/L
Instructor, Occupational Therapy
University of North Dakota
Grand Forks, North Dakota

Estelle B. Breines, Ph.D., OTR, FAOTA
Former Program Chair, Department
    of Occupational Therapy
Seton Hall University
South Orange, New Jersey

Catherine C. Brennan, MA, OTRL/L, FAOTA
Consultant
St. Paul, Minnesota

William R. Croninger, MA, OTR/L
Associate Professor, Occupational Therapy
University of New England
Biddeford, Maine

Anne E. Dickerson, Ph.D., OTR/L, FAOTA
Program Chair and Professor, Occupational
    Therapy
Eastern Carolina University
Greenville, North Carolina

Hahn C. Edwards, MA, MS, OTR
Assistant Professor, Occupational Therapy
    Assistant Program
University of Southern Indiana
Evansville, Indiana

Maria Hinds, JD, MS, OT
Assistant Professor, Occupational Therapy
Florida A&M University
Tallahassee, Florida

Joyce H. McCormick, MS, OTR/L
Fieldwork Coordinator, Occupational Therapy
    Program
Pennsylvania State University—Mont Alto
Mont Alto, Pennsylvania

Deane B. McCraith, MS, OTR/L, LMFT
Clinical Associate Professor, Occupational
    Therapy
Boston University
Sargent College of Health and Rehabilitation
    Science
Boston, Massachusetts

Nichelle L. Miedema, OTR/L
Program Coordinator, Occupational Therapy
    Assistant Program
Kirkwood Community College
Cedar Rapids, Iowa

Candice Jones Mullendore, MS, OTR
Assistant Professor and Academic Fieldwork
    Coordinator, Department of Occupational
    Therapy
Creighton University
Omaha, Nebraska

Kathy Nielson, MPH, OTR/L
Professor and Director, Division of Occupational
    Science
The University of North Carolina at Chapel Hill
Chapel Hill, North Carolina

Karen B. Smith, OTR/L
Program Director, Occupational Therapy
    Assistant Program
Stanly Community College
Albermarle, North Carolina

Kathy Clark Tuminski, MA, OTR/L
Assistant Professor, Occupational Therapy
Eastern Kentucky University
Richmond, Kentucky

Joanne Wright, Ph.D., OTR/L
Program Director, Division of Occupational
    Therapy
University of Utah
Salt Lake City, Utah

INTRODUCTION: THE WHO, WHAT, WHERE, WHEN, AND WHY OF DOCUMENTATION

As occupational therapy practitioners, we work with a variety of clients in a variety of settings. In every setting in which we use our skills as trained professionals, we are asked to document what we do in some way. We may do clinical documentation that becomes part of a medical record. We may contribute to the development of an Individual Education Program (IEP) for a grade school student. We may write a report summarizing our activity as a consultant to a company. It is imperative that our writing demonstrates a high level of professionalism.

▼ WHO ▼

The key to professional writing is to know who we are writing for as well as who we are writing about. As indicated earlier, we write for multiple audiences. Some potential audiences include the intervention team, the client and/or surrogates (caregivers, family, or guardians), facility quality management personnel, third-party payers, peer reviewers, accreditation surveyors, administrators, and lawyers. Because the potential audience for our documentation extends far beyond our peers, it is important that we choose our words very carefully. I know of one occupational therapist who mentally says to herself before putting pen to paper, "Ladies and gentlemen of the jury, . . . " Then she begins her documentation. It forces her to think about how her words may be interpreted by others.

▼ WHAT ▼

On my first occupational therapy job, a director of nursing told me repeatedly, "If it's not documented, it didn't happen." It was like her personal mantra. As much as I got tired of hearing it, I have to admit she was right. It was good advice. If I had to be absent from work, and a substitute had to step in for me, I wanted the substitute to be fully informed about what things have been tried already and in what direction I wanted the intervention to proceed. In order for this to happen, there must be accurate, complete, and clear documentation of what has transpired in occupational therapy thus far. Also, documentation that is written at the time of an event is stronger evidence in a court of law than one's memory. How many of you can remember exactly what you did last Tuesday at 10:00 in the morning? A month ago? Eighteen months ago? Who were you with? What were you doing? Were you successful at whatever you were doing? How much force did you use? You get the picture?

Not only do you want to document what was done, but you also want to document the client's reaction to the intervention. Think of it as painting a verbal picture of the occupational therapy session for the reader. You want to document what instructions were given (e.g., for a home program, splint use and care, adaptive equipment use and care, or instructions to caregivers) and whether the person receiving instructions appeared to understand those instructions. Finally, you want to document what the plan is for future occupational therapy service delivery.

With so much to document, it might become somewhat of a balancing act between working hands-on with a client and documenting that intervention. Most occupational therapists go into the profession because they want to help people. I doubt any become occupational therapists because they love to write notes all day long. In addition, increasing competition for health care dollars have pushed some clinics to develop productivity standards for the amount of billable services each clinician needs to provide each day. This results in less time available for doing documentation. Today, a clinician in a clinical setting will generally spend 6 hours or more (out of an 8-hour day) with clients. The rest of the time is usually for meetings and documentation. In educational or community settings, the time spent with clients may be 7 hours or more in an 8-hour day. However, needing to document so much of what we do does not mean we have to spend a lot of time doing it. Sections III and IV of this book will show you some ways of documenting in an efficient and effective manner.

▼ WHERE ▼

In clinical settings, each client has his or her own clinical record (chart). The chart may be electronic or paper based. Occupational therapy practitioners may document in a section of the chart dedicated to rehabilitation or therapies. In some settings, integrated notes are done, so that each profession documents progress in a progress note section of the chart that is compiled chronologically regardless of which professional is writing. It is important to follow facility standards for where and when to write in the client's chart, regardless of whether the chart is on a computer or is paper based. Standards for good documentation do not change when the format (electronic or paper) changes.

In educational settings, the Individualized Education Program (IEP) or Individualized Family Service Plan (IFSP) is written annually and reviewed every 6 months. The evaluation report, present levels of performance, and occupational therapy goals are integrated into those documents. The IEP or IFSP then goes into the student's educational record. If the school district is billing third-party payers for occupational therapy services, additional documentation may be required. The school district will have policies for the occupational therapist regarding where any other documentation will be filed and retained.

In addition to the official clinical or educational record, some occupational therapy departments retain copies of everything that is in the official record in a departmental file. These departmental files may also contain test forms, attendance records, and other nonofficial documents. Chapter 5 will go into more detail about records retention.

▼ WHEN ▼

Documentation is typically done as close to the time of service as possible. Some occupational therapists reserve the last 5 minutes or so of the intervention session to document in the client's chart. This works fine for contact or progress notes, but may not be sufficient for doing larger documents such as evaluation or discontinuation reports. These documents are usually done when there are no clients being treated such as at the beginning or end of the day or over the lunch hour. In some settings, the occupational therapist will dictate evaluation or discontinuation notes to be transcribed by secretarial staff. Others write them out longhand or on a desktop, laptop, or handheld computer.

The longer the time span from when the evaluation or intervention occurred to when the occupational therapist sits down to write about it, the more the chance that something will be forgotten. When possible, writing directly in the client's chart at the time of service delivery is best. However, this is not always possible. Some occupational therapists carry small notebooks or pieces of paper with them in their pockets, and jot quick notes about the clients they see during the day. Others use handheld computers. This does help them remember more clearly what happened with each client. As you can imagine, if an occupational therapist sees 12 clients in a day, by the end of the day it can be difficult to remember who said or did what.

Occupational therapists document for many reasons. We document to show what has happened to the client in a chronological sequence. We want to show what happened first, then second, then the next thing, and so on. Some regulatory and accrediting bodies want to see that things happened in a clinically sound sequence. For example, if you were working with a client recovering from a severe head injury, you would want to show that the client is aware of safety precautions to take when using a knife before you work on how to use a knife. The client's chart will tell any third-party reviewer the story of that client's recovery following an illness or injury, or a client's development in the case of a developmental delay.

We document to show our high level of clinical reasoning. Someone walking by the occupational therapy clinic could see the occupational therapist watching a client make buttered toast. That person might think, "She went to college for how many years to teach that? I could do that without any training." If that person could read the chart, he or she would see that the occupational therapist was really working on sequencing a task, manipulating utensils, safety awareness, and/or energy conservation. The task of buttering toast represents many different learning opportunities for the client. There is often more to occupational therapy than meets the eye.

We document to inform others on the intervention team about what happened during an intervention session. Everyone is busy, we work different shifts, and there is not always time for each of us to talk to other caregivers about each client. By writing down the essence of what happened in the intervention session, others on the team can be informed in their own time. By the same token, we can read the chart and find out what happened that day in other therapy services, or in the lab, medical imaging, or nursing.

We document to demonstrate the effectiveness of occupational therapy for third-party payers. This is a critically important reason to document well, as payment is often based on the quality of the documentation. Third-party payers such as the government (Medicare, Medicaid, CHAMPUS, and other programs) and private insurers (managed care, worker's compensation, indemnity) want to be sure that they are getting what they paid for—results. A payer virtually never observes the client directly, but relies on the documentation of the services delivered to determine effectiveness. If the payers cannot see progress in the documentation, they will often terminate payment, which in effect terminates services, even if you believe the client could still benefit from further services.

Last, but not least, we document for legal reasons. As stated earlier, the medical record, anything written at the time, is stronger evidence of what happened than anything we can remember from a year or two ago. In many states, a client can bring forward a malpractice case up to 2 years after the incident occurred. In those 2 years, we could have treated more than a hundred other clients. Will we remember exactly what we did with that client on that day, or will all the other clients we have seen since then cloud our memory? Depending on what we write, and how well we write it, the clinical record can be used to protect, or to hurt, us as practitioners. There are ways to ensure that what we write is more likely to help than hurt us, and this book addresses them.

▼ STRUCTURE OF THE BOOK ▼

Section I of this book deals with some of the mechanics of writing. It includes tips on word usage, the use of frames of reference, abbreviations, and jargon. It also takes a broad look at how the language of the profession is ever evolving and describes both internal and external influences on the use of language. This section also includes pointers on professional communication in general.

The second section focuses on the ethical and legal issues around documentation, such as confidentiality, record retention, fraud, and plagiarism. This provides a different yet necessary perspective on documentation: payers, reviewers, and attorneys.

Section III deals with the documentation of the occupational therapy process in a clinical setting. Clinical settings include all occupational therapy practice venues where third-party reimbursement is sought, such as in a hospital, nursing home, clinic, or psychiatric program. Usually, in a clinical setting, there is a physician order or referral, and services are billed for in some way. This is a very broad description of a clinical setting. It excludes services that are paid for with grant money or other funding sources that do not require physician oversight. This section takes you through the occupational therapy process and explains the types of documentation completed at each step of the process. Each chapter describes a type of documentation and includes sections on role delineation and Medicare standards as they apply to that type documentation.

The fourth section is about documentation in school systems. While many school systems are now billing third-party payers to recoup the costs of some therapy services, there are also requirements for certain types of documentation that are unique to school-based services. This chapter addresses only the documentation requirements of school systems.

The last section deals with administrative documentation. Examples of administrative documentation include policies and procedures, incident reports, meeting minutes, job descriptions, grant writing, and job descriptions. Occupational therapy staff write some of these types of documents, while supervisors and managers generally write others.

If you are reading this book as a required text for a course in an occupational therapy educational program, do not be surprised if your instructor does not require you to read each chapter and do each exercise, in the order in which the chapters appear in this text. In an introductory course in occupational therapy, you may only be assigned the first three or four sections. However, I hope that at some point in your educational program, you will have a chance to work with chapters in the rest of the book. That means that you should hang on to this book even when the course is over. You will undoubtedly have opportunities to practice documentation in several courses in your curriculum, and this book will be a good reference to look back at as you draft your assignments.

If you are a clinician reading this book, I congratulate you on your dedication to the profession and to continuing competence. Depending on how long it has been since you were in school, some of the information in the book will be new to you, some merely a refresher. Each chapter of the book can stand on its own, and you can choose the chapter or chapters on which you want to concentrate. You will also find the material in the appendices especially helpful.

Throughout the book there are exercises to help you develop your skills in documentation. Answers to selected exercises are included in Appendix A. While comparing your answers to those in the book can be a good learning experience, it may be even more helpful to get feedback on your answers from an instructor or colleague. An experienced occupational therapist can provide feedback on the subtle nuances that different wording can have on a reader.

As you work through the sections of this book, you will become familiar with principles of good documentation in clinical and educational settings. You will also learn about other types of documentation that occupational therapists may be called on to write during their careers. People form opinions about you as a professional based on how well or how poorly you write. If you want to be thought of as a talented, competent, and skilled professional, you must write like one.

SECTION I

Use of Language

▼ INTRODUCTION ▼

Documentation requires the use of written words. To document well, one must write well. This involves selecting words that will have meaning to the reader and making the documentation clear, accurate, and relevant to the situation. In the first section of this book, general issues about writing are discussed.

How well you write is one way that others will judge your professionalism. If you write poorly, use outdated terms or excessive jargon, use too many abbreviations, or leave out words, people will think you are either careless or lacking in skill. Appendix B contains a review of general grammar and spelling considerations that may be a good review for some readers. The American Occupational Therapy Association (2002; 2008) has developed a framework for occupational therapy practice that can provide some guidance on the use of terms. Different models or frames of reference used in occupational therapy will shape the way occupational therapists write about clinical or educational progress.

▼ PROFESSIONAL DOCUMENTATION ▼

When documenting occupational therapy practice, it is essential to use language appropriately. Occupational therapy practitioners work in many settings. Some settings, such as hospitals, long-term care, school systems, or home health have very specific standards for content. Other settings, such as homeless shelters, prisons, or consulting do not have setting-specific standards, so occupational therapy practitioners may have to create documentation systems to fit the needs of the setting. The American Occupational Therapy Association (AOTA) has guidelines for documentation that can be used in any setting (AOTA, 2007).

In clinical settings such as hospitals, long-term care facilities, home health, outpatient clinics, and psychiatric programs, each step of the occupational therapy process is documented. A referral or physician's order for occupational therapy intervention is typically the first item documented in a clinical record. If an occupational therapy practitioner conducts a screening or makes initial contact with a client, it is documented as a contact note. The occupational therapy evaluation is documented as an evaluation report or evaluation summary. Next, an intervention plan is created. As occupational therapy intervention is provided to the client, the occupational therapy practitioner records progress notes. When occupational therapy intervention is finished, the outcome of that intervention is documented in a discontinuation summary. Section III of this book details these documents.

In educational settings, occupational therapists contribute to team-based documentation of services provided to children with special needs. The services provided to infants and toddlers are documented in an Individualized Family Service Plan (IFSP). The services provided to children between the ages of 3 and 21 are documented in an Individual Education Program (IEP). In addition, every time a team meeting is called, every time a change in the IEP or IFSP is proposed, and every time a child is referred for special education intervention, there are notice and consent forms which document that the child's family has been kept informed of the process. Section IV of this book discusses these documents.

▼ STRUCTURE OF THIS SECTION OF THE BOOK ▼

Chapter 1 presents an overview of the types of written communication one might use on the job, including memos, letters, and e-mails. This chapter discusses the importance of using the proper tone, voice, and language when communicating with other professionals in the workplace. While memos, letters, and e-mails are not generally considered documentation for the purpose of documenting occupational therapy practice, they are an essential part of the work of occupational therapy practitioners. Effectively communicating in writing with referral sources, co-workers, supervisors and supervisees, and colleagues is a skill everyone needs to master.

Chapter 2 will deal with use of language, including buzzwords, jargon, and abbreviations. Lists of common abbreviations are included. This chapter is very specific to occupational therapy practice. Just as certain phrases used in everyday conversations can be trendier than others, so can certain phrases used in occupational therapy.

Chapter 3 relates the language used in documentation to the language used in the primary documents that guide the profession of occupational therapy. These documents are written by the American Occupational Therapy Association and the World Health Organization.

Chapter 4 suggests that the words chosen for documenting occupational therapy services will reflect the model or frame of reference used with a particular client. It includes a brief summary of several different models and frames of reference.

Finally, Chapter 5 includes a checklist for ensuring careful documentation. It deals specifically with documenting clearly and accurately, making the documentation relevant and documenting any exceptions to the way the therapist expected things to go.

The lessons learned in these chapters will help improve documentation regardless of the setting in which the occupational therapy clinician or student works. What is important to remember is that you must always choose your words carefully.

REFERENCES

American Occupational Therapy Association. (2002). Occupational therapy practice framework: Domain and practice. *American Journal of Occupational Therapy, 56,* 609–639.

American Occupational Therapy Association. (2007). *Guidelines for documentation of occupational therapy.* Retrieved June, 16, 2008, from http://www.aota.org/Practitioners/Official/Guidelines/41257.aspx

American Occupational Therapy Association. (2008). Occupational therapy practice framework: Domain and process (2nd ed.). *American Journal of Occupational Therapy, 62,* 625–683.

CHAPTER 1

Professional Communication

Occupational therapy practitioners communicate with others in the workplace using several methods including face-to-face discussions, letters, memos, e-mails, and phone calls. The word choices and tone of the writing or speech used in professional, or formal, communication are very different from those used with friends.

Professional communication requires a level of respect and formality that is not required while e-mailing or talking to friends (Sames, 2008). Professional communication uses complete sentences, and avoids slang or emotionally charged words. Informal communication often uses slang and emotionally charged words, may use phrases and emoticons, and is usually directed toward someone known by the speaker/writer (Sames, 2008). Professional writing is more serious in tone, and more polite (Online Writing Laboratory [OWL] at Purdue University, 2004). When writing a letter to appeal a denial of coverage, an evaluation report, a notice and consent form, or a discontinuation summary, the writer may or may not know the person reading it, so this is where first impressions count (Sames).

Specific standards may govern the contents of formal documentation. For example, the Individuals with Disabilities Education Act (IDEA) requires that specific items be included on the IFSP, and Medicare requires specific documentation elements for occupational therapy reimbursement in long-term care. The Joint Commission on Accreditation of Health Organizations (JCAHO) recommends avoiding the use of certain abbreviations because of the likelihood of medical errors caused by misreading abbreviations that are remarkably close in appearance to each other (JCAHO, 2009). In addition, one's employer may further direct the method (electronic or paper and pen), timing, placement, and word choices of the documentation (Sames, 2008).

▼ TONE ▼

Tone is the most important consideration in professional communication, whether it is spoken or written. In writing, the message has to stand alone, without the benefit of facial expression or gestures that convey meaning in oral communication. Readers will interpret what is written through their own lens, depending on their own practice setting, educational level, and cultural background (Sames, in press). The writer has to consider how the reader is likely to interpret the message. Try to be honest and respectful but, at the same time, not condescending (OWL at Purdue University, 2004). For example, which of the following statements sounds more professional?

- I am appealing this coverage determination because, based on my clinical judgment, it is critical that Mrs. Rameriz receive additional occupational therapy services. I know when a client has reached her full potential, and this client has NOT yet reached her full potential.
- I am appealing this coverage determination because this client has not achieved her goal of independence in meal preparation, which is essential if she is to return to her previous living situation.

Clearly, the second statement is less condescending, yet honest and respectful. The first statement screams that the writer knows more than the reader, and has some underlying angry feelings toward the person who made the initial coverage decision.

The above example also shows emphasis in the form of a word in all capital letters. Using all capitals in writing is like shouting in oral communication (Yale University, n.d.). If you want to emphasize a word or a point, some people suggest putting an *asterisk* around the word or words (Yale University). Another way to show emphasis is to put the most important idea first in the letter, paragraph, or sentence (OWL at Purdue University, 2004). The amount of space you devote to a particular idea also conveys importance (OWL at Purdue University).

▼ ACTIVE VOICE ▼

In professional writing, an active voice is preferred to a passive voice. Using active voice in a sentence means that the person doing the action comes first, then the action (O'Conner, 1996). Active voice is usually more direct and clear than passive voice. Typically, a sentence written in passive voice will have a verb phrase using a "be" word (e.g., have been) (OWL at Purdue University, 2004). Following are two sentences that say essentially the same thing; the first is written in a passive voice, whereas the second uses an active voice.

- Self-care skills have been a concern of this client.
- This client is concerned with his self-care skills.

▼ NONDISCRIMINATORY LANGUAGE ▼

It is important to use nondiscriminatory language in professional writing (American Psychological Association, [APA], 2001 Lunsford, 2005; OWL at Purdue University, 2004). This may seem like an obvious statement, but sometimes words creep into our speech or our writing that reflect personal biases in subtle ways. All professional writing, whether it is a progress note, thank you letter to a referral source, or policy and procedure needs to be free of language that might be interpreted as sexist, racist, ageist, or otherwise biased on such factors as ethnicity, religion, disability, or sexual orientation (OWL at Purdue University). Avoid broad categorizations such as *hemiplegics*, *stroke victims*, or *the blind* when discussing a population (APA). "Person first" language (e.g., people with hemiplegia, people with visual deficits) is preferred when discussing a population with a disability. Use the adjective form of population descriptors rather than the noun form (e.g., elderly people rather than the elderly).

It is no longer acceptable to use masculine pronouns (e.g., he, his) to refer to both sexes, or to refer to all occupational therapists as she (APA, 2000). Using *he/she, s/he,* or *he or she* can be cumbersome and tedious (APA). Other pronouns that can be substituted include *person, one,* and *individual*. Another way to get around this difficulty is to restructure the sentence to use plural forms of pronouns such as *they, their,* and *them* (APA; Lunsford, 2005). The last option is to simply eliminate the pronoun, or replace it with an article (APA; Lunsford)—for example, a departmental policy that says, "Shoes must be removed before jumping in the ball pit." Of course, if you are writing in a specific person's clinical or educational record, and you know the person's gender, it is fine to use the appropriate sex-specific pronoun.

What is the best way to refer to occupational therapists and occupational therapy assistants? When referring to them in combination, the term occupational therapy practitioner may be used (AOTA, 2005). Some people prefer to spell out both levels of practice, and that is fine; it just takes a second or two longer to write out both terms. Be cautious about dropping the adjective *occupational* when talking about occupational therapy practitioners or occupational therapy program. The term therapist can refer to a psychologist, a social worker, a marriage and family counselor, and a variety of other professionals. The term therapy can refer to physical therapy, psychotherapy, nutrition therapy, or any number of other therapy programs. If, as a profession, we want other disciplines to know and respect us, we need to use our complete title at all times.

▼ MEMOS ▼

Sometimes, an occupational therapy practitioner needs to communicate with people who work on another shift or who are not available at the time the critical information needs to be conveyed, or the occupational therapist wants to confirm in writing a conversation that took place. The best way to do this is through a memo. The overall purpose of a memo is to convey information in an effective way (OWL at Purdue University, 2004). A memo may also be used in place of a cover letter when sending a packet of documents to people you know to tell them what is in the packet and why you sent it (Sabath, 2002). A formal letter is preferred if the packet is going to people you do not know.

The first part of a memo is the heading. This is what makes the memo different from a letter. According to OWL at Purdue University (2004), the heading usually contains four elements:

To: (reader's full name, sometimes includes job titles with proper capitalization)
From: (your name, sometimes includes job title)
Date: (month, day, year the memo was written)
Subject or Re: (brief explanation of the point of the memo; re is the abbreviation for regarding.)

Some word processing programs have templates for writing memos that automatically enter the date. Be sure to check the spelling of names, and be sure that you are writing to the right person. Make sure the subject is concise, and cannot be construed to mean something other than what you intended. You do not want to unnecessarily alarm the reader, but you also do not want to put the entire content of the memo in the subject line (OWL at Purdue University).

Bravemen (2006) suggests a basic five-paragraph structure for memos:

Introduction: explain the reason for the memo.
Background: establish the context.
Recommendation or request: what you want the reader to do or what you want to have happen.
Rationale: explain your reasoning behind your recommendation or request.
Conclusion: restate your position.

Make the memo both look good and sound good (Sabath, 2002). Pay attention to the rules of good grammar, such as capitalization, punctuation, and sentence construction. Use one reasonably sized font style that looks professional. Be consistent in your format, such as the indentation of the first line of each paragraph, throughout the document. Although it is generally a good rule to limit a memo to one page, do not squish everything together, decrease font size, or use smaller margins, just to make it fit on one page. If it does not look good on one page, then make it two, well-spaced pages (Sabath). It is most common for a memo to be written with 1-inch margins on all sides, and to use 10- to 12-size font. Font style is a matter of personal preference. But if you want to be viewed as professional in the workplace, use fonts that are common, such as Ariel, Verdana, Cambria or Times New Roman.

▼ LETTERS ▼

Much of the advice for writing memos also applies to writing formal letters. Because the recipient of the letter may not be an acquaintance of the writer, letters often take on an even more formal tone. In a formal letter, the heading is replaced by more detailed information.

Often a letter is written on company or organization letterhead. When writing a letter on a word processor, make sure that you start the letter down far enough on the page that what you write will not print over the letterhead. A good rule of thumb is that you should start the letter at least 2 inches down the page when using letterhead. The first line of print on a formal letter is the date on which the letter was written or completed. It should be left justified (OWL at Purdue University, 2004).

The next part of the formal letter is the sender's address. This is optional, because if the letter is printed on letterhead, the address may already be there. If you do choose to type in your address, leave one empty line between the date and your address (OWL at Purdue University, 2004).

After the sender's address, or date if the sender's address is not typed in, include the name, title, and address of the person to whom the letter is addressed (OWL at Purdue University, 2004). Sometimes this is called the inside address. According to OWL at Purdue University, the inside address is typed one line below the sender's address or 1 inch below the date, and it is always left justified. Make sure you use the proper title of the person to whom you are sending the letter.

Between the inside address and the body of your letter, you need to greet your reader. This is called the salutation (OWL at Purdue University, 2004). If you know the person to whom you are sending the letter, it is fine to greet the person by starting the letter with Dear Maria (or whatever the person's first name is). If the letter is going to someone you do not know, or to someone who holds a higher position than yours, then use the person's full name, including Mr., Dr., Ms, Professor, or other personal title. In a business letter, use a colon after the name rather than a comma. Things get a little dicey when you do not know the gender of the person to whom you are writing, and therefore do not know whether to say Mr. or Ms. When this happens, you have two choices. You can just leave off the personal title and use the person's whole name, or you can use a generic term like "To Whom it May Concern" (OWL at Purdue University).

There are several formats for business letters; the important thing is to be consistent in the format (Sabath, 2002). A block format uses a blank line between paragraphs but does not indent the first line of each paragraph (OWL at Purdue University, 2004). A semi-block format also used a blank line between paragraphs, but the first line of each paragraph is indented (OWL at Purdue University). A less formal format indents first lines of each paragraph but does not include a blank line between paragraphs.

Because a letter does not include a subject line in the heading, it is good to get right to the point and state the purpose of the letter in the first paragraph (OWL at Purdue University, 2004). The following paragraphs can include justification for the main point, and background information the reader needs. The last paragraph restates the purpose of the letter, and may include the action you are requesting the reader take (OWL at Purdue University).

The closing begins one line below the last paragraph (OWL at Purdue University, 2004). A typical closing would simply be the word "Sincerely," but "Thank you," or "Respectfully," could also be used. Notice that there is a comma after the closing word(s), and that only the first word is capitalized. Leave 3–4 lines of blank space, then type in your name and title. This allows room for your signature (OWL at Purdue University).

If you are including other documents with the letter, it is helpful to list those at the bottom of the letter. Underneath the signature, type Enc., which is short for enclosures (OWL at Purdue University, 2004).

▼ E-MAIL ▼

When time is limited, one of the fastest ways to communicate is by e-mail. E-mail has opened up a whole new way to communicate. E-mail, instant messaging, and text messaging have evolved to create new words, phrases, acronyms (e.g., LOL or CU), and emoticons (e.g., :-) [smile] or <g> [grin]), which are fine to use among friends but may be inappropriate in the workplace (Braveman, 2006; OWL at Purdue University, 2004). Professional communication, as stated earlier, is more formal. E-mails to colleagues for work purposes need to follow certain conventions.

Sabath (2002, p. 55) suggests five e-mail commandments:

1. E-mail only those people to whom your messages actually pertain (rather than entire address groups).
2. Make a point of responding to messages promptly.
3. Always use spell-check and grammar-check before sending messages.
4. Include your telephone number in your messages.
5. Learn that e-mail should be used for business rather than personal use.

E-mail is so fast and easy that it is often used in place of memos, letters, phone, and face-to-face conversations; however, it can create as many problems as it can solve in the workplace. E-mails allow the reader to interpret the message in ways the sender never intended. Box 1.1 lists some tips that can help minimize the potential for misunderstandings. A final consideration is that every e-mail system is different, and what looks properly formatted on one system may look different on another system (Sherwood, n.d.).

BOX 1.1   E-mail Tips

- Include a clear subject heading, so your message gets attention. "Update" is pretty vague unless it is followed by a description of what is being updated.
- Address the recipient in the body of the message by starting the message with the person's name.
- Create a signature that includes your name, title, and contact information. You may also include the organization's vision or slogan, or an appropriate quote.
- Be concise but clear.
- When replying to someone's message, include part or all of the sender's message to help the originator remember what he or she said. Do not include entire back-and-forth conversations.
- Respect the confidentiality of the sender. Remove unnecessary names and e-mail addresses before forwarding it on to someone else.
- Use proper spelling and grammar. Many e-mail systems have a spell-checker option.
- Respond in a timely manner. A good habit to get into is to check your work e-mail at least twice a day.
- Don't shout by using all capital letters. Don't underutilize capital letters, either. If a word or name would be capitalized in printed material, it should be capitalized in e-mail.
- Use Cc and Bcc appropriately. Cc is for including people in the message who have a stake in the topic of discussion; everyone who gets the message knows who else got a copy of the message. Bcc is for e-mailing several people who do not know each other. It is a way to protect each person's confidentiality by not sharing their e-mail addresses with strangers.
- Don't use "Reply to All" unless everyone really does need to see your response. If you are part of a listserv and want to reply just to the sender of a message, do not hit reply at all. Copy the sender's e-mail address and paste it into the To: line of a new message.
- Be careful about sending attachments, especially large ones that take up a lot of space on the system. Some people will not accept attachments from people they do not know. When you are replying to an e-mail that contained an attachment, use the "Reply without attachment" option if you have it. If that is not an option on your system, at least delete the attachment before you hit "send." The person who sent you the attachment already has a copy of the document, so he or she does not need another copy of it. It just wastes cyberspace and system resources.
- Never put something in an e-mail at work that would embarrass you if your boss read it.
- Do not overuse the "highest priority" option. It ceases to be a priority if it is used daily.

(continued)

- Keep business e-mails short, a paragraph or two, with sentences that are less than 20 words each. Use bullet points or numbered lists to make the messages easy to read.
- If you are angry when writing an e-mail, save it as a draft and go back and edit it when you have calmed down. Once it's sent, you can't take it back. Expression of extreme emotion in an e-mail is called flaming. Flaming is never a good business practice.
- Keep a copy of the e-mails you send. You can set your e-mail system to automatically save all sent mail.

Sources: Braveman, (2006); Kallos, (2006); OWL at Purdue University, (2004); Sabath, (2002); Sherwood, n.d.; Yale University, n.d.

REFERENCES

American Occupational Therapy Association. (2005). Standards of practice for occupational therapy. *American Journal of Occupational Therapy, 59,* 663–665.

American Psychological Association. (2001). *Publication manual of the American Psychological Association.* Washington, DC: Author.

Braveman, B. (2006). *Leading and managing occupational therapy services: An evidence-based approach.* Philadelphia: F. A. Davis.

Joint Commission on Accreditation of Healthcare Organizations. (2009). *Official "do not use" list.* Retrieved 4-19-09 from http://www.jointcommission.org/NR/rdonlyres/2329 F8F5-6EC5-4E21-B932-54B2B7D53F00/0/dnu_list.pdf

Kallos, J. (2006). *NetManners: Business email basics.* Retrieved March 21, 2006 from http:// www.onlinenetiquette.com/business-email-basics.html

O'Conner, P. T. (1996). *Woe is I: The grammarphobe's guide to better English in plain English.* New York: Riverhead Books.

Online Writing Laboratory at Purdue University and Purdue University. (2004). *Email etiquette.* Retrieved March 22, 2006 from http://owl..english.purdue.edu/handouts/ print/pw/p_emailett.html

Online Writing Laboratory at Purdue University and Purdue University. (2004). *The basic business letter.* Retrieved March 22, 2006 from http://owl..english.purdue.edu/ handouts/print/pw/p_basicbusletter.html

Online Writing Laboratory at Purdue University and Purdue University. (2004). *Memo writing.* Retrieved March 22, 2006 from http://owl..english.purdue.edu/handouts/print/ pw/p_memo.html

Sabath, A. M. (2002). *Business etiquette.* New York: Barnes and Noble.

Sames, K. M. (2008) *Documentation in practice.* In E. Crepeau, E. Cohn & B. B. Schell (Eds.) Willard and Spackman's occupational therapy (11th ed., pp. 403–410). Philadelphia: Lippencott, Wilcott & Williams.

Shamus, E. & Stern, D. (2004). *Effective documentation for physical therapy professionals.* New York: McGraw-Hill.

Sherwood, K. D. (n.d.). *Context.* Retrieved March 22, 2006 from http://www.webfoot.com/ advice/email.top.html

Yale University (n.d.). *Netiquette.* Retrieved March 22, 2006 from http://www.library.yale .edu/training/netiquette

CHAPTER 2

Buzzwords, Jargon, and Abbreviations

INTRODUCTION

The longer you write progress notes and intervention plans, the more you fall into certain patterns. You learn what words get the attention of reviewers in positive and negative ways. There are lists floating around, developed by experienced occupational therapists, containing words one should never use, and other lists with words that one should be sure to use. If your supervisor hands you such a list, he or she will expect you to use it. Go ahead and use these lists. Do not, however, depend on them as your sole source for good words. If you do, all your documentation will sound the same.

▼ BUZZWORDS ▼

Buzzwords are words that are currently popular or trendy. They let the reader or listener know that you are up-to-date. Buzzwords in the early 21st century include "collaborative," "embedded," "function," "hands-on," and "community." On the basis of the proposed International Classification of Function (World Health Organization [WHO], 2002) language, one could expect the phrases "activity limitation," "participation restriction," and "participation in life" to become buzzwords very soon. The problem with buzzwords is that as quickly as they become fashionable, they become unfashionable.

"Function" is a special buzzword. It is a necessary word to occupational therapy practice. Occupational therapy practitioners must show that their services result in functional changes in their clients. This is true of other providers such as physical therapists and speech language pathologists as well. In most settings, demonstrating improvement in function is essential to receiving payment for services. This means that as occupational therapists document their services, it is not enough to say that someone's range of motion increased. So what? Just because Mrs. Smith can bend more at the elbow, it does not automatically mean that she can do more because of it. Can she now feed herself or fasten the top button on her blouse? If a person can now follow three-step directions, what does it mean? Can this person now prepare a meal? Function is the difference between a client tolerating being in water for 3 minutes and taking a bath. Documentation must be explicit in its descriptions of functional activities.

"Evidence" or "evidenced-based" are becoming buzzwords, but they may be buzzwords that appeal to third-party payers. When an occupational therapy practitioner says that the evidence says such and such, it gives credibility to the rationale for choosing a particular intervention. This is good. Payers are calling for evidence-based practice. A practitioner should be ready to support the claim of evidence, if asked to show the payer the evidence. Although the most current definitions of evidence-based practice include not only the best research evidence but also clinician expertise and client preferences, a payer is most likely to expect evidence to be found in the literature. Upon request, a payer will expect to see well-designed clinical studies that demonstrate the effectiveness of the intervention rather than anecdotal evidence.

"Sustainable" is another buzzword. This word became popular during the US invasions of Iraq and Afghanistan. Applied to occupational therapy practice, sustainable means that the outcomes of the interventions will last beyond the duration of the occupational therapy service provision. Payers want to pay for services that will make a lasting difference in the client's life. For example, an occupational therapy practitioner in a clinic setting worked for months with a 4 year old with autism, teaching him to dress himself. After several months, this child was successfully dressing himself every time she worked with him, so she discontinued working on that goal. The child's family received reports and instructions throughout those months to assist in carry-over to the home setting. Then, after 2 months of working on other self-care and play skills, the occupational therapy practitioner decided to see if the boy could still dress himself. He could not. The occupational therapy intervention was not sustainable given the child's home situation. If you were responsible for paying this child's therapy bill, would you think it was money well spent?

Just as there are buzzwords, there are what I call "red-flag words." These words will cause the reader to stop and perhaps not read any further. They serve as big signs of trouble. An example of a red-flag word is "continued" or "maintained" when read by a payer who only pays for occupational therapy services as long as there is demonstrable progress.

Some payers will also view documentation with an eye toward discontinuing service if they read that a client was "seen" in occupational therapy rather than "participated in" the occupational therapy session. If the writer says that a client was seen in occupational therapy today, the payer may interpret it to mean that the client was seen in the room but did not necessarily do anything while in the room. "Participated" implies some action on the part of the client.

For years, clinicians have refrained from writing goals that deal with the client's need to participate in cultural, religious, or spiritual activities. It seemed that culture, religion, and spirituality were red-flag words. Clinicians were hesitant to address issues of participation in cultural, religious, or spiritual activities, primarily because they were sure payers would not pay for such services (they may be viewed as diversionary activities, which are usually not reimbursable). One occupational therapist told me that even though she was working with an elderly priest who had had a stroke, the payer would not pay for her to work toward the goal that he be able to conduct the mass, so she never tried to get any services involving religion or spirituality covered again. While completing the tasks of the mass does relate to religion, perhaps if she had stated the goal in terms of regaining the skills required to return to work, she might have gotten paid for her services.

That was several years ago, and maybe things have changed since then. If what is important to your client is participation in religious or spiritual life, one strategy would be to find ways to dance around those words in setting goals. Instead of setting a goal that Mrs. Smith propel herself in her wheelchair to the chapel each week, the goal could be that she propel herself to all the places she needs to access in the building. Or instead of a goal that a client will be able to kneel on the ground to offer praise to Allah several times a day, the goal can be that the client be able to engage in activities that are personally meaningful.

That strategy can work, but there is something about writing vague goals that does not sit well with me. Instead of anticipating the reaction of payers to red-flag words, we should use them and then appeal the case if it is denied. We may find that we are no longer being denied coverage; we only think we will be, so we have been avoiding being totally honest and direct. The *Occupational Therapy Practice Framework* (AOTA, 2008) can provide an occupational therapy practitioner with wording that is consistent with best practice. However, just because AOTA says an occupation or intervention activity is within the scope of occupational therapy practice, it does not mean a third-party payer will pay for it.

▼ JARGON ▼

Jargon is terminology widely understood by one profession or group of people but not understood by others outside the group or profession (Lunsford, 2005). Occupational therapy practitioners are notorious for their use of jargon; so are many other health professionals. Sadly, each profession uses jargon unique to itself, and it can create a lot of unnecessary confusion. If we all document using common terminology, we can all help each other carry out interventions that support each other for the good of the client. As mentioned in the introduction to this book, occupational therapy practitioners (and other professionals) need to consider the audience they are addressing. Often, the people making decisions about whether or not to pay for occupational therapy services are not occupational therapy practitioners themselves. Physicians and nurses may be called on to translate our documentation for clients, and if they cannot understand our jargon, then we have put them in a bad spot. Although occupational therapy practitioners know what bilateral integration is, most people do not. A look at the *Occupational Therapy Practice Framework: Domain and Practice* (AOTA, 2008) will give you some idea of the kind of jargon that is frequently used in occupational therapy documentation.

Here is an example of a narrative note written with lots of buzzwords, jargon, and abbreviations:

> *Patient seen for 3 units for ADLs. Patient sat at EOB with min assist. Patient told to perform upper body hygiene/grooming. Needed min assist and setup. Patient showed a poor bilateral integration due to left hemiplegia and left hemianopsia. Patient's significant other instructed by this therapist in compensatory techniques and cuing patterns. SO return demonstration not adequate. Will need additional instruction.*

Here is the same paragraph written in relatively plain English:

> *Patient participated in a 45-minute bedside session this morning for self-care activities. The patient sat at the edge of the bed with minimal assistance. With minimal assistance following setup, the patient washed his face and trunk, brushed his teeth, and combed his hair. He did not wash his left arm or the left side of his face. The patient's wife was instructed in ways to set up tasks and verbally cue the patient to compensate for left visual field cut. She tended to try to do the task for her husband; she will need more instruction.*

Both paragraphs describe the same client doing the same activities. The second one is easier for most people to read and understand. Note that it does not eliminate every abbreviation or word of jargon. To do so would make it sound too simplistic and unprofessional. It is a question of balance and of which terms are likely to be understood by every professional in the program and by payers.

Exercise 2.1

Translate these narrative notes into plain English.

1. Jennifer attended three sessions this week. She needed encouragement to engage in the group discussion. She rarely made eye contact with the therapist or other group members. She mumbled incoherently and occasionally picked at something unseen in the air around her, possibly hallucinating. When given a cognitive task to do, she completely disengaged. Her attention span was < 2 min. She appeared to respond +ly to classical music, the mumbling and picking at the air ceased and she smiled. Pt. oriented x1.

2. Ling was seen for a three-unit session today. She selected the 30-inch ball as the first thing she wanted to try. She positioned herself prone on the ball and proceeded to rock in a linear pattern. Then she went to the bolster swing and engaged in circular vestibular stimulation. Ling alternated between these two activities for 15 minutes. Next she asked to draw in the shaving cream on a mirror. She attended to this task for 10 minutes, then ran to the sink to wash and dry her hands. Next she wrapped herself up tightly in a parachute. Following that, she quietly played with puzzles. She is demonstrating improved tactile and vestibular processing. Plan is to continue working on sensory integration activities to improve sensory processing as outlined in plan of care.

▼ ABBREVIATIONS ▼

One way to shorten the time it takes to write notes is to use abbreviations. It takes less time to write "bid" than it does to write "two times per day." However, the problem with abbreviations is that not everyone knows what the abbreviations mean. Sometimes the same abbreviation can mean different things. In one setting "hoh" might mean hard of hearing, but in another it could mean hand over hand (as a form of assisting a client to complete a task). Most facilities have a list of acceptable abbreviations for use at that facility. It is important to use such a list if it exists, and not assume that other people understand your abbreviations.

Here is a narrative note written by a practitioner, using abbreviations when possible and then rewritten using as few abbreviations as possible. Using abbreviations saved two lines of type, but made it harder to read.

Client partic. in OT bid 5x/wk. He partic. in a w.u. Ax consisting of ROM ex. for BUE including ✓/–, ab/ad, & IR/ER. Client shows ↑ in ROM and # reps all directions. He worked coop. c̄ 2 other clients in a ball game, throwing and catching the ball 4/5 trials. The ball game required him to use bilat integ. skills & social interaction skills. Client is showing ↑ in these skills & abilities. Plan to ↑ # and complexity of BUE Ax.

Client participated in OT twice daily for 5 days this week. He participated in a warm-up activity consisting of ROM exercises for both arms including flexion/extension, abduction/adduction, and internal/external rotation. Client shows increase in ROM and number of repetitions of movements in all directions. He worked cooperatively with 2 other clients in a ball game, throwing and catching the ball on 4 out of 5 trials. The ball game required him to use both hands together & socially interact. Client is showing an increase in these skills & abilities. The plan is to increase the number and complexity of upper extremity activities per session.

In some instances, people expect abbreviations to be used. When signing your name on any formal documentation, it is common practice to identify yourself by putting your professional credentials after your name in the form of an abbreviation. Common abbreviations for professional credentials are listed in Box 2.1. There are many others, but these are the most common. Abbreviations are also used to document the frequency with which something occurs. Box 2.2 shows a list of such abbreviations. Abbreviations can refer to parts of the body, injuries, or illnesses. Box 2.3 is a partial list; however, inclusion in this list does not guarantee that anyone who reads these abbreviations knows what they mean. There are other abbreviations referred to in the jargon of the profession as the "x" abbreviations (Box 2.4). These have varied use and acceptability in different parts of the country. Occupational therapists and other medical professionals use a variety of abbreviations to identify types of range of motion, as shown in Box 2.5. Clinical procedures and common clinical terminology are abbreviated in letters and with symbols (Box 2.6). The first part of Box 2.6 contains those terms with letter abbreviations and the symbols follow. Box 2.7 shows abbreviations most commonly used when payment is being discussed. Finally, Box 2.8 contains a list of abbreviations related to education. Please note that not all possible abbreviations are included in these lists and, conversely, inclusion in this book mean that an abbreviation is acceptable in all settings.

BOX 2.1 Professional Credentials and Job Titles

AP	advanced practitioner, for OTAs or COTAs only
APE	adaptive physical education
ATC	athletic trainer certified
CCC	certificate of clinical competence [for speech-language pathologists]
CCM	certified case manager
CEO	chief executive officer
CFO	chief financial officer
CHT	certified hand therapist

CI	clinical instructor
COO	chief operating officer
COTA	certified occupational therapy assistant
COTA/L	certified occupational therapy assistant, licensed
CPE	certified professional ergonomist
CST	craniosacral therapist
D/APE	developmental and adaptive physical education
DC	doctor of chiropractic
DDS	doctor of dental surgery
DMD	doctor of medical dentistry
DO	doctor of osteopathy
DPT	doctor of physical therapy
EBD	emotional or behavioral disorder
EdD	doctor of education
FACP	Fellow of the American College of Physicians
FACS	Fellow of the American College of Surgeons
FAOTA	Fellow of the American Occupational Therapy Association
FWS	fieldwork supervisor
HHA	home health aide
LD	learning disabled
LMFT	licensed marriage and family therapist
LP	licensed psychologist
LPN	licensed practical nurse
MAOT	master of arts in occupational therapy
MD	medical doctor
MOT	master of occupational therapy
MPH	master of public health
MSW	master of social work
OT/L	occupational therapist, licensed
OTA	occupational therapy assistant
OTA/L	licensed occupational therapy assistant
OTAS	occupational therapy assistant student
OTD	occupational therapist, doctor of [clinical doctorate]
OTD/L	doctor of occupational therapy, licensed
OTIP	occupational therapist in independent practice—Medicare
OTR	occupational therapist, registered
OTR/L	occupational therapist, registered and licensed
OTS	occupational therapy student
PA	physician's assistant
PCA	personal care attendant
Pharm D	doctor of pharmacy
PhD	doctor of philosophy
PT	physical therapist
PTA	physical therapist assistant
QMHP	qualified mental health professional
QMRP	qualified mental retardation professional
QRC	qualified rehabilitation consultant
RD	registered dietician
RN	registered nurse
ROH	Roster of Honor
RT	recreation therapist, respiratory therapist
RRT	registered recreation therapist, registered respiratory therapist
ScD	doctor of science
SLP	speech-language pathologist

BOX 2.2 Abbreviations Related to Frequency

qd	once a day
bid	twice a day
BIN	twice at night
tid	three times a day
qid	four times a day
eod	every other day
i	once a day
ii	twice a day
iii	three times a day
1x/wk	once a week
2x/wk	twice a week
3x/wk	three times a week
continues up to 7x/wk	
1x/mo	once a month
2x/mo	twice a month
3x/mo	three times a month
continues	

BOX 2.3 Abbreviations Related to Body Parts and Diagnoses

AA atlantoaxial; adjusted age; or active
   assist
AAA abdominal aortic aneurysm
AAOX3 alert, awake, and oriented to
   person, place and time [times three]
ABG arterial blood gasses
AC joint acromioclavicular joint
ACA anterior communicating artery;
   anterior cerebral artery
ACL anterior cruciate ligament
ACVD acute cardiovascular disease
ADD attention deficit disorder
ADHD attention deficit hyperactivity
   disorder
Adm admitted on; admission
AE above elbow
AEA above elbow amputation
AF atrial fibrilation
AGA appropriate for gestational age
AI aortic incompetence
AIDS acquired immunodeficiency
   disorder
AK above knee
AKA above knee amputation;
   also known as
ALS amyotrophic lateral sclerosis
ant. anterior
AP anterior-posterior
ap before dinner
APGAR appearance, pulse, grimace, activity,
   respiration

ARDS acute respiratory distress syndrome;
   adult respiratory distress syndrome
ARF acute renal failure; acute respiratory
   failure
AS aortic stenosis; ankylosing spondylitis
As & Bs apnea and bracycardia
ASIS anterior superior iliac spine
ASCVD arteriosclerotic cardiovascular
   disease
ASD atrial septal defect
ASHD atherosclerotic heart disease
ATNR asymmetrical tonic neck reflex
AV arteriovenous; atrioventricular;
   aortic valve
BBB bundle-branch block; blood brain–barrier
BE below elbow
BEA below elbow amputation
BK below knee
BKA below knee amputation
bl blood; bleeding
BLE both lower extremities
BMI or bmi body mass index
BMR basal metabolic rate
BP blood pressure
BPD bronchopulmonary disease
bpm beats per minute
BS breath sounds; blood sugar;
   bowel sounds
BUE both upper extremities
BUN blood urea nitrogen
bw birth weight

CA or Ca cancer
CABG coronary artery bypass graft
CAD coronary artery disease
CBC complete blood count
CAD coronary artery disease
Cal calories
cath catheter
CBC complete blood count
CBI closed brain injury
CC or C/C or cc chief complaint; carbon
    copy
CCU cardiac care unit
CF cystic fibrosis
CFS chronic fatigue syndrome
CHF congestive heart failure
CHI closed head injury
CICU cardiac intensive care unit
CLD chronic liver disease
CMV cytomegalovirus
CN cranial nerve, usually followed by the
    number of the nerve using Roman
    numerals
CNS central nervous system
CO cardiac output; carbon monoxide
    c/o complains of
COD co-occurring disorder [psychiatric
    diagnosis with a chemical misuse
    diagnosis]
COLD chronic obstructive
    lung disease
Cont. or cont. continued
COPD chronic obstructive pulmonary
    disorder
CP cerebral palsy; chest pain
CRF chronic renal failure
C&S culture and sensitivity
CSF cerebrospinal fluid
CT chest tube; computerized axial
    tomography
CTR carpal tunnel release
CTS carpal tunnel syndrome
CVA cerebral vascular accident—stroke
DD developmental disabilities; dual
    diagnosis
DDD degenerative disc disease
DDH developmental dysplasia of the hip
DF dorsiflexion
DIP distal interphalangeal joint
DJD degenerative joint disease
DM diabetes mellitus
DMD Duchenne muscular dystrophy
DOB date of birth
DOE dyspnea on exertion
DT delirium tremons
DTR deep tendon reflex

DVT deep vein thrombosis
EBV Epstein Barr virus
ECG or EKG electrocardiogram
ECHO or echo echocardiogram
ED erectile dysfunction
EEG electroencephalogram
EENT ears, eyes, nose, and throat
EID easily identified depression
ELBW extremely low birth weight
EMG electromyelogram
ER emergency room; external rotation
ESRD end-stage renal disease
ETOH alcohol [use or abuse]
FAE fetal alcohol effects
FAS fetal alcohol syndrome
FBS fasting blood sugar
FTT failure to thrive
FUO fever of unknown origin
G good
G-tube gastrostomy tube
GA gestational age
GB gall bladder
GBS Guillain-Barré syndrome
GCS Glasglow coma scale
GERD gastroesophoageal reflux disease
GI gastrointestinal
G#P#A# number of births, pregnancies, and
    abortions
Grava gravida [number of births]
GSW gunshot wound
GU genitourinary
GYN gynecologic; gynecology
H/A or HA headache
Hams hamstrings
HB or Hb or Hgb hemoglobin
HBP high blood pressure
HBV hepatitis B virus
HC heel cords
HCVD hypertensive cardiovascular
    disease
HEENT head, ear, eyes, nose, throat
HIB haemophilus influenza B [vaccine]
HIV human immunodeficiency virus
HLT heart lung transplant
HNP herniated nucleus pulposus
HOH hard of hearing; hand over hand
H & P history and physical
HPI history of present illness
HR heart rate
HSV herpes simplex virus
Ht height
HT heart transplant
HTN hypertension
IBS irritable bowel syndrome
ICA internal carotid artery

(Continued)

BOX 2.3 Continued

ICH intracranial hemorrhage; intracerebral hemorrhage

ICP intracranial pressure

ICU intensive care unit

ID infections disease

IDDM insulin-dependent diabetes mellitus

Ig immunoglobulin

IM intramuscular

imp. impression

Indep independently

inf inferior

IP interphalangeal

IQ intelligence quotient

IR internal rotation

IVC inferior vena cava

JRA juvenile rheumatoid arthritis

jt joint

KUB kidneys, ureter, bladder

lap laparoscopy; laparotomy

lat lateral

LBBB left bundle branch block

LBP low back pain

LBW low birth weight

LCA left carotid artery

LD learning disability

LE lower extremity—leg

LG limb-girdle dystrophy

LLE left lower extremity

LLQ left lower quadrant [abdomen]

LMN lower motor neuron

LMP last menstrual period

LOC loss of consciousness

LP lumbar puncture

LT lung transplant

LUE left upper extremity

LUQ left upper quadrant [abdomen]

MAP main arterial pressure

MCA middle cerebral artery

MCL medial collateral ligament

MCP or MP metacarpal phalangeal

MD muscular dystrophy

med medial

mets metastisis

MH mental health

MI myocardial infarction in some settings, mental illness in others

MRSA methicillin resistant staphylococcus aureus

MS multiple sclerosis or mitral stenosis

MV mitral valve

MVA motor vehicle accident

MVP mitral valve prolapse

MVP mitral valve prolapse

N normal; nausea

N/A not applicable; not available

NAD no appreciable disease; nothing abnormal detected; no acute distress

NG nasogastric

NGT nasogastric tube

NICU neonatal intensive care unit

NIDDM non-insulin-dependent diabetes mellitus

NKA no known allergies

NKDA no known drug allergies

nl normal

nn nerve

NSAID nonsteroidal anti-inflammatory drug

NSR normal sinus rhythm

N & V nausea and vomiting

OA osteoarthritis

OB obstetrics

OBS organic brain syndrome

OD overdose

OI osteogenisis imperfecta

OM otitis media [ear infection]

ORIF open reduction, internal fixation

PA pulmonary artery

PARA or para paraplegia

PCL posterior cruciate ligament

PD Parkinson's disease

PDD pervasive developmental disorder

PE pulmonary embolus; pulmonary edema

PEEP positive end expiratory pressure

PET positron emission tomography

PERRLA pupils equal, round, reactive to light, and accommodation

PFT pulmonary function test

PH past history

Phys Dys physical disabilities

PI present illness

PICA posterior inferior cerebellar artery; posterior inferior communicating artery

PICU pediatric intensive care unit

PID pelvic inflammatory disease

PIP proximal interphalangeal joint

PKU phenylketonuria

PLF prior level of function

PMH past medical history

PNI peripheral nerve injury

post posterior

PSIS posterior superior iliac spine

Psych psychology; psychiatry; psychiatric

PTCA percutaneous transluminal coronary angioplasty

PTSD posttraumatic stress disorder
PVC premature ventricular contraction
PVD peripheral vascular disease
PWA person with AIDS
PWB partial weight bearing
QUAD or quad quadriplegia;
    quadriplegic
RA rheumatoid arthritis; right atrium
RAS reticular activating system
RBBB right bundle branch block
RBC red blood count
RCA right carotid artery
RD retinal detachment
Resp respiration
RF renal failure
RHD rheumatoid heart disease
RLE right lower extremity
RLQ right lower quadrant [abdomen]
r/o rule out
ROS review of symptoms
rr respiratory rate
RSD reflex sympathetic dystrophy
RSV respiratory syncytial virus
RUE right upper extremity
RUQ right upper quadrant [abdomen]
RV right ventricle
SAD season affective disorder
SC subcutaneous
SC joint sternoclavicular joint
SCD sickle cell disease
SCI spinal cord injury
SCM sternocleidomastoid [joint]
SD seizure disorder
SED seriously emotionally disturbed in
    some settings, suberythemal dose in
    others
SF-36 short-form 36
SICU surgical intensive care unit
SIDS sudden infant death syndrome

SIJ sacroiliac joint
SLE systemic lupus erythematosus
SOB shortness of breath
S & S signs and symptoms
STD sexually transmitted disease
STNR symmetrical tonic neck reflex
str strength
sup superior; supine
SVC superior vena cava
Sz schizophrenia
T & A tonsils & adenoids; tonsillectomy and
    adnoidectomy
TB tuberculosis
TBI traumatic brain injury
TD tartive dyskinesia
THA total hip arthroplasty
THR total hip replacement
TIA transient ischemic attack
TKA total knee arthroplasty
TKR total knee replacement
TMJ temporal mandibular joint
TNR tonic neck reflexes [ATNR, STNR]
TPR temperature, pulse & respiration
TSA total shoulder arthroplasty
TUR transurethral resection
TV tidal volume
UA urine analysis
UE upper extremity—arm
UMN upper motor neuron
URI upper respiratory infection
UTI urinary tract infection
VC vital capacity
VD venereal disease
vent. ventilator
VLBW very low birth weight
VSD ventricular septal defect
VT ventricular tachycardia
v.s. vital signs
WBC white blood count

Sources: Borcherding, S. (2005); Jacobs (1997); Kettenback, G. (2004); Shamus & Stern (2004).

BOX 2.4 "X" Abbreviations

Ax	activity
Dx	diagnosis
Fx	fracture
Hx	history of
PMHx	past medical history
Px	physical examination
Rx	therapy
Sx	symptom
Tx	treatment or traction

BOX 2.5   Range of Motion Abbreviations

AAROM	active assisted ROM
AROM	active ROM
CPM	continuous passive motion
FROM	functional ROM
PROM	passive ROM
ROM	range of motion
RROM	resisted ROM

BOX 2.6   Abbreviations for Clinical Procedures

(A) assist; assistance
A assessment
ABD or abd abduction
ABR absolute bedrest
ac before meals
ADD or add adduction
ADL activities of daily living
ad lib at liberty, as desired
AFO ankle-foot orthosis
ALF assisted living facility
ALOS average length of stay
a.m. or AM morning
ama or AMA against medical advice
amb ambulation; ambulates
amt or am't amount
ASA aspirin
ASAP as soon as possible
assist assistance
AT assistive technology
(B) or bilat. bilateral or both
BADL basic activities of daily living
b/c because
b/4 before
bm body mechanics
BP bed pan
bpm beats per minute
BRP bathroom privileges
B/S bed side
C centigrade
cal calories
CAT computer-assisted tomography
CBR complete bed rest
CBT cognitive behavioral therapy
cc chief complaint
CGA contact guard assist
cm centimeter
c/o complains of
cont. continue
CP cold pack
CPAP continuous positive airway
    pressure

CPM or CPMM continuous passive motion
    machine
CPR cardiopulmonary resuscitation
CVP continuous venous pressure
DAFO dynamic ankle foot orthosis
D/C discontinuation; discharge
Dept. department—may also be written
    with a small d
DME durable medical equipment
DNR do not resuscitate
DOB date of birth
DOE dyspnea on exertion
DRS disability rating scale
EBP evidence-based practice
e.g. for example; such as
eob edge of bed
ES or e-stim electrical stimulation
etc. et cetera, and so forth
eval evaluation
ex exercise
ext. extension
F or f fair
f female
FCE functional capacity evaluation
FES functional electrical stimulation
FEV_1 forced expiratory volume in 1 second
FIM functional independence measure
flex flexion
FRG functional related groups
ft feet; foot as in a measurement, not a body
    part
f/u follow-up
FW I fieldwork one
FW II fieldwork two, also called affiliation
    experience
FWB full weight bearing
G good as in muscle strength
g gram
GM&S general medicine and surgery
GSR galvanic skin response
GT gait training

h or hr. hour
H&P history and physical
Hemi hemiplegia
HEP home exercise program
HH home health; hand held
HHA hand hold assist
HKAFO hip knee ankle foot orthosis
HME home medical equipment
HOB head of bed
HOH/hoh hand over hand;
    hard of hearing
HP hot pack
HR heart rate
hr. hour
hs at night, hours of sleep
ht height
Ⓘ independently
ICU intensive care unit
I & O intake and output
IADL instrumental activities of daily living
ICD-9 International Classification of
    Diseases, Ninth Edition
ICF Intermediate care facility; International
    Classification of Function
ICU intensive care unit
i.e. that is; in other words
ILC independent living center
IM intramuscular
imp impression
in. inches
inhal inhalation
Inj injection
IP inpatient
ITB intrathecal baclofin
IV intravenous
KAFO knee-ankle-foot orthosis
kg. kilogram
KJ knee jerk
Ⓛ left
L or l liter
l/m liters per minute
LAD language acquisition device
lb. pound
LBQC large-based quad cane
LLB long leg brace
llq left lower quadrant
LOS length of stay
LP lumbar puncture
LTC long-term care
LTG long-term goal
LUQ left upper quadrant
L&W living and well
m male
MAO monoamine oxidase
max maximum or maximal

MED minimal effective dose; minimal
    erythemal dose
meds medications, medicines
MET metabolic level; maximal
MFR myofascial release
MFT or mft muscle function test
mg milligram
MH moist heat
MHP moist hot pack
min minutes; minimum
ml milliliter
mm millimeter
mm-Hg millimeters of mercury
MMSE Mini-Mental Status Exam
MMT manual muscle test
mo. month
mob mobility; mobilization
mod moderate
MRI magnetic resonance imaging
MSQ mental status questionnaire
MVC maximum voluntary contraction
N normal, as in muscle grade
na or N/A not applicable; not available
NaC normal saline
NBQC narrow-based quad cane
NDT neurodevelopmental treatment
neb nebulizer
neg. negative
NICU neonatal intensive care unit
NKA no known allergy
NKDA no known drug allergy
NMES neuromuscular electrical stimulation
noc nocturnal, at night
NPO nothing per mouth
nt not tested
NWB non-weight bearing
O objective
O_2 oxygen
OBS observation
od once daily; right eye
OH occupational history
OOB out of bed
OP outpatient
OR operating room
os left eye
OTC over the counter
ou both eyes
Ox3 oriented times three [person,
    place, time]
Ox4 oriented times four [person,
    place, time & situation]
oz. ounce
P plan; poor; pulse
PADL personal activities of daily living
PAMS physical agent modalities

(Continued)

BOX 2.6   Continued

para paraplegic
pc after meals
PEDI Pediatric Evaluation of Disability
    Index
per by or through
PLOF past level of function
PLOP present level of performance
p.m. or PM between noon and midnight
PMR or PM&R physical medicine and
    rehabilitation
PNF proprioceptive neuromuscular
    facilitation
po per mouth, orally
P/O or post-op after surgery
POC plan of care
POD post-op day number
POMR problem-oriented medical record
pos positive
poss possible
post posterior
post-op after surgery
PPE personal protective equipment
PRE progressive resistive exercise
pre-op before surgery
pro or pron pronation
PRN or prn per as needed
Pt or pt. patient; pint; point
PTA prior to admission
PTB patellar tendon bearing [prosthesis]
PVE prevocational evaluation
PWB partial weight bearing
q every
qt. quart
quad quadriceps
Ⓡ right
RA reasonable accommodation
Re: or re: regarding
rehab rehabilitation
REM rapid eye movement
reps repetitions
RET rational emotion therapy
resp respiratory, respiration
rlq right lower quadrant
RM repetition maximum
RPE rating of perceived exertion
RTC return to clinic
RTI Routine Task Inventory
RTO return to office
ruq right upper quadrant
RW rolling walker
S subjective
SBA stand by assist
SE side effects

sec seconds
SH social history
SI sensory integration
sig directions for use, give as follows
SLB short leg brace
SLR straight leg raise
SNF skilled nursing facility
SOAP subjective, objective, assessment, plan;
    progress note format
SOB shortness of breath
SOC start of care
SOP standard operating procedure
SPEM smooth pursuit eye movement
stat immediately
STG short-term goal
STM short-term memory
STNR symmetrical tonic neck reflex
sup supination
SWD short wave diathermy
T trace as in muscle strength; temperature
Tbsp. or tbsp. tablespoon
TCU transitional care unit
TDD telecommunications device for the deaf
TDWB touch down weight bearing
TEDS thrombo-embolic disease stockings
TENS, TNS transcutaneous electrical nerve
    stimulation
ther ex therapeutic exercise
TLSO thoracic lumbar spine orthosis
TO or t.o. telephone order
TOS thoracic outlet syndrome
TPN total pareteral nutrition
trng. training
tsp. teaspoon
TTWB toe touch weight bearing
TWB total weight bearing
un unable
US ultrasound
UV ultraviolet
VC vital capacity
v.o. verbal order
vol. volume
VS or v.s. vital signs; vestibular stimulation
W walker
WB weight bearing
WBAT weight bearing as tolerated
WBQC wide base quad cane
W/C or w/c wheelchair
WFL within functional limits
Wk week
WN well nourished
WNL within normal limits
w/o without

WP or wpl whirlpool   % percent
wt. weight   Δ change
X or x times   ♀ female
x̄ except [for]   ♂ male
y/o or y.o. year old, as in a 5 y/o girl   # number, pound
yd yard   & and
yr year   @ at or each
° degree   / per
' feet   < less than
" inches   > greater than
↑ increased, up   ✓ flexion
↓ decreased, down   / extension; per
→ toward   c̄ with
↔ to and from   p̄ post, after
+ positive, plus, and   s̄ without
– negative, minus   1° primarily, primary
= equal   2° secondary, secondary to
~ or ≈ approximately   ψ psychology; psychological

Sources: Borcherding, S. (2005); Jacobs (1997); Kettenback (2004); Shamus & Stern (2004).

BOX 2.7   Abbreviations Related to Payment and Administration

ADA	Americans with Disabilities Act
BBA	Balanced Budget Act
BCBS	Blue Cross Blue Shield
CARF	Commission on Accreditation of Rehabilitation Facilities
CDC	Centers for Disease Control and Prevention
CHAMPUS	Civilian Health and Medical Program of the Uniformed Services
CMS	Center for Medicare and Medicaid Services, formerly HCFA
COLA	Cost of living adjustment
CORF	certified outpatient rehabilitation facility
CEU	Continuing Education Unit [10 contact hours]
CQI	Continuous Quality Improvement
CPT	Current Procedural Terminology, a coding system used to bill for medical procedures
DHHS	Department of Health and Human Services
DOE	Department of Education
DOL	Department of Labor
DOT	Dictionary of Occupational Titles
DRG	diagnostic-related group
DSM-IV	Diagnostic and Statistical Manual, Fourth Edition
FDA	Food and Drug Administration
FI	fiscal intermediary
GAO	Governmental Accounting Agency
HCFA	Health Care Financing Administration [part of the U.S. Department of Health and Human Services, now the Centers for Medicare and Medicaid Services]
HCPCS	Health Care Procedures Coding System
HMO	Health maintenance organization
HHA	Home health agency
HIPAA	Health Insurance Portability and Accountability Act
ICD-9	International Classification of Diseases, Ninth Edition
IDEA	Individuals with Disabilities Education Act

(Continued)

BOX 2.7 Continued

IEP	Individualized education program
IFSP	Individualized family service plan
IPA	Independent Practice Association
IPO	Independent Practice Organization
IRB	Institutional Review Board
JCAHO	Joint Commission on Accreditation of Health Organizations
MCH	Maternal and Child Health [DHHS]
MDS	Minimum Data Set
NCLB	No Child Left Behind
NBCOT	National Board for Certification in Occupational Therapy
NIH	National Institutes of Health
NIOSH	National Institute for Occupational Safety and Health
OASIS	Outcome and Assessment Information Set
OBRA '87	Omnibus Budget Reconciliation Act of 1987
OCR	Office of Civil Rights [DHHS]
OIG	Office of the Inspector General
OMB	Office of Management and Budget
OOT	Outpatient occupational therapy
OSEP	Office of Special Education Programs [DOE]
OSERS	Office of Special Education and Rehabilitation Services [DOE]
OSHA	Occupational Safety and Health Administration
OTPP	Occupational Therapist in Private Practice
PDR	Physicians' Desk Reference [medication information]
PHI	Protected Health Information
PPO	Preferred Provider Organization
PPS	Prospective Payment System
PSRO	Professional Standards Review Organization
QA	Quality Assurance
QI	Quality Improvement
QM	Quality Management
RBRVS	Resource-Based Relative Value Scale [Medicare]
RSA	Rehabilitation Services Administration [DOE]
RUGS	Resource Utilization Groups
SAMHSA	Substance Abuse and Mental Health Services Administration [DHHS]
SSA	Social Security Administration [DHHS]
SSN	Social Security number
TEFRA	Tax Equity and Fiscal Responsibility Act
TQM	Total quality management
UR	Utilization Review
URQA	Utilization Review Quality Assurance
VA	Veterans Administration
VAMC	Veterans Affairs Medical Center
WHO	World Health Organization

*Sources: Administrative and Management Special Interest Section (2000); Jacobs (1997); Meyer &
Schiff (2004).*

APE	adapted physical education
AT	assistive technology
CFR	Code of Federal Regulations
D/APE	developmental and adaptive physical education
DOE	Department of Education
ECFE	early childhood family education
ECSE	early childhood special education
EI	early intervention
FAPE	free and appropriate public education
IDEA	Individuals with Disabilities Education Act
IEP	Individualized Education Program
IFSP	Individualized Family Service Plan
LD	Learning disability
LEA	local education agency
LRE	least restrictive environment
NCLB	No Child Left Behind
OHI	other health impaired
OSEP	Office of Special Education Program, U.S. Department of Education
OSERS	Office of Special Education and Rehabilitation Services [DOE]
PI	physically impaired
PLEP	present level of educational performance
RSA	Rehabilitation Services Administration [DOE]
SEA	state education agency
SI	sensory integration
USC	United States Code

Source: Jackson (2007).

Exercise 2.2

Translate these notes into plain English.

1. Jacques is 4 weeks s/p surgical repair of tendons around his Ⓡ first MCP joint. He wears a thumb immobilizer splint, but is now allowed to remove it tid for 5 minutes of movement, within 20° of midline in ✓/ and ab/ad. Reports pain has decreased during Ⓡ thumb movements. No swelling evident, wound has healed nicely. He has begun to swing a bat, gripping it fully with his left hand and gripping with his fingers only, thumb immobilized on his Ⓡ. Maintaining upper arm strength is important for him to be able to return to finish the baseball season (plays outfield for the Chicago Cubs). Plan to continue ROM exs as prescribed, ice, e-stim., and fnct'l Ax.

2. Andrea has been ref. to OT for work on ADLs, following a TBI, Fx Ⓛ clavicle and humerus, and fx Ⓛ pelvis. Visited Andrea in her room to introduce her to OT and explain the schedule of visits. She has no mem. of accident or 1st wk. in the hospital. She is D in all ADLs. In the 5 min. I spent with her, she asked my name 6X. Knows she is married, but cannot remember the names of her 4 children. She appears to tire easily, yawning often. She is agreeable to tx, but states she has no idea what she'd like to accomplish in OT; does not know what would be realistic for STGs. For a LTG, she would like to go home and live life like she did b/4 her accident.

SUMMARY

Buzzwords, jargon, and abbreviations can give the appearance that you are on top of things, that you know what you are doing. However, they can also become barriers to effective communication. As with most things in life, using buzzwords, jargon, and abbreviations in moderation is fine, but do not overdo it.

In documenting occupational therapy practice, regardless of the setting, choosing your words carefully is a critical step in the writing process. There are words that are trendy or send positive messages to the reader, and there are other words that send up red flags to the reader. Sometimes occupational therapists get so involved in describing things so accurately that only another occupational therapist can make any sense out of it. Other times, occupational therapists use abbreviations to the extent that they make the note hard to read. Always remember who the readers of the documentation could be so that you write for all audiences.

REFERENCES

Administration and Management Special Interest Section. (2000). *Occupational therapy administrative reimbursement algorithm.* Retrieved January 5, 2000, from www.aota .org/members/area2/docs/industrial.pdf.

American Occupational Therapy Association. (1994). Uniform terminology (3rd ed.). *American Journal of Occupational Therapy, 48* (11), 1047–1059.

American Occupational Therapy Association. (2008). Occupational therapy practice framework: Domain and process (2nd ed.). *American Journal of Occupational Therapy, 62,* 625–683.

Borcherding, S. (2005). *Documentation manual for writing SOAP notes in occupational therapy* (2nd ed.). Thorofare, NJ: Slack.

Jackson, L.L. (Ed) (2007). *Occupational therapy services for children and youth under IDEA* (3rd ed.). Bethesda, MD: American Occupational Therapy Association.

Kettenback, G. (2004). *Writing SOAP notes* (3rd ed.). Philadelphia: F. A. Davis.

Lunsford, A. A. (2005). *The everyday writer.* Boston: Bedford/St. Martin's.

Sabath, A. M. (2002). *Business etiquette.* New York: Barnes and Noble.

World Health Organization. (2002). *International classification of function.* Geneva, Switzerland: Author. Retrieved May 22, 2002, from http://www3.who.int/icf

CHAPTER 3

The Occupational Therapy Practice Framework and Other Documents

INTRODUCTION

The language of the profession of occupational therapy is ever evolving. As the leaders and great thinkers of the profession review and revise the documents that guide the profession, the terminology used to describe occupational therapy changes. In addition, organizations external to occupational therapy, such as the World Health Organization, change the way words are used to describe the human condition. In this chapter, we explore the changes that have occurred in the last 10 years.

▼ INTERNATIONAL CLASSIFICATION OF FUNCTIONING, DISABILITY, AND HEALTH ▼

The World Health Organization (WHO) has changed the way in which it looks at disability and functioning. With this new look comes a new set of words to describe disability and functioning. Instead of looking at the source of the dysfunction, WHO is looking at the outcomes of the dysfunction, the body structures and functions, activities and level of participation in life, and the environmental factors affecting performance (WHO, 2002). WHO suggests that instead of diagnosing a person with a particular disease, condition, or injury, the clinician should describe the client's level of functioning, demonstrating the impact of the disease, condition, or injury. This will enable health professionals and payers to determine if progress is being made. The document *International Classification of Functioning, Disability and Health* (ICF) issued by WHO is intended to standardize the terminology used across health professions the world over. This document provides a numerical coding system for every possible body part, body function, activity one can participate in, and environments and personal factors that can affect a person's ability to actively participate in life situations. This system is seen as more universal (not specific to any particular culture), more integrative (not just medical or social), more context inclusive (not just the person), and more interactive (not linear) than previous models (WHO).

There are two parts within the structure of the ICF. The first part highlights functioning and disability, and the second focuses on contextual factors. Table 3.1 shows the basic structure of the ICF.

The ICF identifies more than 1,400 terms that can help clinicians think globally while labeling the tasks and activities that their clients engage in on a daily basis. At the WHO website there is a sample checklist to aid in gathering data about a client's function (http://www.who.int/classifications/icf/training/icfchecklist.pdf). The American Occupational Therapy Association (AOTA) used the ICF during the development of the *Occupational Therapy Practice Framework*, which helps illustrate the importance of this document (AOTA, 2008).

TABLE 3.1 Structure of the International Classification of Functioning, Disability and Health (ICF)

Components	Body Functions and Structures	Activities and Participation	Environmental Factors	Personal Factors
Examples	Structures • nerves • muscles • lungs Functions • vision • hearing • breathing	• Learning • Self-care • Interpersonal interactions • Community, social and civic life	• Products and technology • Natural environment • Attitudes • Systems and policies	• Gender • Age • Coping style • Education
Constructs	Functions Structures	Capacity Performance	Barriers Facilitators	
Qualifiers	Structure: Nature of the change • No change • Total absence • Partial absence • Additional part • Aberrant dimensions • Discontinuity • Deviating position • Qualitative changes • Not specified Function: Extent of impairment • No impairment • Mild • Moderate • Severe • Complete	Capacity: • No problem • Mild • Moderate • Severe • Complete Function: • No problem • Mild • Moderate • Severe • Complete	Barriers • No barriers • Mild • Moderate • Severe • Complete Facilitators • No facilitator • Mild • Moderate • Severe • Complete	

▼ UNIFORM TERMINOLOGY ▼

For many years, the AOTA had a document called *Uniform Terminology for Reporting Occupational Therapy Services, Third Edition* (AOTA, 1994). This document was commonly referred to as *Uniform Terminology* or simply *UT*. It contained a list of the domains of concern for occupational therapy; it defined terms that outlined the scope of practice for the profession. However, by the late 1990s it became apparent that major revisions in the document were necessary. In 2002, AOTA officially rescinded the document.

Uniform Terminology was useful for teaching about the profession, and many occupational therapists grew up speaking about occupational therapy in terms recognized by the document (AOTA, 1994). One concept that was taught at many college and university programs was looking at occupational therapy in terms of performance areas, performance components, and contexts. Performance areas were observable occupations in which a person might engage, including those occupations necessary for the care of oneself, the care of others, work and productive activities, and play/leisure activities. Performance components were the skills and abilities needed to perform occupations such as muscle strength, sensory perception, reflexes, sequencing skills, and memory. Contexts were those environmental factors and internal characteristics that influenced performance of occupation such as age, living situation, point in the disease process, support systems, and the availability of tools and equipment. These concepts were useful because an instructor could ask students to summarize an evaluation, being sure to address performance areas, performance components, and contexts, or that students write goals addressing client needs in performance areas (AOTA, 1994).

It is likely that in some settings, *Uniform Terminology* is still used. This may be because not every occupational therapy practitioner is a member of AOTA and therefore might not know that *Uniform Terminology* has been replaced. Those who are members of AOTA may not read the *American Journal of Occupational Therapy* (AJOT) cover to cover each month. It may also be used because some occupational therapists really liked its clean delineation of the occupational therapy scope of practice.

The reason that AOTA replaced *Uniform Terminology* is that it had become outdated as the practice of occupational therapy expanded and new terminology was being incorporated into the profession. The most glaring deficit of *Uniform Terminology* was that the term "occupation" was not mentioned in the document, yet occupation is at the core of the profession (AOTA, 2002). In addition, it was silent on the concept of spirituality, and the terminology was not consistent with ICF.

▼ OCCUPATIONAL THERAPY PRACTICE FRAMEWORK ▼

In 2002, AOTA withdrew *Uniform Terminology* as an official document of the association. It was replaced by a document called the *Occupational Therapy Practice Framework: Domain and Process* (AOTA, 2002). Often referred to simply as *The Framework*, the document describes the domain (scope of practice) of occupational therapy and the processes involved in interactions between occupational therapists and clients. It described the process of occupational therapy with an emphasis on the use of occupations as a therapeutic agent. *The Framework* began with an understanding of the occupational needs of any client (a client can be an individual, a family, a group, or a community) and ended with achieving occupational therapy outcomes that are focused on the client's "engagement in occupations to support participation in context or contexts" (AOTA, 2002, p. 610).

In 2008, *The Framework* was revised (AOTA, 2008). It still describes the domain and process of occupational therapy, but presents a revised overarching statement. In the *Occupational Therapy Practice Framework: Domain and Process, Second Edition,* the overarching statement is "supporting health and participation in life through engagement in occupation" (AOTA, 2008, p. 626). This change was made to put the emphasis on engagement in occupation as the vehicle by which occupational therapy helps people achieve health and participation in life (AOTA, 2008).

While *The Framework,* 2nd ed., is summarized here, it is not a sufficient substitute for the original document. *The Framework* is available from AOTA through its online store (www.aota.org), in the November/December 2008 issue of AJOT, and at some campus bookstores and libraries.

The Framework, 2nd ed., no longer makes a distinction between occupations and activities, but rather it states that occupations include activities (AOTA, 2008). *The Framework,* however, recognizes that some occupational therapy scholars do differentiate between the terms.

One point that *The Framework,* 2nd ed., makes is that the concept of independence may be viewed differently by occupational therapy practitioners and others outside the profession (AOTA, 2008). To an occupational therapy practitioner, a client may be considered independent when performance of a given occupation is controlled by the client, regardless of whether any assistance is needed. It recognizes that some occupations are done by one person and some are done with others. It also recognizes the concept of co-occupation, in which two or more people share an occupation, which requires interaction between the people engaged in it. Co-occupation is also used to describe engagement in multiple occupations at once, integrating and enfolding occupations. Examples of co-occupation include

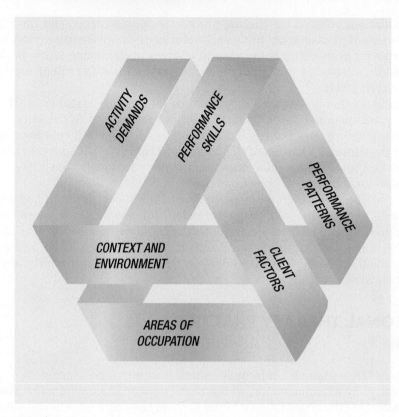

FIGURE 3.1 Domain of Occupational Therapy. *Source: AOTA (2008).*

preparing a meal while simultaneously giving a child words to spell so the child can practice for an upcoming spelling test, playing a team sport, or discussing finances with one's spouse while carpooling to work.

In *The Framework,* 2nd ed., the term client means a person, an organization, or a population (AOTA, 2008). Occupational therapy practitioners use the power of engagement in occupations when working with individuals, families, groups of people, or communities. A client can be a person who has been injured on the job, the family of a child with a disability, a group of residents of a group home learning to plant a garden, a company seeking to reduce the incidence of workplace injuries, or a city developing ways to safely shelter people in the wake of a natural disaster.

Domain of Occupational Therapy

The Framework, 2nd ed., uses the phrase "supporting health and participation in life through engagement in occupation" (AOTA, 2008, p. 626) to represent the domain of occupational therapy practice. There are six areas in the domain of occupational therapy, and no one area is of greater importance than any other. The areas are illustrated in Figure 3.1.

Areas of occupation are the observable acts that a person wants or needs to do in order to participate in life situations (AOTA, 2008). Within these areas are eight categories:

- Activities of daily living: Those things we do to take care of ourselves, including, bathing/showering, bowel and bladder management, dressing, eating, feeding, functional mobility, personal device care, personal hygiene and grooming, sexual activity, and toilet hygiene.

- *Instrumental activities of daily living:* Those things we do in our daily life at home and in the community such as care of others, care of pets, childrearing, communication management, community mobility, financial management, health management and maintenance, home establishment and management, meal preparation and cleanup, safety and emergency maintenance, and shopping.
- *Rest and sleep:* Those things we do to restore ourselves such as resting, sleeping, sleep preparation, and sleep participation.
- *Education:* Those things we do as students or to participate in a learning environment, including exploring and participating in both formal and informal learning situations.
- *Work:* Those things we do to engage in paid employment or volunteer experiences such as exploring, identifying, seeking, and obtaining paid work; performing at work; preparing for and adjusting to retirement, and exploring and participating in volunteer experiences.
- *Play:* Those things we do simply for "enjoyment, entertainment, amusement, or diversion" (Parham & Fazio, 1997, as cited in AOTA, 2008, p. 632), including both exploration and participation in play.
- *Leisure:* Those things we do when we are not obligated to do anything else, including both exploration and participation in leisure.
- *Social participation:* Those things we do when we are interacting with others, whether that interaction takes place between friends/peers, family, or community.

In *The Framework,* 2nd ed. (AOTA, 2008), performance skills and performance patterns enable a person's performance in areas of occupation. Performance skills are the building blocks of activities and occupations. They are small, observable, and purposeful. In *The Framework*, there are five categories of performance skills:

- *Motor and practice skills* are those skills involved in moving, such as bending, reaching, turning, pacing, coordination, balancing, maintaining posture, and manipulating objects.
- *Sensory-perceptual skills* are those used to recognize, interpret, organize, and use sensations, such as "visual, auditory, proprioceptive, tactile, olfactory, gustatory, and vestibular" (AOTA, 2008, p. 640) for purposeful activity.
- *Emotional regulation skills* are those things we do to recognize, interpret, use, and express feelings, such as identifying emotions of others, use strategies to help us control our emotions, persevere when we are tired, forgive others for hurting us, or show appropriate emotional reactions to a variety of situations.
- *Cognitive skills* are those used to plan or manage an activity, such as organizing, prioritizing, selecting, creating, sequencing, or carrying out an activity.
- *Communication/interaction skills* are those that are required for getting one's wants, needs, and intentions across to others and understanding the wants, needs, and intentions of others, including verbal and nonverbal communication, giving and receiving messages, and participating in appropriate relationships.

Performance patterns reflect the ways in which behavior occurs including habits, routines, roles, and rituals (AOTA, 2008). *Habits* are things we do without thinking; they are automatic. Some habits are useful in that they contribute to life satisfaction; others are dominating and interfere with daily life, as in obsessive–compulsive disorder. Impoverished habits either do not support daily life, or need practice to improve. *Routines* are sequences of behavior that occur in the same way each time they are done, providing structure for one's daily life. An example of this might be always putting the right shoe on before the left, or always taking a particular route to work, regardless of traffic delays. *Roles* are "sets of behavior expected by society, shaped by culture, and may be further conceptualized by the client" (AOTA, 2008, p. 641). Examples of roles include those of parent, teacher, coach, or patient, and are tied very closely to a person's sense of identity. *Rituals* are symbolic actions associated with spiritual, cultural, or social meaning. Habits, routines, roles, and rituals can, depending on the circumstance, be helpful or hinder health and well-being. *The Framework,* 2nd ed., describes habits, routines, roles, and rituals at the individual, organization, and population levels (AOTA, 2008).

Contexts are conditions that exist within or around a person and have an influence on the individual's performance (AOTA, 2008). Environments surround a client in the physical and social realms; they are the people, spaces, and objects with whom people interact. While some people use the terms *context* and *environment* interchangeably, *The Framework,* 2nd ed., uses both so as to capture the widest possible interpretations of the terms. *The Framework* names seven kinds of contexts and environments:

- *Cultural contexts* represent the customs, beliefs, activity patterns, and behavioral expectations and standards of the community in which the client is a member. They can include health, political, legal, economic, educational, and employment opportunities.
- *Physical environments* are natural and human-made space, terrain, buildings, objects, plants, and animals.
- *Social environments* concern groups of people and the influences that they have on the performance of each other. People can include relatives, friends, caregivers, and members of an organization in this context.
- *Personal contexts* are unique to the individual and include age, gender, economic status, employment status, educational status, and living situation.
- *Temporal contexts* include aspects of performance that relate to time, such as developmental age, life stages, seasonal considerations, and time of day.
- *Virtual contexts* are those where communication takes place without physical contact between people, such as via computers, radio, or telephone.

The demands of an activity are defined as those aspects of an activity that are needed to carry out that activity (AOTA, 2008). For example, some demands of the activity of grocery shopping include mobility enough to push a grocery cart, remove items from store shelves, and put them in the cart; money management to purchase items; and an understanding of social expectations for behavior in a public space. The aspects of activity demands identified by AOTA (2008) in *The Framework* include:

- Objects and their properties (things needed to carry out the activity such as tools and the inherent properties [weight, size, etc.] of the objects)
- Space demands (aspects of the physical environment such as temperature, lighting, noise, room size and color, etc.)
- Social demands (aspects of social and cultural contexts related to that activity such as rules for social conduct, social interaction, etc.)
- Sequence and timing (being aware of the order in which things happen, how quickly or slowly they happen)
- Required actions and performance skills (the "doing" part of the activity, in terms of physical, process, and interaction skills; what any performer of the activity must do)
- Required body functions (what the body and mind do during the activity including mobility, cognitive processes, sensory functions, and functions of other body systems)
- Required body structures (parts of the body that are needed to engage in the activity)

The difference between activity demands and client factors is that activity demands are based on a particular activity and include conditions external and internal to the client. Client factors are identified regardless of the activity and are internal to the client (AOTA, 2008).

In *The Framework,* there are three main client factors (AOTA, 2008). One client factor is the set of body structures—anatomical parts and systems that make up the person. Body functions are the mental, sensory, neuromuscular, cardiovascular, vocal, digestive, genitourinary, and skin-related processes that occur inside a person. Specific examples of body functions include, but are not limited to, orientation, temperament, memory, proprioception, and muscle tone and reflexes. Values, beliefs, and spirituality are the third client factor. These factors help us understand what clients find meaningful, what they think is important, and what they hold as true (AOTA, 2008). A more detailed breakdown of *The Framework* can be found in Appendix I.

Process

The process of occupational therapy, at its most simple, involves evaluation, intervention, and outcomes (AOTA, 2008). The process is intended to be "fluid and dynamic" (AOTA, 2008, p. 647), rather than linear. While there is a fixed starting point (the occupational profile), the other parts of the process interact with and influence the other parts throughout occupational therapy service delivery. The focus of the occupational therapy process is to "support health and participation in life through engagement in occupation" (AOTA, 2008, p. 646). Figure 3.2 shows the occupational therapy process as outlined by *The Framework*.

The evaluation process has two substeps: the occupational profile and the analysis of occupational performance (AOTA, 2008). The occupational profile helps the occupational therapist understand "the client's occupational history and experiences, patterns of daily living, interests, values and needs" (AOTA, 2008, p. 646). The analysis of occupational performance uses information gathered from assessment tools to more fully understand the nature of the occupational performance problem (AOTA, 2008).

The occupational profile starts when the occupational therapist engages in a shared process of data gathering with the client or client's surrogate (e.g., a parent when the client is a child or the adult child of an older adult with Alzheimer's disease). Clients bring information about their history, interests, values, wants, and needs, and the occupational

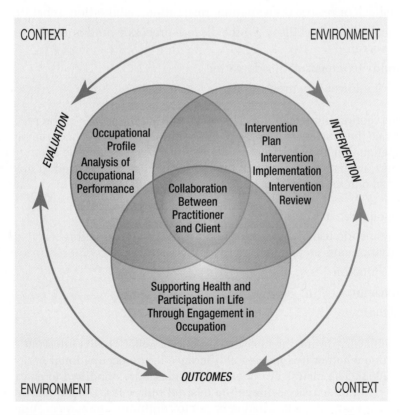

FIGURE 3.2 Process of Occupational Therapy. *Source: AOTA (2008).*

therapist brings information about the power of engagement in occupation, disease or conditions, theoretical perspectives, and clinical reasoning, to the discussion. The type of questions the occupational therapist might ask is influenced by the frame of reference and/or theories employed by the occupational therapist. Knowledge of disease processes, medical and psychiatric conditions, and human anatomy and physiology are also used to help guide the occupational therapist in gathering information and forming a hypothesis about the client. While the occupational profile is the first step in the evaluation process, it is adjusted as the client moves through the process and new data comes to light (AOTA, 2008). You can see that this is a very client-centered process.

The second step of the evaluation is the analysis of occupational performance (AOTA, 2008). In this step, more data is gathered about the client in relation to the domains of occupational therapy practice. The process of analyzing occupational performance includes identifying both barriers and facilitators to successful engagement in occupations. The frame of reference and/or models used by the occupational therapist will influence the type of and method by which this data is gathered. A more thorough description of the evaluation process is described in Chapter 10 of this text.

There are three substeps in the intervention process: the intervention plan, intervention implementation, and intervention review (AOTA, 2008). First, the plan is developed using the data gathered in the evaluation process. The intervention plan is influenced by the frames of reference and/or models used by the occupational therapist and must be directed by goals established in collaboration with the client (AOTA, 2005, 2008). Other influences on the intervention plan include care for the well-being of the client, the setting, and the domains of occupational practice (AOTA, 2008).

The intervention plan requires identifying specific strategies to help the client achieve desired outcomes (AOTA, 2008). There are five strategic approaches to intervention that an occupational therapist could take in developing the plan (AOTA, 2008; Harvison, 2003):

1. Create or promote (health promotion)
2. Establish or restore (remediation, restoration, habilation, rehabilitation)
3. Maintain (retain skills when the disease process would normally result in deterioration of function)
4. Modify (compensation, adaptation)
5. Prevent (disability prevention)

Intervention implementation involves putting the words of the plan into action (AOTA, 2008). Once the strategy and kinds of intervention are established, the occupational therapist or occupational therapy assistant works in collaboration with the client to execute the plan.

There are five main kinds of interventions that can be used to help the client achieve established outcomes (AOTA, 2008; Harvison, 2003):

1. Therapeutic use of self
2. Therapeutic use of occupations and activities (occupation-based activities, purposeful activities, and preparatory methods)
3. Consultation
4. Education
5. Advocacy

Periodically during the intervention implementation, the intervention must be reviewed to determine whether it is making a difference in the occupational performance of the client (AOTA, 2008). The plan is evaluated and, if necessary, modified to enable the client to most efficiently and effectively achieve the desired outcomes. During the intervention review, a determination is made as to whether or not to continue to provide occupational therapy intervention or to make referrals to other professionals. This substep may include a reevaluation of the client as well as reevaluation of the plan (AOTA, 2008).

The last step in the process is the outcome; the end result of the occupational therapy process (AOTA, 2008). Remember that the overarching outcome of occupational therapy is "supporting health and participation in life through engagement in occupation" (AOTA, 2008, p. 660). Three concepts that will be used to determine the success of the occupational therapy process are health, participation, and occupational engagement (AOTA, 2008). Has the client's health improved from the client's perspective? Is the client actively participating in meaningful occupations?

Early in the occupational therapy process, the occupational therapist identifies the outcomes and selects the outcome measures (AOTA, 2008). There are nine types of outcomes that concern occupational therapy practitioners:

1. Occupational performance
2. Adaptation
3. Health and wellness
4. Participation
5. Prevention
6. Self-advocacy
7. Role competence
8. Quality of life
9. Occupational justice

During the occupational therapy process, the occupational therapist uses the identified outcomes to measure 32progress and make adjustments to client goals and interventions, and to make recommendations about whether or not to continue occupational therapy services (AOTA, 2008). Outcomes may also influence decisions about discharge disposition for an individual client.

When documenting any phase of the occupational therapy process, using the terminology reflected in *The Framework* shows that you are up-to-date and on top of your profession. While it is not necessary to memorize each term within each of the six aspects (areas of occupation, performance skills, performance patterns, activity demands, client factors, contexts and environments) of the domain of occupational therapy, it is useful to understand the differences between the types of items in each aspect. Some clinicians suggest that goals be written only to address areas of occupation; others write goals for performance skills or client factors, depending on the frame of reference the occupational therapy practitioner is using. Some occupational therapy evaluation reports have sections for each of the aspects, so the occupational therapist needs to know what types of terms go into each section.

Exercise 3.1

Using the following key, place the appropriate letter in the blank in front of each phrase.

    A = Area of occupation
    P = Performance skill
    C = Client factor

1. _____ Combing one's hair
2. _____ Elbow range of motion
3. _____ Wheelchair mobility
4. _____ Making one's needs known
5. _____ Hand strength
6. _____ Career exploration
7. _____ Time management

8. _____ Understanding nonverbal communication
9. _____ Posture
10. _____ Endurance
11. _____ Knitting
12. _____ Balancing a checkbook
13. _____ Making eye contact
14. _____ Balancing on one leg
15. _____ Taking turns during a card game
16. _____ Dressing a wound
17. _____ Word processing
18. _____ Changing a diaper
19. _____ Finding items in a hidden picture puzzle
20. _____ Identifying signs of danger

▼ SPECIFIC OCCUPATIONAL THERAPY TERMS ▼

Occupational therapy practitioners often use terms they learn in school. This is usually a good thing. However, sometimes the way in which terms are used changes in official documents of the profession. If a practitioner is unaware of these changes, he or she may be using terms incorrectly in current practice. The following is a list of terms whose meanings have changed over the last decade (AOTA, 2005, p. 1):

Assessment: Specific tools or instruments that are used during the evaluation process.

Client: A person, group, program, organization, or community for whom the occupational therapy practitioner is providing services.

Evaluation: The process of obtaining and interpreting data necessary for intervention. This includes planning for and documenting the evaluation process and results.

Screening: Obtaining and reviewing data relevant to a potential client to determine the need for further evaluation and intervention.

Other professions may use these terms in other ways, and they are not wrong. Each profession has its own standard. For example, in education, assessment is the process and evaluations are the tools. Some facilities may also use terms in certain ways. While it is very important to follow the standards established by your professional organization, it is also important to communicate clearly with coworkers in other professions. If there is any doubt about how a term is being used at a particular facility, ask a department head who has been at the facility for a few years or more. This will be an experienced professional who can advise you on how to best be understood by others at the facility.

SUMMARY

The American Occupational Therapy Association has developed guidelines for the practice of occupational therapy, which in turn influences the words we use in occupational therapy documentation. The *Occupational Therapy Practice Framework* is a document that seeks to describe the process of providing occupational therapy services to clients across practice settings and to describe the domains of occupational therapy practice (AOTA, 2008). The process begins with understanding the occupational needs of any client, and then an analysis of the client's occupational performance. Intervention is then planned and implemented in order to assist the client in achieving his or her desired outcomes. The outcome of any occupational therapy intervention is "health and participation in life through engagement in occupation" (AOTA, 2002, p. 626). The *Practice Framework* describes eight domains of occupational therapy practice: (1) activities of daily living, (2) instrumental activities of daily living, (3) rest and sleep, (4) education, (5) work, (6) play, (7) leisure, and (8) social participation (AOTA, 2008). This document also includes recommended language for discussing the work of occupational therapy practitioners, including a glossary of terms.

Some facilities may still use the *Uniform Terminology* document that AOTA developed years ago (AOTA, 1994). However, the AOTA has rescinded that document, and the terminology used in it is no longer considered correct. *Uniform Terminology* provided a system of organizing the domains of practice, but it did not address the process of providing occupational therapy services (AOTA, 2002).

In addition to AOTA, the World Health Organization has also developed a taxonomy for describing human function and dysfunction called *International Classification of Function* (ICF) (WHO, 2002). The language of that document is also helpful in choosing words that members of other disciplines will understand. The language used by the ICF was influential in the development of the *Occupational Therapy Practice Framework* (AOTA, 2008).

It is critical to use terminology that is understood and accepted by both others in the profession and those outside the profession. The more consistent occupational therapy personnel are in using terminology, the more likely the documentation is to be understood by others. It is equally critical that you stay current in your use of terminology as the profession evolves and changes.

Using the language of the profession can strengthen one's documentation. Your words carry the weight of the best minds in the profession. In addition, you show that you are current in your understanding of the profession by using the words of the professional association. The importance of staying up-to-date with the profession, with best practice, should never be overlooked.

REFERENCES

American Occupational Therapy Association. (1994). Uniform terminology for occupational therapy, 3rd edition. *American Journal of Occupational Therapy, 48,* 1047–1054.

American Occupational Therapy Association. (2002). Occupational therapy practice framework: Domain and process. *American Journal of Occupational Therapy, 56,* 609–639.

American Occupational Therapy Association. (2005). Standards of practice for occupational therapy. *American Journal of Occupational Therapy, 59,* 663–665.

American Occupational Therapy Association. (2008). Occupational therapy practice framework: Domain and process (2nd ed.). *American Journal of Occupational Therapy, 62,* 625–683.

Harvison, N. (2003). Overview of the occupational therapy practice framework: Part 1. *Administration and Management Special Interest Section Quarterly, 19*(1), 1–4.

World Health Organization. (2002). *International classification of functioning disability and health.* Geneva, Switzerland: Author. Retrieved July 27, 2006, from http://www3.who.int/icf/intros/ICF-Eng-Intro.pdf

CHAPTER 4

Impact of Models and Frames of Reference

INTRODUCTION

In Chapter 3 we discussed the ways in which the language of the profession is changing. In addition to staying current on terminology, the words an occupational therapist uses while summarizing evaluation results, planning intervention, reporting progress, and planning discontinuation will also depend on the model or frame of reference being used for a particular client.

▼ DESCRIPTION OF MODELS AND FRAMES OF REFERENCE ▼

Depending on which textbook you read, the definition of a model and of a frame of reference will vary. Both models and frames of reference are based on theory and help organize knowledge so that it can be used to guide an occupational therapist in determining the cause of dysfunction and ways to assist a client to engage in occupations that are meaningful to the client.

According to Mosey (as cited in Christiansen & Baum, 1991), a model integrates theoretical assumptions for use in practice. Mosey describes a model as

> A profession's model is the typical way in which a profession perceives itself, its relationship to other professions, and its association with the society to which it is responsible. The model of a profession is characterized by a description of the profession's philosophical assumptions, ethical code, theoretical foundations, domain of concern, legitimate tools, and the nature of and principles for sequencing the various aspects of practice (as cited in Kielhofner, 1997, p. 325).

Christiansen and Baum (1991) describe a model as referring to ways of structuring or organizing information that is relevant to practice and for the purpose of guiding thinking.

A frame of reference is closely related to a model, but is typically more specific in terms of application of knowledge and information. A frame of reference is a bridge between theory and practice. It takes the knowledge we have and organizes it in such a way that it can be applied to working with clients (Christiansen & Baum, 1997). Frames of reference are based on theory and provide direction for evaluating, planning and implementing intervention, and discontinuing services. According to Mosey (as cited in Christiansen & Baum, 1991), frames of reference are the portions of models that are methodological in focus; they tell the occupational therapist how to use the information in practice. She goes on to say that frames of reference should provide the following: "1) information on the domain of concern; 2) the theories upon which their assertions are based; 3) the nature of function and dysfunction; 4) behaviors which reflect these states;

and 5) the principles regarding intervention on how one can change from a dysfunctional to a functional state" (pp. 12–13).

Think of a frame of reference or model as being the lens through which you see your client. Just as different-colored lenses (i.e., sunglasses) change the way you see your surroundings and what parts of the environment stand out, so do different frames of reference change what parts of the client's situation stand out. For example, a biomechanical frame of reference looks at structural enhancements such as strengthening, decreasing edema, and splinting to improve range of movement in an injured limb while a task-oriented frame of reference looks at finding goal-directed functional behaviors to encourage use of the affected limb (Hagedorn, 1997; Kielhofner, 1997; Neistadt & Crepeau, 1998). In this example, the biomechanical approach has a focus on client factors and performance skills (AOTA, 2008) while the task-oriented approach looks at performance patterns and performance in areas of occupation (AOTA, 2002).

Some models or frames of reference used by occupational therapy practitioners focus on getting at the root cause of the dysfunction, such as the psychoanalytical or neurodevelopmental frames of reference. Others focus on the level of dysfunction and ways to minimize it, regardless of the cause, such as the cognitive disabilities frame of reference or ecological models. Some use a developmental focus, others an environmental one.

In later chapters, the mechanics of writing goals and completing different types of documents will be discussed. This chapter focuses on identifying different models and frames of reference and how the word choices may vary between them.

▼ HOW MODELS AND FRAMES OF REFERENCE ARE REFLECTED IN DOCUMENTATION ▼

Table 4.1 summarizes different frames of reference used in occupational therapy and hints for how that frame of reference can be reflected in one's documentation. Please note that the summaries of these frames of reference are not intended to be comprehensive or all-inclusive. Because of the vast number of new and developing frames of reference, it would be impossible to cover every one. Memorizing this table will not tell you everything you need to know about each frame of reference.

TABLE 4.1 Influence of Frames of Reference on Documentation

Frame of Reference	Description of Key Concepts	How It Is Reflected in Documentation
Behavioral (Skinner, Pavlov)	A person's behavior is the result of feedback from the environment. Insight and personality are not considered. One can unlearn maladaptive behaviors and learn adaptive ones through the use of techniques such as shaping, teaching, and reinforcement. OT works with others on the team to consistently work toward positive changes in behavior.	Evaluation reports contain detailed observations of behavior including frequency of behavior, where and when behavior occurs. Progress notes document behavior modification methods used and the results of these interventions. Measurable goals specify the person, the observable behavior expected, and conditions for the behavior such as where, when, frequency, and any cuing that will occur.

(Continued)

TABLE 4.1 Influence of Frames of Reference on Documentation (Continued)

Frame of Reference	Description of Key Concepts	How It Is Reflected in Documentation
Biomechanical	Focus on "the body as a machine." Improving strength, endurance, and structural integrity will lead to improved function. Use splinting, exercise, massage, biofeedback, and other physical means of intervention. Once range of motion, strength, edema, and endurance are regained, functional use will follow. Pain, loss of sensation, and poor coordination are not of primary concern.	Evaluation reports focus on performance skills/client factors. Progress notes reflect improvements in range of motion, strength, edema, and endurance. Range of motion, strength, edema, and endurance are easily quantified for goal setting. Functional goals would reflect new activities that increased movement will allow.
Canadian Model of Occupational Performance (Law et al.)	The person is in constant interaction with the environment. Client-centered practice Spirituality gives meaning to occupations. Environment influences occupational performance.	Evaluation reports focus on activities of daily living, play, spirituality and work. Progress notes focus on the client's level of ability and satisfaction in performing meaningful occupations. Goals relate to level of ability and satisfaction in the performance of meaningful occupations.
Cognitive-Behavioral Therapy (Bandura; Rotter; Ellis and Beck)	Maladaptive behaviors are the result of cognitive distortions and self-defeating thinking. People have automatic thoughts that they tell themselves internally. "Core schemas" are the thoughts people tell themselves that color the way they perceive themselves and their environment. Clients are taught to repeat positive "self-talk" to alter the core schemas. Clients are taught to challenge logically the core schemas and automatic thoughts they had.	Evaluation reports focus on client report of feelings and thoughts about oneself. Progress notes reflect client's report of feelings and thoughts, which lead to changes in behavior. Goals suggest the positive statements the client will repeat to oneself, use of stress management techniques, and identify desired behavioral outcomes.
Cognitive Disabilities (also called Cognition & Activity) (Allen)	Neurological problems lead to limitations in cognitive capacity, which lead to a performance deficit.	Evaluation reports identify the current cognitive level as supported by descriptions of functional performance in everyday occupations.

(Continued)

TABLE 4.1   Influence of Frames of Reference on Documentation (Continued)

Frame of Reference	Description of Key Concepts	How It Is Reflected in Documentation
	Cognitive limitations occur as six cognitive levels on a continuum. Occupational therapy cannot change cognitive levels that are the result of brain pathology. Palliative treatment attempts to reduce symptoms by changing the tasks (adapting) a patient is asked to do. Expectant treatment means that nature takes its course, and the role of the OT is to document and monitor the patient's functional abilities. Supportive treatment is like maintenance treatment; the goal is to sustain strength during illness and recovery, using things like diversionary activities. Tasks and activities are analyzed for fit with a person's cognitive level; they are adapted to remove obstacles to performance and use a person's available cognitive capacity.	Progress notes describe the client's response to adaptations in the task or environment and any changes noted in cognitive level (based on observations). Goals are established to identify desired performance within the context of the client's environment, and relate to palliative, expectant or supportive treatment.
Contemporary Task-Oriented (Haugen & Mathiowetz)	Focus on the interaction between the characteristics of a person and the contexts in which the person exists. The personal and environmental characteristics have no hierarchy in terms of their influences on performance. The client's perspective is the focus of evaluation and intervention; it is client-centered. Intervention involves practice and experimentation.	Evaluation reports center on the client's unique characteristics, contexts, and motivations. Recording observations is essential in progress notes. Goals relate to functional performance.
Developmental (Piaget, Freud, Erickson, Kohlberg and many others)	Humans normally develop in a sequential fashion. Each new gain in structure enables a gain in function; each new gain in function enables further development. Physical, sensory, perceptual, cognitive, social, and emotional development are interconnected and affect the whole person.	Evaluation reports focus on comparing a child's performance to that of a typically developing child of the same chronological age to identify areas in need of intervention. Progress reports show the child has made gains in functional performance of daily occupations.

(Continued)

TABLE 4.1   Influence of Frames of Reference on Documentation (Continued)

Frame of Reference	Description of Key Concepts	How It Is Reflected in Documentation
	Stress can cause regression to earlier levels of adaptation. Focus on seven developmental areas: Perceptual–Motor, Cognitive, Drive–Object, Dyadic Interaction, Group Interaction, Self-Identity, and Sexual Identity.	Goals identify desired occupations to enable the child's maximum participation in life situations.
Ecology of Human Performance (Dunn)	Ecology is the interaction between a person and contexts (the environment). The person, the context, and task performance interact with and affect one another. Performance is improved by establishing/restoring the person's skills or abilities, or altering/adapting the context or the task to support performance in context.	Evaluation reports look not only at the person but also at contexts and tasks and the person–context match. Progress reports describe what interventions/alterations have been tried and their results. Goals reflect the person's participation in occupations and performance in context.
Model of Human Occupation (Kielhofner)	Volition, habituation, and performance are hierarchical subsystems within a person that regulate choice, organization, and performance. Personal and environmental factors influence choice, organization, and performance. Change is a holistic process. Individuals are given the opportunity for guided participation in life tasks to improve organization, function, and adaptation as demonstrated by successful role performance. Occupations must be relevant and related to a person's roles, habits, and the environment.	Evaluation reports focus on the client's performance in areas of occupation, choices (volition), habits, and roles. Progress notes focus on the client's choices (volition), habits, and roles during meaningful occupations. Goals relate to performance in occupations, choices (volition), habits, and roles that are meaningful to the client.
Neurodevelopmental Treatment (NDT) (Bobaths)	Spasticity and hypotonia are the major barriers to normal movement. The trunk and proximal joints need stability to enable limb movement. The brain is plastic and capable of new learning.	Evaluation reports focus on observations of movement patterns and barriers to normal movement. Progress notes need to reflect frequent clinical observations. Goals relate to patterns of movement that enable occupational performance.

(Continued)

TABLE 4.1 Influence of Frames of Reference on Documentation (Continued)

Frame of Reference	Description of Key Concepts	How It Is Reflected in Documentation
	Work toward inhibiting abnormal reflexes and synergies to enable learning of normal movement. Bilateral focus; use positioning, handling, and sensory stimulation to facilitate normal movement patterns.	
Occupational Adaptation (Schkade & Schultz)	As clients become more adaptive, their ability to function improves. The ability of clients to adapt can be overwhelmed by stressful life events, including illness, injury, or disabilities. When a client's ability to adapt is challenged so much that performance demand cannot be satisfactorily met, dysfunction occurs. Internal and external factors continually interact resulting in an occupational response; the observable outcome of the person-environment interaction.	Evaluation reports focus on the environmental demands, internal resources, occupational roles, and occupational adaptation abilities of the client. Progress notes focus on the client's ability to adapt to changing demands. Goals may begin with the client learning adaptive skills, and then evolve into the client using adaptive skills and occupational mastery.
Occupational Behavior (Reilly)	Active participation in tasks can lead to development of mastery and, therefore, permit successful role performance. Focus is on activities of daily living, play, and work. Role fulfillment provides positive feedback to the person and enables that person to go on to new skills, more complex tasks. Skills become habits through repetition. Through the continuum of work–play, a person learns the roles needed to become competent in mastery.	Evaluation reports focus on activities of daily living, play, and work. Progress notes focus on the client's performance during meaningful occupations. Goals relate to performance in occupations and roles that are meaningful to the clients, and address the different environments in which the client spends time.
Person–Environment–Occupational Performance (Christiansen & Baum)	Many intrinsic (neurobehavioral, physiological, cognitive, psychological, and spiritual) and extrinsic (social support, social and economic systems, culture and values, built environment and technology, and natural environment) factors contribute to occupational performance.	Evaluation reports reflect the client's assets and limitations in relation to his or her occupational performance as well as the supports and barriers in the environment. Progress reports demonstrate the client's occupational performance within environmental contexts.

(Continued)

How Models and Frames of Reference are Reflected in Documentation   **41**

TABLE 4.1   Influence of Frames of Reference on Documentation (Continued)

Frame of Reference	Description of Key Concepts	How It Is Reflected in Documentation
	Adaptation is the process used by people to meet challenges in daily living through the use of personal resources. The characteristics of the person, environment, and the nature/meaning of actions, tasks, and roles are considered when trying to understand occupational performance. Focus is on the person's wants and needs rather than on dysfunction.	Short-term goals may relate to intrinsic factors inhibiting occupational performance. Long-term goals may relate to functional performance of daily life tasks and roles.
Proprioceptive Neuromuscular Facilitation (PNF) (Knott & Voss)	Weakness and lack of voluntary control over movements are the main obstacles to normal movement patterns. Frequent repetition and stimulation of the proprioceptors support the learning of new motor abilities. Movements are more often diagonal than linear. Vision, breathing, and verbal commands all play a strong role in movement.	Evaluation reports emphasize observable movement patterns. Progress notes reflect client responses to inhibition and facilitation techniques. Goals relate to the client's movements during activities of daily.
Psychoanalytic (Freud); Object Relations (Fidler)	Intrapsychic (unconscious) conflicts are at the heart of the problem. The major areas of concern are the psychodynamics, level of psychosexual and psychosocial development, and alterations of intrapsychic content. Goal is to resolve these inner conflicts. Use of activity to resolve intrapsychic conflict and reality orientation such as psychodrama, projective art, creative writing and poetry therapy, and guided fantasy.	Evaluation reports focus on the affect of the client, symptoms of psychopathology, and how these interfere with daily life functions. Progress reports often reflect the client's subjective report of feelings as well as observations of client behavior. Goals reflect the client's self-expression of feelings.
Rehabilitative (Compensatory)	Through the continuum of work–play, a person learns the roles needed to become competent in mastery.	Evaluation reports emphasize both strengths and areas in need of improvement.

(Continued)

TABLE 4.1 Influence of Frames of Reference on Documentation (Continued)

Frame of Reference	Description of Key Concepts	How It Is Reflected in Documentation
		Progress notes document what types of adaptations have been tried and the results of each trial. Goals do not specify specific techniques, tools, or equipment. Goals reflect functional outcomes, what the client will do.
Spatiotemporal Adaptation (Gilfoyle, Grady, & Moore)	Movement and activity influence a person's development. Movement is important for physical, psychological, and social development of a child. Development occurs in an ever-widening spiral that represents increasing skills as influenced by experiences with the environment. Emphasis on integration of old behaviors with new ones. Emphasis on integration of old behaviors with new ones.	Evaluation reports focus on the movements of the child in relation to environmental demands. Progress reports reflect the increasing complexity of the movement–environment interactions of the child. Goals can be structured to reflect prevention, remediation, and/or adjustment to dysfunction.
Sensory Integration (Ayers)	Sensory integrative dysfunction is a result of a failure of the brain to properly organize and interpret sensory input. There is interaction between brain organization and adaptive behavior. People have an inner drive to participate in sensory motor activities and seek out organizing sensations. Play is self-directed, within an environment carefully set up by the OT to meet that client's needs. Environment provides the opportunities to experience needed sensations in a safe, nonthreatening atmosphere, and includes access to sensory input to all sensory processing systems of the body, including vestibular.	Evaluation reports focus on identifying areas of sensory processing deficits and how these impact participation in everyday life experiences. Progress notes reflect the child's responses to different sensory experiences, qualities of movement, and changes in the child's participation in everyday life experiences. Goals focus on increased duration or repetitions of an activity, or the quality of movements during an activity.

Sources: Christiansen, C. & Baum, C. (1997); Hagedorn, R. (1997); Kielhofner, G. (2004); and Neistadt, M. S. & Crepeau, E. B. (1998).

The reader is referred to the sources used in developing this chapter for more information on each frame of reference. Having a good understanding of the frame of reference you are using will help you in writing reports and notes and in establishing goals. Often the frame of reference will suggest the use of certain terminology.

There are two primary approaches to occupational therapy that are reflected in the models and frames of reference. One approach is referred to as the top-down approach, and the other is referred to as the bottom-up approach (Weinstock-Zlotnik & Hinijosa, 2004; Trombly Latham, 2008). According to Weinstock-Zlotnik and Hinijosa, using a top-down approach, you would begin by considering the client's performance in areas of occupation and the other aspects of the domain of occupational therapy (client factors, performance skills, performance patterns, activity demands, and contexts and environments) later. The primary concern is the client's ability to engage in meaningful occupations. Trombly Latham takes a slightly different view of the top-down approach. She suggests that when considering performance in areas of occupation, the client's roles and contexts are a necessary part of the process. Once the occupational therapist has a clear picture of the roles, contexts, and occupations that are meaningful to the client, the causes of the current problems in occupational performance are evaluated, including the specific client factors, performance skills, and performance patterns (Trombly Latham). The *Occupational Therapy Practice Framework* (2nd ed.) takes a top-down approach by suggesting that the occupational profile be completed first, then the analysis of occupational performance (AOTA, 2008).

An assumption of the bottom-up approach is that if you improve the performance skills (motor, cognitive, sensory perceptual, communication, or emotional regulation skills) and client factors, then the client's performance in areas of occupation will take care of itself (Weinstock-Zlotnik & Hinijosa, 2004). This approach holds some appeal for practitioners in medical settings where time is limited and pressure from third-party payers to produce measurable results is strong. In these settings, the occupational therapy practitioner may receive a physician order to see a client to increase range of motion following surgery, or increase strength following an injury.

Weinstock-Zlotnik and Hinijosa argue that bottom-up approaches are useful because of the number of standardized assessment tools available leading to more measurable outcomes. They also argue that top-down approaches are more broad and difficult to measure but provide a stronger professional identity for occupational therapy. In the end, Weinstock-Zlotnik and Hinijosa suggest that the profession needs both approaches and that using only one or the other approach does a disservice to the profession.

Occupational therapy began by using occupation-based, top-down approaches, then, following the lead of the medical community, became reductionistic, using a more bottom-up approach (Keilhofner, 2004; Weinstock-Zlotnik & Hinijosa, 2004). Coming full circle, the profession of occupational therapy now favors top-down, occupation-based approaches (Keilhofner, Weinzstock-Zlotnik & Hinijosa). Each of these approaches has generated the formation of models and frames of reference to explain dysfunction and suggest intervention strategies.

Exercise 4.1

For each of the models and frames of reference in Table 4.1, tell whether it is a top-down or bottom-up approach.

1. Behavioral

2. Biomechanical

3. Canadian Model of Occupational Performance

4. Cognitive-Behavioral Therapy

5. Cognitive Disabilities (also called Cognition & Activity)

6. Contemporary Task-Oriented

7. Developmental

8. Ecology of Human Performance

9. Model of Human Occupation

10. Neurodevelopmental Treatment (NDT)

11. Occupational Adaptation

12. Occupational Behavior

13. Person–Environment–Occupational Performance

14. Proprioceptive Neuromuscular Facilitation (PNF)

15. Psychoanalytic (Freud); Object Relations

16. Rehabilitative (Compensatory)

17. Spatiotemporal Adaptation

18. Sensory Integration

People who work together at one facility tend to all use the same model or frame of reference, or the same mix of them. When you start working (or go on fieldwork) at a new place, be sure to ask which models or frames of reference are acceptable to use. Usually, but not always, more than one frame of reference is used at a facility or program. When multiple models or frames of reference are blended together, it is sometimes called an eclectic approach. Hopefully, this blending occurs in a thoughtful way, based on the collective experiences of the occupational therapy staff and the types of clients being served in that program or facility. However, sometimes occupational therapists say they are eclectic in their approach when they are unable to name a specific model or frame of reference.

Exercise 4.2

Are the following goals compatible with the frame of reference cited?

1. In the next 30 days, the client will increase range of motion of shoulder flexion from 40° to 60°. (Bobath)

2. Arwan will eat at least one meal per day, for 5 consecutive days, that contains at least three different textures without screaming, spitting, or turning away by June 15, 2007. (Sensory integration)

3. Robert will consistently brush his teeth twice per day, without cues from his parents, by November 24, 2007. (Model of human occupation)

4. In 1 month, Sonja will independently ride the bus from home to work. (Behavioral)

5. In 6 months, DeNeda will demonstrate the self-care and home-maintenance skills necessary for her to return home to independent living. (Psychoanalytical)

6. In 6 weeks, Christianne will word-process at a rate of 60 words per minute with two or fewer errors. (Cognitive behavioral therapy)

7. Xia will place eight knobs in a bag, with the use of an adapted jig if necessary, by July 7, 2007. (Cognitive disabilities)

8. Rosita (age 6) will print her name legibly with each letter touching the line by December 12, 2007. (Canadian model of occupational performance)

SUMMARY

Models and frames of reference are ways to organize one's thinking about how to approach a client, and guide the way an occupational therapist evaluates, plans, and implements interventions and determines when a client has achieved desired outcomes. Both models and frames of reference are based on theory.

The model or frame of reference that you choose to work from with a given client needs to be reflected in the way you document about that client. Often the words used in documentation are suggested by the model or frame of reference being used. A model or frame of reference is used to help you select an appropriate evaluation method, set goals, and describe progress. You can use Table 4.1 to help in ensuring that your documentation is reflective of the model or frame of reference being used. Some facilities or programs use multiple models or frames of reference.

REFERENCES

American Occupational Therapy Association. (2008). Occupational therapy practice framework: Domain and process. *American Journal of Occupational Therapy, 62*, 625–683.

Christiansen, C., & Baum, C. (1991). *Occupational therapy: Enabling function and well-being.* Thoroughfare, NJ: Slack.

Christiansen, C., & Baum, C. (1997). *Occupational therapy: Enabling function and well-being* (2nd ed.). Thoroughfare, NJ: Slack.

Hagedorn, R. (1997). *Foundations for practice in occupational therapy* (2nd ed.). London: Churchill Livingstone.

Kielhofner, G. (1997). *Conceptual foundations of occupational therapy* (2nd ed.). Philadelphia: F. A. Davis.

Kielhofner, G. (2004). *Conceptual foundations of occupational therapy* (3rd ed.). Philadelphia: F. A. Davis.

Trombly Latham, C. A. (2008). Conceptual foundations for practice. In M.V. Radomski & C.A. Trombly Latham, *Occupational therapy for physical dysfunction* (6th ed., pp. 1–20). Philadelphia: Lippencott, Williams, & Wilken.

Neistadt, M. S., & Crepeau, E. B. (1998). *Willard & Spackman's occupational therapy* (9th ed.). Philadelphia: Lippencott-Raven.

Weinstock-Zlotnik G. & Hinijosa, J. (2004). *Bottom-up or top-down evaluation: Is one better than the other?* American Journal of Occupational Therapy, 58, 594–599.

CHAPTER 5

Document with CARE: General Tips for Good Documentation

INTRODUCTION

If you have read the previous chapters, you know that careful wording in documentation is essential. There is a system for double-checking your documentation so that you can be assured that it will be well written. This system is called "Document with CARE" (Sames & Berkeland, 1998). CARE is an abbreviation for:

Clarity: The reader can understand what you are saying.
Accuracy: The documentation reflects what actually happened.
Relevance: The documentation relates to identified needs and purposes.
Exceptions: Any unusual occurrences, noncompliance, or changes are documented.

Let's examine each of these criteria one at a time.

▼ CLARITY ▼

In order for the reader to understand what you have written, it has to be written in clear, concise, unbiased language (Sames & Berkeland, 1998). Abbreviations and jargon need to be kept to a minimum and, when used, must be approved by the facility in which they are used. Grammar and spelling should not interfere with the professional appearance and intended message of the documentation. Usually, simple, shorter sentences are clearer than long ones. In some settings, it is acceptable to use phrases or incomplete sentences to keep the note brief. While computers are often used for formal documentation, any handwritten notes must be legible. People who are not familiar with the jargon of the profession must be able to read and understand your notes. These seem like commonsense things, but you would be amazed at some of the documentation that is out there (Sames & Berkeland, 1998).

Remember the discussion about the use of jargon in Chapter 2. Too much jargon makes documentation less clear to people outside the profession, but over simplifying the language may make the documentation sound less than professional. How specific or technical your documentation is depends on the setting, the types of people who are most likely to read your documentation, and the type of service being documented (Sames, 2008). If you are writing an Individualized Family Service Plan (IFSP) for the family of an infant with whom you are working, you would use as little jargon as possible. If you are writing a detailed evaluation report in a teaching hospital, you might use more technical terms and more jargon (Sames).

▼ ACCURACY ▼

Your documentation needs to be factually correct (Sames & Berkeland, 1998). Documentation is almost always done chronologically, that is, what happens first is written about first, and then events are recorded in the order in which they happen. Documentation also needs to be consistent with the protocols of the institution or agency involved. Documentation written away from the client's clinical or educational record is placed in the correct file, and in the correct place within the file. Never document about another client by name in your client's record. For example, if Mr. Smith and Mr. Jones play checkers, and you are writing in Mr. Smith's chart, you may say that Mr. Smith played checkers with another client, but do not put Mr. Jones's name in Mr. Smith's note (Sames & Berkeland, 1998).

Another aspect of accuracy is distinguishing between what you observe and what you think it means (Sames & Berkeland, 1998). This will be addressed more completely in Chapter 10. In the meantime, think about the following. You observe a client with a plate of food in front of her and a fork in her right hand. She uses her right hand to scoop up the food and begins to raise the food to her mouth. The fork tips and the food falls off. She lowers her fork to the plate and scoops at the food, pushing the food off her plate. She then drops the fork and picks up the food with her fingers. If in your note you write, "The client made two attempts to feed herself with a fork, then proceeded to feed herself with her fingers," you are truly describing what you saw. If in your note you write, "The client is unable to feed herself with a fork. She gets frustrated and starts using her fingers," then you are interpreting what you saw. You are generalizing a short, one-time observation into applying to every time she eats. There are times when your interpretation is as important as, or more important than, your description, but you must be careful to identify when you are describing and when you are interpreting a client's performance (Sames & Berkeland, 1998).

▼ RELEVANCE ▼

The reader must see, on the basis of what you write, why occupational therapy was initiated, continued, and discontinued (Sames & Berkeland, 1998). In other words, the documentation must demonstrate the need for skilled service. By skilled service, I mean services requiring the expertise of an occupational therapist or an occupational therapy assistant under the supervision of an occupational therapist. The reader needs to see that what you are doing in occupational therapy is something that uses the unique skills and abilities of occupational therapy practitioners. When the occupational therapy practitioner is working in a transdisciplinary model (a model of service delivery in which several professionals from different disciplines all fulfill the same role, and there is little or no differentiation between what each person does), then the documentation needs to reflect the client's need for the program's services (Sames & Berkeland, 1998).

When the client's chart or file is read from beginning to end, it should be clear that the results of the screening (if there is one), the referral, the evaluation, the intervention planning, the intervention, and the discontinuation have a common theme. In other words, if an adult with chronic schizophrenia is referred to occupational therapy to learn to live independently, then the evaluation summary should be centered on independent living skills, the intervention plan should address independent living skills, the progress notes should demonstrate work on independent living skills, and the discontinuation summary should also reflect the client's skills in independent living. If a child is referred to you to improve handwriting skills, then the documentation should reflect work on handwriting skills. This does not mean that you cannot document work on any other domain of concern, but other domains are documented only after demonstrating additional needs in those areas. For every problem or need identified, there should be written evidence that the problem or need was addressed or an explanation of why it was left unaddressed (Cathy Brennan, MA, OTR/L, FAOTA, personal communication, June 21, 2006).

Documentation should always be timely (Sames & Berkeland, 1998). This means the documentation, in order to be relevant, needs to be done as close to the time as the event occurred. Generally, evaluation reports are done within a day or two of completing the evaluation; intervention plans are done according to the schedule of the facility (annually, bimonthly, or monthly); progress notes are often done at the close of each visit to occupational therapy; and discontinuation summaries are usually completed within 2 days of discharge. Each facility will have standards related to timeliness. These standards are to be taken seriously, not as general targets, but as deadlines (Sames & Berkeland, 1998).

Other relevant information needs to be available in the client's record. If there are precautions or contraindications that must be observed, they need to be documented (Sames & Berkeland, 1998). It is not necessary to include them on every piece of documentation, as long as they are easy to find in the client's chart. These can be very relevant to the activities and tasks selected during intervention (Sames & Berkeland, 1998).

There can be a tendency to overdocument. Out of fear of lawsuits, fear of forgetting something, or just plain verbosity, some people write very long documents. Time is precious, and time spent documenting is time spent away from clients. Eliminate all but the most necessary information (Sames & Berkeland, 1998). Ask yourself, is this relevant? If you are working with a client on managing a checkbook, is it necessary to document what the client is wearing? Is it necessary to document what the client says about the weather? Is it necessary to document about how the client holds the pen? The answers are no, no, and maybe. You would only document about how the client holds the pen if the act of writing was important to the case. If you were working on managing a checkbook because of cognitive deficits, then how the client holds the pen is not particularly relevant, unless the client used to know what a pen was and how to hold it and today he or she looked at it like it was a new and strange object (Sames & Berkeland, 1998).

▼ EXCEPTIONS ▼

Any unusual occurrences or events need to be documented (Sames & Berkeland, 1998). In the example above, if the client had suffered a traumatic brain injury, was progressing nicely, then suddenly did not recognize a pen, this would be unusual, and possibly indicate some bleeding on the brain. It would be essential to document this event, as well as inform nursing or the client's doctor verbally about what transpired. This might require immediate medical attention, and it is up to you to see that the proper people are informed as quickly as possible. It is also up to you to see that this critical event is documented in the chart. You are the one who saw what happened. It should be in your words. The doctor or nurse might also document what you told them, but when they do so, they are documenting secondhand information. In most courts of law, secondhand information is considered hearsay.

Client noncompliance is also something that should be documented (Sames & Berkeland, 1998). If you have prescribed a home exercise program, and the client reports not following through with it, you need to document that. It might explain why a client is progressing more slowly than you would like.

Since the clients we work with are human, unpredictable things can happen. New problems surface. When you deviate from your original intervention plan, there needs to be a brief explanation of why you are doing something new (Sames & Berkeland, 1998). In other words, you need to provide justification for deviating from the original plan (Cathy Brennan, MA, OTR/L, FAOTA, personal communication, June 21, 2006). Many clients have multiple complications; for example, a person with schizophrenia may have a stroke, a person with rheumatoid arthritis may have diabetes and depression, and a child with Asperger's syndrome may suffer a traumatic amputation. This may mean that the intervention plan you develop may differ from your typical plan of action. A depressed client who rented an apartment could lose her lease and become homeless. This change in the client's environment would likely cause a change in plan.

Figure 5.1 is the Document with CARE checklist. This is a handy, one-page document that you can use to help evaluate your report and note writing.

```
┌──────────────────────────────────────────────────────────────────────┐
│                    ▼ DOCUMENT WITH CARE ▼                              │
│                                                                        │
│  Clarity: The reader can understand what you are saying.               │
│  ❑ Free from jargon                                                    │
│  ❑ Concise                                                             │
│  ❑ Only facility-approved abbreviations                                │
│  ❑ Readable/legible                                                    │
│  ❑ Grammar and spelling do not interfere with the professional         │
│    appearance and the intended message of the note                     │
│  ❑ Understandable to all readers                                       │
│                                                                        │
│  Accuracy: The documentation reflects what actually happened           │
│  ❑ Chronologically, technically, and factually correct                 │
│  ❑ Instructions are specific and individualized                        │
│  ❑ Reflect the behavior observed, interpretations are labeled as such  │
│  ❑ Consistent use of terminology                                       │
│  ❑ Adheres to protocol of facility, agency, or school                  │
│  ❑ Preserve confidentiality of all involved                            │
│                                                                        │
│  Relevance: The documentation relates to identified needs and purposes │
│  ❑ Clear why OT is initiated, continued, and discontinued              │
│  ❑ Consistency between referral, evaluation, intervention plan,        │
│    ongoing intervention, discontinuation planning, and follow-up       │
│  ❑ Documentation reflects the skilled service being provided           │
│  ❑ Description of changes in function relates to treatment goals       │
│  ❑ Timely                                                              │
│  ❑ Precautions and contraindications are clearly outlined for the      │
│    individual                                                          │
│  ❑ Include information necessary for quality management and research    │
│    projects                                                            │
│  ❑ Eliminate all but necessary information                             │
│                                                                        │
│  Exceptions: Any unusual occurrences, non-compliance, or changes are   │
│  documented                                                            │
│  ❑ Deviations from original intervention plan are justified            │
│  ❑ Deviations from evaluation and intervention protocols are described │
│    and explained                                                       │
│  ❑ Client noncompliance is noted                                       │
│  ❑ Unusual occurrences and events are described                        │
│  ❑ Complications and responses are documented                          │
└──────────────────────────────────────────────────────────────────────┘
```

FIGURE 5.1 Document with CARE. *Source: Sames & Berkeland (1998).*

Exercise 5.1

Evaluate the following narrative progress notes using the Document with CARE checklist.

Case 1: This involves a 3-year-old child with cerebral palsy in a preschool setting. Her areas of concern are in hand use, balance, and using sign language.

Anoushka participated in three 30-minute sessions this week. She participated in group activities, snack, and playground activities each day. She played catch with another child on Monday. She signed "more" during snack. Anoushka loved balancing on the big ball. Wednesday she refused to go down the slide. Plan to continue seeing Anoushka per plan of care.

C:

A:

R:

E:

Case 2: This case involves a teenager in a chemical dependency program.

Paul attended group as scheduled. He seems to be opening up and talking more. He still does not reveal much about his own feelings, but is identifying feelings in others. When confronted on any issue, he deflects the comments back to the person who made the comment. For example, when a member of the group accused him of being dishonest about the strength of his addiction, he shouted, "As if you people are saints! Your problems are way bigger than mine!" He recognizes that he had enough of a problem to land himself in this program, but he says that he really does not need any intervention; he can quit on his own anytime he wants. He says he is only here because it is better than going to jail.

C:

A:

R:

E:

Case 3: This case involves a 34-year-old man recovering from a massive hand injury from an on-the-job accident. He has had surgical repair of three tendons on the palm of his hand and an amputation of the distal joint of his index finger.

Ivan has been receiving hard therapy for his injuries for 3 weeks. He is making steady progress. The postsurgical edema is almost gone. He has greater AROM in each finger than at this time last week. Refer to flow sheet for detailed ROM of each joint. Bruising has faded to pale yellow. He is able to squeeze lightweight putty and spread his fingers inside a ring of the same-weight putty. Plan to continue therapy 3x/wk for 45–60 min to work on strengthening of hand and fingers, increased ROM, and functional use of hand and fingers.

C:

A:

R:

E:

Case 4: This case involves a 93-year-old woman recovering from a hip fracture. Up until she fell, she lived independently in an apartment in a large metropolitan area.

Mrs. Nguen was seen today for 30 minutes in the OT clinic. She is partial weight bearing. Although she has been instructed to use her quad cane every time she takes a step, she refuses to use the quad cane in the kitchen. She reports that she prefers to hold on to the counter or a chair back when she is preparing meals in her kitchen, and demonstrated her technique in the OT kitchen. Kim from physical therapy saw her do this and scolded her. Plan to continue 2x/wk for IADLs.

C:

A:

R:

E:

SUMMARY

Documentation is a complex process; there are many things you must consider all at once when writing about a client. The *Document with CARE* checklist is one way to check to see that your documentation is on the right track. It can help you see if you are writing about the right things, and if you are writing them well. CARE stands for clarity, accuracy, relevance, and exceptions. If you document with CARE, you will be a good documenter of occupational therapy practice.

REFERENCE

Sames, K., & Berkeland, R., (1998). *Document with CARE.* Checklist and oral presentation at the Sister Genevieve Cummings Colloquia, June 19, 1998, St. Paul, MN.

Ethical and Legal Considerations

▼ INTRODUCTION ▼

If an attorney ever asks to see your documentation, it is usually because you, a client/patient, student, or coworker, are involved in some kind of litigation. Section I of this book talked about general principles for good documentation. In this section, we will talk about ethical and legal considerations in documentation. If the records you write get called into court, the attorneys will likely tell the jury how they would like your writing to be interpreted. Your mistakes might be accidental, but an attorney may not see it that way. Table II.1 is a list of what your documentation might look like, and how an attorney could interpret it (Ranke, 1998).

▼ AVOIDING LEGAL ACTION THROUGH DOCUMENTATION ▼

Some, but not all, errors in documentation may be violations of laws, rules, or regulations. A client's clinical (or educational) record can be called into court by either or both sides in a legal case (Fremgen, 2006). The best defense is to document appropriately and competently

TABLE II.1   Ways an Attorney Could Interpret Documentation

What You Said or Did	What the Attorney Will Say About It
Erasures, cross-outs, or other alterations to original documentation	Writer was unsure of what to say, careless, or incompetent; writer is trying to cover up or hide something.
Poor grammar or spelling	Writer is not competent, is careless.
Negative statements by one provider toward another provider or toward the facility/ administration	Providers not coordinated in care of client; blaming others might indicate decreased quality of care; client is caught in a fight between caregivers.
Negative statements toward the client	Words like "fat," "lazy," "abusive," "faking," "stupid," "goofy," etc., indicate that the provider disliked the client and therefore gave inferior service.
Gaps in documentation or documentation out of sequence	Writer is careless; problems in staffing, in adequate staff to care for client; writer is hiding something.

Sources: Fremgen (2006); Ranke (1998).

every day. Always be sure you are writing in the right chart (Fremgen). Be sure the client is named on every page of the clinical or educational record; a good electronic record keeping system will do this automatically.

Ranke (1998) lists three criteria for avoiding legal action. First, be careful and objective in your documentation. Base your documentation on firsthand information, things you see and hear. When you write that something occurred, you are identifying yourself as a witness in the eyes of an attorney. Do not assume something must have happened if you did not see it happen or write what someone else tells you happened. For example, do not document that the patient fell unless you saw the patient fall. Instead, you could say that you found the patient sprawled on the floor and that the patient said she fell. Documentation should never be derogatory toward the client or a coworker, or defensive in tone (Fremgen, 2006).

Be brief, but be complete (Borcherding, 2005; Fremgen, 2006; Shamus & Stern, 2004). If you do something, but leave it out of your documentation, a court will determine that it never happened. Be sure to document the reason(s) for any missed evaluation, intervention, or follow-up sessions.

When you give instructions to a client, carefully document those instructions and whether the client was able to demonstrate understanding of the instructions (Ranke, 1998). The same is true when you are instructing family members or other caregivers in ways to follow through on an occupational therapy program for a specific client. Documenting that the client, or caregiver, nodded to indicate understanding is not enough (Ranke, 1998). Document any telephone conversations or other correspondence that relates to the client, as well as any actions you take as a result of those conversations or correspondence (Fremgen, 2006).

Second, Ranke (1998) says documentation should be timely, grammatically correct, legible, and correctly signed. All documentation should be in chronological order, and done as close to the time as possible (Fremgen, 2006). The longer the lag time between when the service was provided and when the documentation occurred, the less reliable it will be considered in court. In addition to recording the date of the entry into the record, many facilities require the time be recorded as well (Ranke). Use only facility-approved abbreviations. Use proper grammar and spelling to ensure understandability, accuracy, and clarity. Write legibly (printing is preferred to cursive), word process or use an electronic medical record system program to generate the documentation. Illegible notes can lead—and have indeed led—to improper care. Sign and date all documentation with at least your first initial, full last name, credentials (i.e., OTR/L, OTA/L) and the date it was written.

Finally, Ranke (1998) says your documentation should be tamper-free, which means you should not change, remove, add to, or write over any documentation. Always correct your errors with a single line through the mistake with your initials above or next to the error (Fremgen, 2006; Ranke). Then make the correction. Never correct someone else's documentation in a client's record, only your own. Never sign anyone else's documentation, except in a supervisory situation. Do not leave blank lines or large blank spaces. Fill the blank areas with a line. Never use correction fluid or erasers. Always use ink in a permanent or official record. The American Occupational Therapy Association (AOTA) has established guidelines to help occupational therapists document properly; see Appendix D to read the guidelines.

Exercise II.1

Potential Problems with Documentation

   For each potential problem with documentation listed on the left, identify a potential solution or way to prevent the problem in the first place.

Problem	Solution
Illegibility	
Cannot tell which patient the note is about	
Notes written out of sequence	
Pencil or colored ink	
Erasures or white out	
Blank spaces	
Incomplete signatures	
Notes written by students are not cosigned by supervisor	
Poor grammar/spelling	
Poor word choices	
Unknown abbreviations	
Missing documents	
Computer screen with client information displayed left unattended	
Chart left unattended	

Sources: AOTA (2006); Ranke (1998); Shamus & Stern (2004).

▼ STRUCTURE OF THIS SECTION OF THE BOOK ▼

In this section of the book, we explore the ethical and legal considerations that impact documentation. For the purposes of this book, ethical considerations are defined as those actions that reflect doing the right thing. The principles outlined in the AOTA Code of Ethics (2005) will be the guide. While situations involving questionable ethics exist in many ways in clinical practice, we focus on those that involve documentation. Examples of these ethical considerations include, but are not limited to, confidentiality, fraud, plagiarism, and retention of records.

   Chapter 6 presents considerations in confidentiality and records retention. This includes issues such as how to protect your client's confidentiality and where and for how long to retain client documentation. Specific standards from the AOTA Code of Ethics (2005) that apply to these issues as well as the Health Insurance Portability and Accountability Act (HIPAA), a federal law designed to protect the rights of recipients of health care services, are discussed.

In Chapter 7, situations that could be construed as fraud are discussed. There is an emphasis on Medicare fraud and abuse, since the government has recently been cracking down on this. You will learn what the penalties are for engaging in fraud. Standards that apply to these situations from the AOTA Code of Ethics (2005) are described.

The last chapter in this section, Chapter 8, takes us in a slightly different direction. While it is less about documentation and more about writing papers, plagiarism can be considered a form of fraud. As students, you will write numerous papers, and colleges seem to be paying more attention to issues of plagiarism these days. As a clinician, you will put together handouts for in-services, home exercise programs, and general information for your clients. In every case, you must give credit where credit is due. The AOTA Code of Ethics (2005) standards will be presented along with strategies for avoiding plagiarism.

REFERENCES

American Occupational Therapy Association. (2005). Occupational therapy code of ethics. *American Journal of Occupational Therapy, 59,* 639–642.

American Occupational Therapy Association. (2006). Guidelines to the occupational therapy code of ethics. *American Journal of Occupational Therapy, 60,* 652–658.

Borcherding, S. (2005). *Documentation manual for writing SOAP notes in occupational therapy* (2nd ed.). Thorofare, NJ: Slack.

Fremgen, B. F. (2006). *Medical law and ethics* (2nd ed.). Upper Saddle River, NJ: Prentice Hall.

Ranke, B. A. E. (1998). Documentation in the age of litigation. *OT Practice, 3*(3), 20–24.

CHAPTER 6

Confidentiality and Records Retention

INTRODUCTION

Occupational therapists have access to very personal information about clients. There are rules that have to be followed in order to protect clients' rights to privacy. Confidentiality refers to keeping information to oneself, not releasing information about a client without the written permission of that client. Recently, the Health Insurance Portability and Accountability Act (HIPAA) has tightened rules concerning protection of client privacy. These rules include the kinds of information protected, when written consent is needed, and who may give consent (AOTA, 2003; Meyer & Schiff, 2004). In addition to issues of disclosure of information, in order to further protect confidentiality, how records are stored and who has access to stored records also need consideration.

▼ CONFIDENTIALITY ▼

When you write anything that identifies a specific client by name, you are ethically responsible for ensuring that the information remains confidential (AOTA, 2005). This means that you take all reasonable precautions to make sure that only the people who have permission to read the record actually read it. When sending confidential information via the mail, you first need permission from the client or responsible party to share the document, and then the envelope should be marked "confidential." When sending documents via fax, include a cover sheet marked "confidential", and make sure the person to whom you are sending the fax is there to receive it (Fremgen, 2006). In other words, no one except those who have written consent of the client or the client's guardian should have access to a client's medical record in any form (electronic or paper).

The client or the client's guardian has the right to see what is written in the clinical or educational record (Fremgen, 2006; United States Department of Health and Human Services [USDHHS], 2002). This is another reason to choose your words carefully, to remain objective and nonjudgmental. Most facilities have specific policies and procedures for allowing clients to read their own records. In some cases, a physician, nurse, or other professional needs to be present to provide immediate answers to any questions that arise, or a physician must also sign a release (Fremgen). Other facilities will provide photocopies of medical records to the client (they may charge a fee for the copying). Again, find out the rules at your facility before you share the clinical record with anyone.

The electronic medical record has made the accessing of private health information more efficient, but has opened new possibilities for violating the confidentiality of clients (Fremgen, 2006). One way to minimize the potential for breaches of confidentiality is to carefully limit the number of people who have access to individual client information through the use of passwords and other user verification methods. Only those caregivers who have a need to know should be assigned user names and passwords on the electronic medical record system. Position computer screens so that no unauthorized people, such as clients or visitors to the clinic can see it (Fremgen). Never walk away from a computer screen that is displaying confidential information; close out of the program or record before even taking a step away from the computer. Facilities using electronic record keeping systems will have clearly established policies and procedures to protect the confidentiality of the clients (Shamus & Stern, 2004). These policies must address not only the protection of the record in electronic form, but the backing-up, storage and safe-keeping of discs, tapes, and other electronic media storage devices (Meyer & Schiff, 2004).

▼ ETHICAL RESPONSIBILITY ▼

The American Occupational Therapy Association (2005) has ethical standards that address issues of confidentiality. Occupational therapists are ethically responsible for protecting the confidentiality of all client information regardless of the format of the communication.

> Principle 3. Occupational therapy personnel shall respect recipients to assure their rights (AUTONOMY, CONFIDENTIALITY). Occupational therapy personnel shall:
>
> D. Protect all privileged confidential forms of written, verbal, and electronic communication gained from educational, practice, research, and investigational activities unless otherwise mandated by local, state, or federal regulations. (AOTA, 2005, p. 640)

Ethical responsibility for occupational therapy practitioners is further articulated in the *Guidelines for the Occupational Therapy Code of Ethics* (AOTA, 2006).

> 5. CONFIDENTIAL AND PROTECTED INFORMATION: Information that is confidential must remain confidential. This information cannot be shared verbally, electronically, or in writing without appropriate consent. Information must be shared on a need-to-know basis only with those having primary responsibilities for decision making.
>
> 5.1 All occupational therapy personnel shall respect the confidential nature of information gained in any occupational therapy interaction. The only exceptions are when a practitioner or staff member believes that an individual is in serious, foreseeable, or imminent harm. In this instance, laws and regulations require disclosure to appropriate authorities without consent.
>
> 5.2 Occupational therapy personnel shall respect the clients' and colleagues' right to privacy.
>
> 5.2 Occupational therapy personnel shall maintain the confidentiality of all verbal, written, electronic, augmentative, and nonverbal communications (e.g., HIPAA).

It is important to note that while AOTA can only enforce these ethical standards with AOTA members, an attorney could present these standards in court as representing prevailing community standards, regardless of whether the occupational therapy practitioner is a member of AOTA or not.

▼ STATE LAWS ▼

Breaches of confidentiality can invite lawsuits. Many states have laws governing the protection of medical records. It is considered an invasion of privacy to allow unauthorized access to the clinical record or to disclose information about a specific patient/client in any way (Liang, 2000). Some types of information, such as HIV infection or drug/alcohol addiction, are protected to an even greater degree (Fremgen, 2006; Liang, 2000). For example, releasing HIV status of a patient without permission to release that specific information can result in both civil and criminal penalties. A client can make claims of "intentional infliction of emotional distress" (Liang, 2000, p. 51). Check the website for your state Department of Health or Department of Human Services for state regulations on confidentiality and release of information.

Occupational therapists are required by law to comply with the privacy sections of the Health Insurance Portability and Accountability Act (HIPAA). This law covers many topics, including protections for American workers regarding health insurance, standardization of electronic patient records, and a section on protection of privacy rights of individuals (Centers for Medicare and Medicaid Services [CMS], 2002; Fremgen, 2006; Meyer & Schiff, 2004; Shamus & Stern, 2004). HIPAA was enacted in 1996; however, the section on privacy did not take effect until 2003 (USDHHS, 2002).

Individuals are guaranteed certain rights by the HIPAA privacy rules. They can request an accounting of the people to whom personal health information was disclosed and the dates of the disclosures (Meyer & Schiff, 2004). Individuals have the right to read and copy their health information. They can also request that disclosure of their health information be restricted in some way. While individuals have the right to view their medical record, they do not have an automatic right to access their entire medical record. Psychotherapy notes; information on a criminal, civil, or administrative action or proceeding; and information that "a qualified provider has determined would endanger the life of the individual if he had access to it" (Meyer & Schiff, p. 23) may be withheld from the individual.

Usually, when a client is seen in an institutional setting (e.g., hospital, nursing home, school, etc.), the institution has established policies regarding access to patient/client information. The occupational therapist must comply with these policies. These may vary somewhat from place to place, but generally all must be consistent with the language and requirements of HIPAA. Staff involved in direct caregiving, supervisors, medical records personnel, billing personnel, and insurance representatives usually are allowed access to a client's record provided it is necessary for "treatment, payment, or health care operations" (Office for Civil Rights [OCR], 2002, p. 8 [§ 164.502 (a)(1)(ii)]).

Clients must sign a form stating they have been informed of their rights, specifically how the health information will be used, what will be disclosed, and how the client can get access to this information (OCR, 2002). This form, called a HIPAA Privacy Notice, must be written in plain language so that it is readable by most adults, yet meets all the legal requirements of the law (Health Resources and Services Administration [HRSA], 2003). The required topics are (HRSA, 2003, p. 2):

- Header with specific language
- Uses and disclosures
- Separate statements for certain uses and disclosures
- Individual rights
- Covered entity's duties
- Complaints
- Contact

Box 6.1 lists some suggestions from the HRSA (2003) for making the notice easier to read. The HRSA also has a thesaurus to aid in the translating of terms in the law into "plain language words and phrases" (HRSA, 2003, p. 9). For example, the HRSA suggests that "authorizing disclosures" can be translated into "allowing us to share information" (p. 9). Many of the principles for making the notice more readable, and the thesaurus, are also useful tools in creating any written materials for client education.

HIPAA protects all health information "that relates to past, present, or future physical or mental health condition" (Meyer & Schiff, 2004, p. 9). Under HIPAA, deceased persons have the same right to confidentiality and protection as a living person (Meyer & Schiff). Protected health information (PHI) must be held in the strictest confidence. This means that copies of documentation are not left on a therapist's desk where others can see them. Client charts or records should not be left where any identifiable information is exposed to

---

BOX 6.1   Increasing the Readability of a HIPAA Privacy Notice

Wording

- Translate the rules into a conversational style.
- Use short sentences (15 words or fewer).
- Do not use hyphens or compound words.
- Use examples to explain concept, category, or value-judgment words.
- Use lowercase letters wherever possible.
- Give context first, then giving new material.

Appearance

- Allow white space (blank areas or wide margins).
- Break long lists into "chunks."
- Use visuals (pictures, drawings, and symbols).
- Use large fonts.
- Use high contrast.
- Do not use high-gloss paper.
- Cue the reader (use arrows and captions for visuals).

Source: HRSA (2003).

---

public view (OCR, 2002). Documentation is also not left on computer screens when a therapist steps away from his or her desk. Computers, whether desktop, laptop, or handheld, should be password protected for each user, again to protect the confidentiality of client information (Fremgen, 2006). Occupational therapists should not discuss clients in public areas of the facility (especially in hallways, the cafeteria, and in elevators) where they can be overheard. You can imagine what would happen if you were talking to a coworker in the cafeteria about Mrs. Johnson's rolls of fat getting in the way of her being able to clean herself while her daughter was at the next table listening in on your conversation! Or telling a coworker how sassy little Timmy is while, unknown to you, his aunt is riding in the elevator with you. Besides being unethical and illegal, it is rude and unprofessional.

There are exceptions to this rule. Providers may use and disclose PHI without written authorization from the individual for treatment; victims of abuse, neglect, or domestic violence; judicial and law enforcement purposes; and health oversight (Meyer & Schiff, 2004). PHI may also be released if it has been de-identified. The following information must be removed from the record in order to be considered de-identified:

- Name
- All address information (street as well as email, URL and IP addresses)
- Day and month of dates (year is acceptable)
- Age, although age group is acceptable
- Telephone and fax numbers
- Social security number
- Medical record and health plan numbers
- Vehicle or device identifiers
- Biometric identifiers
- Facial photographs
- Any other unique information such as identification numbers, characteristics or codes (Meyer & Schiff)

For health care providers, HIPAA stipulates that both the medical record and billing record of each client be protected (Federal Register, 2000). Under the act, disclosure is defined as "the release, transfer, provision of access to, or divulging in any other manner of information outside the entity holding the information" (Federal Register, 2000, p. 82489). Health information that is necessary for what the act calls "health care operations" do not require written permission of the client before being shared. Examples of health care operations include

> quality assessment and improvement activities, reviewing the competence or qualifications and accrediting/licensing of health care professionals and plans, . . . training future health care professionals . . . conducting or arranging for medical review and auditing services and compiling and analyzing information in anticipation of or for use in a civil or criminal legal proceeding. (Federal Register, 2000, p. 82490)

Individually identifiable health information is protected under the act (Federal Register, 2000; USDHSS, 2002). This includes any means by which a person could be identified, such as by name, social security number, address, phone number, and the like (OCR, 2002). Examples of prohibited activities include using a client's social security number as a client identifier (i.e., case number) on written or electronic documentation, and listing the full name of a client on a schedule hanging on a wall where anyone could see it.

Penalties for releasing or obtaining individually identified health information can be quite severe. First, a person who releases or obtains such information can be jailed for up to 1 year, fined up to $50,000, or both (CMS, 1996). This increases to not more than 5 years in jail, up to $100,000 in fines, or both, if the violation occurs under false pretenses (e.g., fraud). If the violation occurs in a way that it is clear there was an intent to profit from the sharing of the protected information for personal or corporate gain, or malicious harm, the penalties increase to up to 10 years in jail, fines up to $250,000, or both (CMS, 1996).

If the individually identifiable health information is included in an educational record, it is governed by the Family Education Rights and Privacy Act (Public Law 93-380).

▼ FAMILY EDUCATION RIGHTS AND PRIVACY ACT OF 1974 AND THE INDIVIDUALS WITH DISABILITIES EDUCATION ACT, 2004 REVISION ▼

The Family Education Rights and Privacy Act (FERPA) of 1974 identifies the confidentiality requirements of a student's educational record. It has been revised, as have the regulation that describe how the law should be implemented. The most recent revision of the regulations occurred in 2008, with the final regulations published in December 9, 2008, in the Federal Register (U. S. Department of Education [USDE], 2008). The Individuals with Disabilities Education Act (IDEA), 2004 revision, governs the types of services provided to children with disabilities, and how those services are documented. An educational record includes material written by school district employees and contractors (IDEA Partnerships 1999; Jackson, 2007). If a student is receiving special education and related services (including occupational therapy), FERPA covers all documents that contain the student's name, address, phone number, parents' names, and any other identifying information. The file may be called a "cumulative file, permanent record, or official educational record" (AOTA, p. 128). These files contain documents such as the Individual Education Program (IEP) (see Chapter 17), the Individual Family Service Plan (IFSP) (see Chapter 16), and notice and consent forms (see Chapter 15) required by IDEA, as well as grades, samples of student work, and district- or statewide test results.

The Individuals with Disabilities Education Act (IDEA), 2004 revision, also contains language about privacy of information. IDEA has separate sections that address early intervention services (birth through age 2) and school-age (ages 3–21) services. Both sections specifically define identifying information as including the name of the child, parent, or other family member; the address of the child; any identifier such as a social security number; or a list of characteristics or other information that would result in reasonable certainty of the identity of the child (34 C.F.R. § 303.401[a] and 34 C.F.R. § 300.500[b][3]) (USDE, 2007a; 2007b). IDEA further provides for the opportunity for parents to examine the records of their child (34 C.F.R. § 303.402 and 34 C.F.R. § 300.560-576) (USDE, 2007a; 2007b).

Exercise 6.1

Which of the following constitutes a breach of confidentiality?

1. A client was discharged from the hospital yesterday and was admitted to a transitional care facility. The occupational therapist at the transitional care facility calls to get more information about the client than you can usually find in a discharge summary, nitty-gritty things about the personality of the client and the supportiveness of the family. The transitional care facility has permission to get copies of discharge information from the hospital. Based on that, the occupational therapist at the hospital who has worked most closely with the client answers the questions of the occupational therapist at the transitional care facility over the phone.

2. A client at an outpatient clinic has a work-related injury. As a result of participating in the worker's compensation system, this client is assigned a case manager. The case manager comes by the clinic and asks to review the client's record. The client did sign a release for you to share medical records with the insurer.

3. In a busy nursing home therapy room, a schedule is posted on the wall listing each client's full first and last name and room number. The schedule includes intervention sessions for physical and occupational therapy and speech-language pathology. The rehab aide who transports clients to and from their rooms can look at the schedule to see who needs to go where and when.

4. A parent brings a family friend to the IEP team meeting. No one from the school district has ever met this person before. Since the parent brought the friend, the team assumes that constitutes verbal consent and proceeds with the meeting without obtaining written consent to disclose information from the parent.

▼ RECORDS RETENTION ▼

Records, both educational and clinical, are retained for several reasons. One reason is to provide information about what happened in the past that could contribute to the client's present condition. Another reason is to provide comparative data that might enable a practitioner to identify trends toward improved function or loss of function. Records are retained in case legal questions arise after care is discontinued. Finally, we retain records for quality management purposes. By reviewing records of past clients, medical and educational professionals can learn which practices yield the best results.

Records are generally stored in locked file cabinets in a records office once the client has been discharged from the facility or program. The office is locked whenever it is unattended. Active client charts usually travel with the client (in hospitals), or stay in the nursing department (long-term care facility) or in a therapy office (outpatient clinic). In a school or community setting, records may be kept in a central office. Therapy departments often keep copies of client records. These should be kept in a secure area and be locked when not in use.

Each state has laws that govern clinical records retention. At minimum, these laws require health care providers to retain records for at least as long as the statute of limitations for medical malpractice suits (Fremgen, 2006). A statute of limitation specifies how long a patient or the family of a patient has to file a malpractice claim against a health care practitioner. The statute of limitations may be different for physicians, nurses, and therapists, but generally range from 2 to 6 years.

Official records for adult patients are usually kept for 5 to 10 years after discharge, although some records may be stored off-site when storage space is limited (Fremgen, 2006; Shamus & Stern, 2004). Records for children are kept until the child turns age 21 plus the number of years that state statutes require records to be retained. These are generalities, and some facilities may keep files for as little as 2 years or as long as 15. The American Health Information Management Association (AHIMA) has adopted standards for recommended retention of records (Fremgen, 2006). AHIMA recommends that records be retained for 10 years beyond the last encounter for adult patients, until the age of maturity plus the length of the statute of limitations for a child, and that Medicare and Medicaid records be kept for at least 5 years (Fremgen, 2006; Liang, 2000). The key is that there is a policy and the policy applies to all clients.

When the required length of time for records retention has elapsed, the records must either continue to be retained or be destroyed. Duplicate records, such as those kept in the occupational therapy department, should not be retained after the client is discontinued unless facility policy requires it. Because of the sensitive information in the records, the term *destroyed* means that the records are shredded and/or burned. Information kept on a disc, tape, or other portable storage devices need to be cut up or otherwise destroyed (Meyer & Schiff, 2004). Simply putting them in the trash or in recycling would violate the client's right to confidentiality, since a good gust of wind could blow them into someone's path, or the trash collector could read them.

SUMMARY

Confidentiality is a major concern of all health care providers. As health care providers, we are obligated to protect the confidentiality of our clients. This applies to all settings, to all types of documents, and to spoken words as well. A new federal law, HIPAA, limits the kind of information that can be shared without written permission and protects clients from public disclosure of any information. FERPA protects the educational records of students. Our clients deserve to have their privacy protected to the furthest extent possible without interfering with intervention.

Records are retained for at least the length of each state's statute of limitations, and often longer. These records are also protected and stored where they will be safe and secure. Access to stored records is limited to only those who absolutely need access to them. Once the statute of limitations has expired, the records may stay in a secure and locked site, or be thoroughly destroyed by burning or shredding. Never toss old records into the garbage.

REFERENCES

American Occupational Therapy Association. (2003). *Fact sheet: HIPAA privacy rule web links.* Retrieved March 15, 2003, from http://www.aota.org/members/area5/links/LINK07.asp?PLACE=/members/area5/links/link

American Occupational Therapy Association. (2005). Occupational therapy code of ethics. *American Journal of Occupational Therapy, 59,* 639–642.

American Occupational Therapy Association. (2006). Guidelines to the occupational therapy code of ethics. *American Journal of Occupational Therapy, 60,* 652–658.

Centers for Medicare and Medicaid Services. (1996). *Health Insurance Portability and Accountability Act of 1996 [PL 104-191].* Retrieved July 31, 2006, from http://www.cms.hhs.gov/HIPAAGenInfo/Downloads/HIPAAlawdetail.pdf

Centers for Medicare and Medicaid Services. (2002). *HIPAA insurance reform.* Retrieved March 15, 2003, from http://cms.hhs.gov/hipaa/hipaa1/content/more.asp

Federal Register. (2000). *Final privacy rule.* Retrieved March 5, 2003, from http://www.hhs.gov/ocr/hipaa/finalreg.html

Fremgen, B. F. (2006). *Medical law & ethics* (2nd ed.). Upper Saddle River, NJ: Prentice-Hall.

Health Resources and Services Administration. (2003). *Plain language principles and thesaurus for making HIPAA privacy notices more readable.* Retrieved July 15, 2003, from http://www.hrsa.gov/language.htm

IDEA Partnerships. (1999). *Discover IDEA CD '99* [CD-ROM]. A collaborative project of the IDEA Partnership Projects (through project ASPIIRE at The Council for Exceptional Children) and the Western Regional Resource Center at the University of Oregon.

Jackson, L. L. (Ed) (2007). *Occupational therapy services for children and youth under IDEA* (3rd ed.). Bethesda, MD: American Occupational Therapy Association.

Liang, B. A. (2000). *Health law & policy: A survival guide to medicolegal issues for practitioners.* Woburn, MA: Butterworth-Heinemann.

Meyer, M. J. & Schiff, M. (2004). *HIPAA: The questions you didn't know to ask.* Upper Saddle River, NJ: Pearson Education.

Office for Civil Rights, United States Department of Health and Human Services. (2002). *Standards for privacy of individually identifiable health information (Unofficial version) (45 CFR Parts 160 and 164).* Retrieved March 17, 2003, from http://www.hhs.gov/ocr/combinedregtext.pdf

Shamus, E. & Stern, D. (2004). *Effective documentation for physical therapy professionals.* New York: McGraw-Hill.

United States Department of Education. (2006). *Building the legacy: IDEA 2004.* Retrieved October 1, 2008, from http://idea.ed.gov/explore/home

United States Department of Education. (2007a). *Federal register May 9, 2007 (34 CFR Part 303).* Retrieved October 10, 2008 from http://edocket.access.gpo.gov/2007/pdf/07-2140.pdf

United States Department of Education. (2007b). *Federal register August 14, 2006 (34 CFR Part 303).* Retrieved May 24, 2007 from http://idea.ed.gov/download/finalregulations.pdf

United States Department of Education (2008) *34 CFR part 99: Family educational rights and privacy; Final rule.* Retrieved January 11, 2009, from http://www.ed.gov/legislation/FedRegister/finrule/2008-4/120908a.pdf

United States Department of Health and Human Services. (2002). *Fact sheet: Administrative simplification under HIPAA: National standards for transactions, security and privacy.* Retrieved March 15, 2003, from http://www.hhs.gov/news/press/2002pres/hipaa.html

CHAPTER 7

Fraud

INTRODUCTION

"Fraud is the deliberate concealment of the facts from another person for unlawful or unfair gain" (Fremgen, 2006, p. 125). Fraud can take many forms, but in this book we will only be talking about it in terms of documentation. Fraud can be obvious, as when a therapist documents that a client received services when the services were not provided (Fremgen). It can also be subtle, as when a therapist documents that a client is making slower progress than the client really is in order to keep the client on the caseload longer. Fraud charges can be filed against the practitioner and the facility if the codes used to bill for services do not match the written description of services in the progress notes and related documentation (e.g., log sheets).

▼ MEDICARE FRAUD ▼

According to Kornblau and Starling (2000, p. 27), there are six "acts prohibited by Medicare and Medicare fraud and abuse provisions:

1. Making false claims for payment
2. Making false statements for payment
3. Billing for visits never made
4. Billing for nonface-to-face therapy services
5. Paying or receiving kickbacks for goods and services
6. Soliciting for, making an offer for payment, paying or receiving payment for patient referrals."

Medicare has strict penalties for fraud. It can cost the practitioner money, jail time, and license to practice occupational therapy. There are both civil and criminal penalties (Bailey & Schwartzberg, 2003; Kornblau & Startling, 2000; Liang, 2000). Filing false claims, that is, for services not rendered, can be punishable by fines up to $25,000 and 5 years in jail (criminal sanctions) and up to an additional $10,000 in civil fines for each false claim, as well as an additional $10,000 and payback of triple damages under two additional parts of the law (American Occupational Therapy Association [AOTA], 2000, 2005b; Kornblau & Starling, 2000; Liang, 2000). Besides these costly consequences, a person participating in fraud can be excluded from ever participating in any federal reimbursement program such as Medicare, Medicaid, Veteran's Affairs, Public Health Service Programs, and other government-funded programs (AOTA, 2000; Kornblau & Starling, 2000; Liang, 2000). The standard of proof in Medicare fraud cases does not require a specific intent to defraud the government (AOTA, 2000). If one acts with "deliberate ignorance" or "reckless disregard," in other words, if one does not know or understand the standards, but should know them, then that could be construed as fraud (AOTA, 2000, 2005b). Obviously, the occupational therapy practitioner is best advised to be truthful and accurate in all documentation in order to avoid claims of fraud.

In July 2006, the Tri-Alliance, a group made up of representatives of the American Occupational Therapy Association, the American Physical Therapy Association, and the American Speech-Language-Hearing Association, took the unusual step of sending a letter to members of all three associations, emphasizing the importance of using the highest standards of ethics and clinical reasoning in documenting the justification for Medicare B therapy cap exceptions (AOTA, 2006). The process of obtaining either automatic or manual exceptions to the cap puts the burden on the clinician to attest that the duration and intensity of the service is reasonable and necessary. The concern that prompted this letter is that the Centers for Medicare and Medicaid Services (CMS) stated "they do not believe a large number of services should exceed the cap" (p. 1), and if post-payment reviews show that exceptions exceeded expectations, that could result in a stricter cap being placed on therapy services. It is critical that "documentation is appropriate to justify additional treatment" (p. 1). While not explicitly stating that there is great potential for Medicare fraud in this process, a warning to clinicians is implied. Not only could CMS or Congress decide that stricter regulations are called for, which could hurt entire practice areas, individual clinicians are at risk of accusations of fraud if their documentation fails to demonstrate that the services provided in excess of the cap were reasonable and necessary (AOTA, 2006).

▼ OTHER FORMS OF FRAUD ▼

To avoid allegations of fraud, the therapist must be knowledgeable of the regulations, must follow those regulations, and document with sufficient accuracy and honesty. There have been numerous cases where occupational therapists and others have been accused of fraud because they documented that they provided intervention to a client on a specific date when in fact they did not. Making an honest error on the date of service is one thing; creating fictional progress notes is another. Fraud investigators are trained to know the difference. Over the last several years, Medicare has stepped up efforts to catch occupational therapy practitioners who attempt to obtain Medicare reimbursement through fraud. If you know that someone else has committed fraud, and you do not report it, you can be charged with conspiracy to commit fraud (Kornblau & Starling, 2000).

Fraud can be more subtle. It can be any documentation that is meant to deceive the reader, especially if payment is sought for that service (Fremgen, 2006). For example, under Medicare, only the time the client spends in contact with the therapist is considered billable time. That means the time an aide spends taking a client to and from the clinic, time spent resting in the therapy room, and time the therapist spends documenting care or on the phone talking to other caregivers are not billable time. It also means that documenting slower progress than is accurate in order to justify keeping a client on one's caseload longer, or faster progress than is accurate to look more effective, is considered fraudulent (Bailey & Schwartzberg, 2003).

Another example of fraud could be intentionally using a billing code that you know will be reimbursed, rather than using a more accurate billing code that may not get reimbursed. I had an occupational therapist once tell me that at her clinic, they were using a new intervention that most insurance companies and the American Academy of Pediatrics considered to be experimental. The clinic manager suggested that rather than name the specific intervention in the notes, which she knew would be a red flag for the payers, clinicians should just document that therapeutic sensory experiences were provided. Rather than billing for an unlisted procedure, they used the billing code for therapeutic activities. Fortunately, that clinic manager left, a new one came in, and the practice of vague and misleading documentation stopped. Instead, the clinic began informing parents that the intervention was considered experimental, that insurance would not cover it, and that parents who were interested in intervention would have to pay for it out of pocket. This is a much more honest approach. Now that the intervention can be mentioned by name, fraudulent billing is no longer a concern, and the occupational therapists can do retrospective chart reviews to determine the effectiveness of the intervention.

The AOTA Code of Ethics (2005a) specifically states in Principle 6.C: "Occupational therapy personnel shall refrain from using or participating in the use of any form of communication that contains false, fraudulent, deceptive, or unfair statements or claims." This applies to occupational therapy documentation, advertising and promotional materials, speeches and in-services, or any other form of communication that an occupational therapist might engage in regardless of the setting. This is further elaborated in the AOTA *Guidelines to the Occupational Therapy Code of Ethics:* "All documentation must accurately reflect the nature and quantity of services provided" (AOTA, 2006, 1.5) and, even more explicitly, "Occupational therapy personnel do not make deceptive, fraudulent, or misleading statements about the nature of the services they provide or the outcomes that can be expected" (AOTA, 2006, 2.1). The Guidelines further state, "Documentation for reimbursement purposes shall be done in accordance with applicable laws, guidelines, and regulations" (AOTA, 2006, 2.3), and "Documentation shall accurately reflect the services delivered and the outcomes. It shall be of the kind and quality that satisfied the scrutiny of peer review, legal proceedings, regulatory bodies and accrediting agencies" (AOTA, 2006, 2.4). Finally, the Guidelines explicitly state, "Occupational therapy personnel do not fabricate data, falsify information, or plagiarize" (AOTA, 2006, 2.8).

For example, an occupational therapist in private practice was accused of adding one billed unit of time (usually 15 minutes of direct service) for every visit that the occupational therapists working for her submitted to her for billing. If the therapists documented in a progress note that the client was seen for a 30-minute session, and marked 30 minutes (two units) on the billing record, the owner of the company would submit the bill for 45 minutes (three units). She did this without the knowledge of the therapists. The therapists found out that this was happening because the family of the client brought a copy of the bill in to the occupational therapist to see why they were being billed for 45-minute visits when they were scheduled for 30-minute visits. The therapists started asking questions and the owner said that she was simply adding a unit to account for the time the therapists spent in documenting services, time on the phone with the client's doctor, cleaning up after sessions, and other miscellaneous clinic expenses. The therapists did some more digging and found that the owner was destroying the progress notes when they were 1 month old, or as soon as the next intervention plan was written. The family reported the fraud to the HMO that was paying for services, and the therapists resigned and then reported the fraud to the state regulatory board. If the allegations proved to be true, the owner could face major penalties and will probably lose her license. Insurance fraud is a federal crime. The Federal False Claims Act, 31 U.S.C.A. §3729-3733, allows whistleblowers, those who report fraud and who help in the prosecution of the case, to receive 15–25% of the monies recovered (damages, civil penalties, and treble damages) from a false claim (Kornblau & Starling, 2000).

Exercise 7.1

Which of the following scenarios constitutes fraud, and which is just carelessness?

1. A therapist dates her notes "Jan. 3, 2009" when in fact the date is January 3, 2010.

2. A therapist writes in her note on Monday that the client was weaker on her right side than on her left. On Wednesday she writes that the client was weaker on her left than on her right. On Friday she writes that although the client is showing improvement in function on her right side, it remains weaker than her left.

3. A therapist bills for hot packs when in fact the client soaked her hand in a bowl of warm water.

4. A therapist bills for a 45 minute session when in fact the client was in the room for 45 minutes, although for 20 of those minutes the client rested while the therapist worked with another client.

5. A therapist realizes that she wrote a progress note in the wrong chart, so she uses white-out to cover up her error.

SUMMARY

Fraud is a form of lying that is absolutely illegal. Fraud happens when an occupational therapist documents in such a way as to create a false perception by the reader about what has actually transpired. Examples of fraud include documenting that you spent more time with a client than you really did, describing progress that is faster or slower than reality, or billing for services not rendered. There can be severe criminal and civil penalties for fraud. AOTA, in the *Code of Ethics* (2000), explicitly prohibits occupational therapists from making false statements. The best advice is to document accurately and be truthful in everything you do.

REFERENCES

American Occupational Therapy Association. (2000). *Final civil fraud and abuse penalties rule.* Retrieved August 4, 2006, from http://www.aota.org/members/area5/links/LINK56.asp

American Occupational Therapy Association. (2005a). Occupational therapy code of ethics. *American Journal of Occupational Therapy, 59,* 639–642.

American Occupational Therapy Association. (2005b). *Fact sheet: Fraud and abuse basics.* Retrieved January 11, 2009, from http://www.aota.org/Practitioners/Reimb/Resources/Fraud/37789.aspx

American Occupational Therapy Association. (2006). Guidelines to the occupational therapy code of ethics. *American Journal of Occupational Therapy, 60,* 652–658.

Bailey, D. M., & Schwartzberg, S. L. (2003). *Ethical and legal dilemmas in occupational therapy.* Philadelphia: F. A. Davis.

Fremgen, B. F. (2006). *Medical law and ethics* (2nd ed.). Upper Saddle River, NJ: Prentice Hall.

Kornblau, B. L. & Starling, S. P. (2000). *Ethics in rehabilitation.* Thorofare, NJ: Slack.

Liang, B. A. (2000). *Health law and policy: A survival guide to medicolegal issues for practitioners.* Woburn, MA: Butterworth-Heinemann.

Plagiarism

INTRODUCTION

Plagiarism is a form of cheating and theft that has become very pervasive across the country. The term *plagiarize* is defined as "to steal and pass off (the ideas or words of another) as one's own" (*Merriam-Webster Online,* n.d.). It includes using someone else's exact words or using someone else's ideas, even if the wording is changed, without giving credit to the originator of the idea or words. Because of the availability of sample intervention plans, student papers, and research papers on the Internet, it is appropriate to discuss plagiarism in the context of a book about documentation. In occupational therapy practice, there are times when an occupational therapist has to put together a report, cite evidence to support practice, or present an in-service with handouts. Each of these situations presents an opportunity for plagiarism.

Plagiarism has a cultural element to it. While some cultures believe that no one can "own" words, in many Western cultures, and American culture in particular, words and ideas are considered to be the intellectual property of the writer or publisher, and cannot be used without giving credit to the author (Lunsford, 2005; Purdue University On-Line Writing Laboratory [OWL], 2006).

▼ AMERICAN PSYCHOLOGICAL ASSOCIATION STANDARDS ▼

Since the American Occupational Therapy Association (AOTA) uses the American Psychological Association (APA) standards for writing in the profession, all examples in this book are cited in APA style.

Here is a passage as it appears in the *APA Publication Manual*, Fifth Edition (2001).

Quotation marks should be used to indicate the exact words of another. *Each time* you paraphrase another author (i.e., summarize a passage or rearrange the order of a sentence and change some of the words), you will need to credit the source in the text. (p. 349)

The following is a paraphrase of that same passage in which proper credit is given to the author.

According to the American Psychological Association (2001), the exact words of another should be enclosed in quotation marks. Rearranging the order of a sentence, summarizing a passage, or changing a few of the words is paraphrasing (APA, 2001). A credit for the source needs to be included each time a source is paraphrased (APA).

Here is an example of outright plagiarism:

> *Quotation marks must be used to indicate the exact words of another, along with a citation of the author, year, and page number. Paraphrasing is rearranging the order of a sentence and changing some of the words or summarizing a passage. Each time a source is paraphrased, you need to give credit to the original author.*

In this case, the writer added a few original words, but one cannot tell where any of the ideas come from and whether any of the words are directly taken from a source. Here is the same paragraph with proper citation:

> *"Quotation marks must be used to indicate the exact words of another" (APA, 2001, p. 349) along with a citation of the author, year, and page number. Paraphrasing is rearranging the order of a sentence, changing some of the words, or summarizing a passage (APA). Each time a source is paraphrased, you need to give credit to the original author (APA).*

This paragraph demonstrates a common pitfall that people often fall into: They think that the author of the passage has said what needs to be said in the best possible way, so why paraphrase it? Isn't it safer to quote than to paraphrase? They proceed to write papers that are simply strings of quotes linked with a few transitional phrases in the person's own words. While this may feel like a safe way to go, papers that are strings of quotes are difficult to read; all those quote marks and citations get in the way of the flow of the paper. Also, some professors believe that when a student overuses quotes, the student is not taking proper responsibility for completing the assignment (Hashimoto, 1991).

Quotes can enhance a paper, but only when used to support the writer's idea (thesis of the paper) by adding a new perspective on it. If a writer uses a quote to show that someone else who knows better is thinking the same way as the writer, the quote becomes redundant (Hashimoto, 1991). For example, if I make a thesis statement in a paper that students use excessive quotes, then follow that with the quote "Too often, they use quotations just to restate their own positions" (Hashimoto, 1991, p. 170), I am being redundant and not really adding anything meaningful to my paper.

Another form of plagiarism that can occur happens when students share their work. If you have a friend who took a pediatric occupational therapy course last semester, and you are taking it this semester, your friend might offer you her intervention plans "to look at." If you use them to write your own intervention plans, you are stealing his or her work unless you give credit on your assignment (i.e., "Mary Smith contributed to this assignment"). Most of the time, instructors want you to do your own work, so even if you did give your classmate credit on your assignment, your instructor would probably either make you redo it without help or fail you on that assignment. Using a fellow student's work prevents you from learning and gaining skills needed for the real world. If this was a pattern of behavior, more serious consequences could occur, up to and including expulsion from the program or the school. Disciplinary action can also be taken against the student who did the work herself and then shared it with someone who copied it, because this contributes to the problem of cheating. Clinicians plagiarize when they copy someone else's intervention plan wording. This may be a breach of confidentiality as well. Electronic documentation, which uses standardized phrases that a clinician clicks on to add to the documentation would not be considered plagiarism.

Many people learn to cheat in middle and high school, and by the time they get to college or the workplace it is so commonplace that they do not see the problem with it. According to a survey administered by Duke University's Center for Academic Integrity, 70% of students admit to cheating in college (McCabe, 2005). In that same survey, nearly 40% admit to cutting and pasting words from an Internet site into their own paper, without citing the source, which is up from 10% in 1995. Just over three quarters of all students surveyed did not think cheating was a serious issue (McCabe). Even more astonishing to me is that a poll by *U.S. News* found that 90% of college students believe that those who cheat never get penalized for cheating (Kleiner & Lord, 1999). These are big numbers, and the trend is that they are getting bigger by the decade. Survey results like this have gotten the attention of college administrators everywhere, and faculty are examining their academic integrity policies.

I have heard occupational therapy students complain that occupational therapy instructors make too big a deal about plagiarism. Many try to argue that in other majors, instructors do not appear to care if a student plagiarizes. This is a lousy argument. It is not true that other disciplines do not care. However, in a profession where competence and integrity are essential, catching cheaters at an early stage in their careers can help keep the profession respectable. Plagiarizing in school and getting away with it could start one on a slippery slope toward falsifying documentation and engaging in fraud as a clinician.

Related to plagiarism is the concept of copyright infringement. This occurs when someone copies something that someone else has written without getting permission from the creator or publisher (Nolo, 2009). For example, copying journal articles for everyone in the department or on a committee is copyright infringement unless you have written permission from the publisher. Fair use allows a person to use another person's copyrighted works under certain conditions (Nolo). Under the concept of fair use, you may be able to use someone else's work if you do not profit from its use, you give credit to the originator of the work, and you only use part of the original work; however, there is no guarantee that following these rules will make it fair use (Nolo). The best advice is to ask before you use anyone else's work.

Clinicians seem to want to share what they know with others in the hope that it helps some situation. Often, an occupational therapy department can only afford to send one practitioner to a workshop. When that person comes back from that workshop, he or she copies the handouts for the other members of the department and presents an in-service on it. Unless the practitioner has written permission to copy and distribute those handouts, he or she may be committing copyright infringement (Nolo, 2009). If a clinician copies exercises out of a textbook to give to a client or client's caregiver to use in a home program, it could be considered copyright infringement unless the textbook gives readers permission to copy and distribute material.

By any professional standard, plagiarism is wrong; it is a form of stealing. The American Occupational Therapy Association Code of Ethics (2005) states, "Occupational therapy personnel shall accurately represent the qualifications, views, contributions, and findings of colleagues" (principle 7.B). This is further elaborated in the AOTA *Guidelines to the Occupational Therapy Code of Ethics*: "Occupational therapy personnel do not fabricate data, falsify information, or plagiarize" (2006, 2.8) and "Occupational therapy personnel must give credit and recognition when using the work of others (2006, 2.7). Whether you are a student or a clinician, representing anyone else's work as your own is a violation of professional ethics.

▼ PREVENTING PLAGIARISM ▼

How can you protect yourself against allegations of plagiarism? The first rule of thumb is that when in doubt, cite a source. If reading something someone else wrote puts a thought in your head and it comes out your fingertips onto the paper (or computer screen), then cite it. Things that are general knowledge, such as using sunscreen can prevent sunburn or that more falls happen to elderly people in the winter in Vermont than in the summer, do not need to be cited. One suggestion is that you can call something common knowledge if you find the same information in five different sources, and each time the author did not document a source for it.

To make an allegation of plagiarism against a student, a teacher needs to be pretty sure the work was copied, or at least paraphrased from an identifiable source. New Internet search engines such as Google.com™ and Turnitin.com™ make it easy for instructors to find out if a student has copied someone else's work. The instructor can simply type in a phrase and search the Internet to see if it has been used by someone else on the Internet. If an instructor finds a student has used someone else's work, there can be serious consequences for the student. Some instructors require students to turn in their papers to Turnitin.com™.

To find out what could happen if you got caught cheating or plagiarizing, check out your school's policy on academic integrity, honor code, or plagiarism policy. If you were to get caught using someone else's words when you are a clinician, you would be subject to disciplinary action from your employer, AOTA, the National Board for Certification of Occupational Therapists, and, depending on your state regulations for licensure or registration, disciplinary action from your state regulatory board as well.

This can be scary stuff. It almost makes one afraid to write anything. Chances are that all the good phrases have been taken, that is, "it's all been said before" (author of quote unknown). Bob Newhart had a comedy sketch in which he theorized that if you put a group of monkeys in a room with a typewriter apiece, sooner or later by random efforts they would reproduce all the world's great literature. There are common phrases that everyone uses so that it would be impossible to give credit to any one author. Sometimes two people who have never met can come up with similar word sequences. This cannot be helped.

According to the Georgetown University Honor Council (2002), one way to protect yourself is to allow yourself time to do it right. If you are writing a 12-page paper at 11:59 P.M. the night before it is due at 8:00 A.M., you could inadvertently leave out some quote marks or forget to cite a source. It might seem easier at that point to copy someone else's paper (or buy one off the Internet) than to stay up all night working hard on it. If you find yourself in this kind of situation, it is better to risk a lower grade on the paper (by not being thorough enough, making spelling errors, wandering off topic, etc.) than to risk the disciplinary consequences of an academic integrity violation (http://www.georgetown.edu/honor/plagiarism.html, Section 4). Of course, the best course of action is to not get yourself into this kind of situation in the first place.

Purdue University, On-line Writing Laboratory (OWL) offers a printable handout on their Web page for avoiding plagiarism http://owl.english.purdue.edu/owl/resource/589/01/. In it there are suggestions for what you can do during the writing process and how your finished product should look. They suggest coding your paper during early drafts with "Q" for quote, and then coding the rest with either an "S" when the material comes from any source, and "ME" when it is your own idea or insight. Others suggest that when you make notes on a reading, anytime you write the words of the author, use quotes around those notes (Lunsford, 2005). OWL further suggests summarizing or paraphrasing from memory, rather than while reading the material. Table 8.1 provides some general guidance on when to quote from, paraphrase, or summarize another writer's words or ideas. Remember that proper citation is required in all of these instances.

3. "To protect confidentiality, medical records should not be released to third parties without the patient's written consent" (Fremgen, 2002, p. 160).

4. "The classical form of psychoanalysis is that originated by Freud at the beginning of the twentieth century" (Hagedorn, 1997, p. 85).

5. "Wordiness is every bit as irritating and uneconomical as jargon and can impede the ready grasp of ideas" (APA, 2001, p. 35).

6. "Occupational therapy is the art and science of helping people do the day-to-day activities that are important to them despite impairment, disability or handicap" (Neistadt & Crepeau, 1998, p. 5).

TABLE 8.1   When to Quote, Paraphrase, or Summarize a Source

Type of citation	When to do it	How to do it
Quote	• The wording is so powerful that if you changed it, it would weaken it. • The author is a well-known expert in the field whose opinion you want to emphasize to make a specific point. • The author offers a perspective that is distinctly different from yours, not a restatement of your idea. • The author offers a perspective that is distinctly different that most people's.	• Use quote marks around the words you are quoting for quotes under 40 words, use a block quote format if the quote is over 40 words. • Do not change any of the words, even if they are spelled incorrectly, from the way the original author said it. Use [*sic*] to indicate the error was the original author's. • If you want to shorten the quote to remove extraneous information, use three ellipsis points (. . .) to represent the removed words. • Cite the source, including author's name, year of publication, and page number immediately at the end of the quote.
Paraphrase	• The author's exact words are not as important as the point the author is making.	• If you want to cite the author as part of the same sentence with the paraphrased material, include the year in parentheses immediately after the author's name. • Alternatively, you can cite both the author and year in parentheses at the end of the sentence. • Paraphrase without looking at the original, but check the original afterward to see if you have accurately captured the author's meaning.
Summarize	• The passages are very long, and not every detail is important to you.	• If you want to cite the author as part of the same sentence with the summarized material, include the year in parentheses immediately after the author's name. • Alternatively, you can cite both the author and year in parentheses at the end of the sentence. • Summarize without looking at the original, but check the original afterward to see if you have accurately captured the author's meaning.

Sources: APA (2001); Lunsford (2005); OWL (2006).

Exercise 8.3

Is this plagiarism?

1. You change the verb tense, but otherwise keeping the sentence the same as the original author, but citing the author and year in parentheses at the end of the sentence.

2. You change the order of the sentences in a paragraph and adding one sentence of your own construction to the paragraph, and name the author of the original work as part of one sentence (e.g., According to Garza, such and such).

3. At a conference, the presenter, R. Yount, runs out of handouts, so you ask the presenter to e-mail his or her presentation to you, and then you use it in your own presentation at work. Each slide says © R. Yount, (2006) on the bottom.

4. You write a brilliant paragraph for an evaluation report. You like it so much, you keep pulling it up on the computer whenever you have to write a new evaluation report for a similar client, and change the name, but otherwise use the same wording.

SUMMARY

When you plagiarize, you not only cheat the originator of the material out of his or her proper credit, but also you cheat yourself by not really learning the material. Occasional honest mistakes can usually be tolerated, but repeated instances of the same type of error in citing sources could be used to show a pattern of carelessness that amounts to plagiarism. A student who plagiarizes can expect to fail the assignment or the course, or be expelled from the program. Blatant and repeated plagiarism can lead to expulsion from a school. Plagiarism done by a professional can result in loss of a job or even a career in occupational therapy. There are ways to prevent plagiarism. Allowing plenty of time to complete written work, learning how to properly cite sources, and summarizing or paraphrasing from memory are a few of the ways that plagiarism can be prevented.

REFERENCES

American Occupational Therapy Association. (2005). Occupational therapy code of ethics. *American Journal of Occupational Therapy, 59,* 639–642.

American Occupational Therapy Association. (2006). *Guidelines to the code of ethics. American Journal of Occupational Therapy,* 60, 652–658.

American Psychological Association. (2001). *Publication manual of the American Psychological Association* (5th ed.). Washington, DC: Author.

Avoiding plagiarism. Retrieved May 23, 2002, from http://sja.ucdavis.edu/avoid.htm

Bailey, D. M. & Schwartzberg, S. L. (2003). *Ethical and legal dilemmas in occupational therapy* (2nd ed.). Philadelphia: F. A. Davis.

Fremgen, B. F. (2002). *Medical law & ethics.* Upper Saddle River, NJ: Prentice Hall.

Georgetown University Honor Council. (2002). Retrieved May 5, 2002, from http://www.georgetown.edu/honor/plagiarism.html

Hagedorn, R. (1997). *Foundations for practice in occupational therapy* (2nd ed.). Edinburgh, Scotland: Churchill Livingstone.

Hashimoto, I. Y. (1991). *Thirteen weeks: A guide to teaching college writing.* Portsmouth, NH: Boynton/Cook.

Kleiner, C., & Lord, M. (1999, November 29). The cheating game. *U.S. New and World Report.* Retrieved May 10, 2002, from http://www.usnews.com/usnews/edu/college/articles/cosheata.htm

Lunsford, A. A. (2005). *The everyday writer.* Boston: Bedford St. Martin.

McCabe, (2005). *New CAI Research.* Retrieved August 3, 2006 from http://www.academic integrity.org/cai_research.asp

Merriam-Webster Online. (n.d.). *Definition of plagiarize.* Retrieved on August 3, 2006, from http://www.m-w.com/dictionary/plagiarizing

Neistadt, M. S., & Crepeau, E. B. (1998). *Willard & Spackman's occupational therapy* (9th ed.). Philadelphia: Lippencott-Raven.

Nolo.com. (2009). The *"fair use" rule: When use of copyrighted material is acceptable.* Retrieved January 11, 2009, from http://www.nolo.com/article.cfm/pg/1/objectId/ C3E49F67-1AA3-4293-9312FE5C119B5806/catId/DAE53B68-7BF5-455A-BC9F3D9C9C1F7513/310/276/ART/

Purdue University Online Writing Laboratory. (2006). *Avoiding plagiarism.* Retrieved August 3, 2006, from http://owl.english.purdue.edu/owl/resource/589/01/

Schwartzberg, S. (2002) *Interactive reasoning in the practice of occupational therapy.* Upper Saddle River, NJ: Prentice Hall.

SECTION III
Clinical Documentation

▼ INTRODUCTION ▼

Now that we have some of the basics out of the way, we can get to the actual writing of occupational therapy documentation. This section explores the different types of documentation that occupational therapy practitioners write when working with clients whose ability to participate fully in life is diminished or at risk due to physical, psychological, or developmental issues. Typically, in clinical settings, payment for services is sought from third-party payers such as insurance companies, managed care organizations, government programs, or from the clients themselves. When third-party payers get involved in the care process, it adds an additional layer of requirements that occupational therapy practitioners need to address in their documentation. Clinical settings for occupational therapy services may include medical or psychiatric hospitals, clinics, or long-term care settings as well as in the clients' homes, sheltered workshops, group homes, or other facilities.

▼ CLINICAL DOCUMENTATION ▼

Clinical documentation typically consists of documentation of the client's referral for services, a summary of the evaluation results (including the occupational profile and analysis of occupational performance), intervention plans, documentation of progress, attendance records, discontinuation summaries, and follow-up documentation (if any). Table III.1 shows each step of the occupational therapy process and the corresponding documentation for each step. In essence, for each step of the occupational therapy process there is documentation to go with it. Each of these types of documentation is discussed in the chapters in this section.

Regardless of the type of clinical documentation, certain conventions for good documentation must be followed. While there may be differences between the documentation written by an occupational therapist in a hospital in Los Angeles and an occupational therapy assistant in a sheltered workshop in Bangor, Maine, all documentation must be well written, accurate, and clear.

▼ ROLE DELINEATION FOR DOCUMENTATION ▼

In this section of the book, the term "occupational therapy practitioners" refers to both occupational therapists and occupational therapy assistants. The occupational therapist has primary responsibility for assuring that documentation is completed in compliance with standards. The occupational therapy practitioner who provided the services to the client is the person who should document that service. If the documentation is written by an occupational therapy assistant, the documentation is often cosigned by the supervising occupational therapist as a way to show that supervision has occurred, and that the occupational therapist has read the

TABLE III.1   Occupational Therapy Process and Clinical Documentation

Steps in the Occupational Therapy Process	Types of Documentation
Client identification	Referral or physician's order Contact note
Screening (if required)	Screening report Contact note
Initial evaluation (occupational profile and analysis of occupational performance)	Evaluation report or evaluation summary
Intervention planning	Intervention plan (treatment plan, plan of care)
Intervention	Attendance logs Progress flow sheets Progress notes (SOAP, DAP, or narrative notes) Contact notes
Reevaluation (intervention review)	Revised intervention plans
Discontinuation (discharge)	Discontinuation (discharge) summary
Follow-up	Follow-up note Contact note

Sources: AOTA (2007); Moyers & Dale (2007).

documentation. The American Occupational Therapy Association (2007) does not require that an occupational therapist cosign documentation written by an occupational therapy assistant, unless it is required by state law.

It is important to be familiar with state laws and regulations related to occupational therapy practice. The law that describes how occupational therapy practitioners become licensed or registered to practice in that state is often called the "Occupational Therapy Practice Act." This law will describe the requirements for supervision of occupational therapy assistants including the frequency, type, and how that supervision is documented. Some states not only require a cosignature by the occupational therapist but a log of supervisory visits.

All documentation written by occupational therapy or occupational therapy assistant students need to be cosigned by the student's supervisor. This shows that the supervisor has read the note.

▼ AOTA STANDARDS FOR DOCUMENTATION ▼

The American Occupational Therapy Association (AOTA) has standards for documentation. The AOTA document *Guidelines for Documentation of Occupational Therapy* (2007) lists 13 elements that must be present in any and all clinical documentation:

1. *Client identification:* The client's full name should be mentioned on every page, along with the client's case number, if there is one (see also Fremgen, 2006; Borcherding, 2006). The case number may be a medical records number or room/bed number, whichever is used at a particular facility or program.

2. *Date and type of contact:* Each document should be dated with the day, month, and year (see also Fremgen, 2006; Ranke, 1998). Documentation of occupational therapy sessions (evaluation or intervention) often includes the time of day and sometimes the length of the session (see also Ranke). Dates and times are used to show the chronological order of events. The type of contact (i.e., screening, evaluation, intervention plan, etc.) should be specified.

3. *Type:* The type of documentation should be clearly stated, as should the name of the facility/agency and department. For example, the type of document may appear at the top of the page, and the name of the department may be under the signature line.

4. *Signature:* The writer should sign the document using at least his or her first initial and full last name followed by the appropriate professional designation (e.g., OTR, COTA, OT/L, OTA/L, etc.) (see also Fremgen, 2006; Borcherding, 2006; Ranke, 1998). Using initials only is usually not sufficient. In some cases, such as on an attendance log, the occupational therapist might simply place his or her initials in the space for each day. At the bottom of the page there should be multiple signature lines so that for each set of initials appearing on the page, there is a full name and credentials written out to clearly identify the person who worked with the client.

5. *Placement of signature:* Notes should be signed directly at the end of the note; there should be no space between what is written and the signature (see also Ranke, 1998). This can help prevent someone else from tampering with your documentation. Some facilities have the staff draw a wavy line where there is blank space between the end of a note and the signature.

6. *Countersignature:* As required by state or facility regulations, occupational therapists must countersign the signatures of occupational therapy assistants and students. This countersignature signifies that the occupational therapist has read the document and is in agreement with the conclusions drawn by the writer. This also provides documentation of supervision, which is required by law.

7. *Terminology:* All terminology used, including abbreviations, must be recognized by the facility as acceptable (see also Fremgen, 2006; Borcherding, 2006; Ranke, 1998). Official documents of the profession may be used to define terms, or the facility may specify terminology to be used by all professionals at the facility.

8. *Abbreviations:* Use only abbreviations approved by the facility/agency (see also Borcherding, 2006; Fremgen, 2006; Ranke, 1998). There is usually a list that is used by all disciplines. Some common abbreviations are listed in Chapter 2 of this book. However, just because an abbreviation is listed in this book does not mean that it will be recognized at your facility or in your program.

9. *Corrections:* Follow facility rules for correcting errors. Correct errors by drawing one line through the word(s) in error and initialing your error (see also Borcherding, 2006; Fremgen, 2006; Ranke, 1998). No erasures or correction fluid should be used. Do not scribble out a word or cross out a single letter or part of a word. Some facilities want errors dated. For example:

    KMS 8/21/03

    Client completed 15 ~~repititions~~ repetitions of bicep curls.

10. *Technology:* Follow professional standards and agency/facility policies and procedures for use of technology in documentation.

11. *Record Disposal:* Follow federal and state laws as well as agency/facility policies and procedures for proper disposal of records. (See Section II of this book.)

12. *Confidentiality:* All federal, state, and agency/facility rules and regulations for confidentiality must be obeyed. (See Section II of this book.)

13. *Record Storage:* All federal, state, and agency/facility rules and regulations for storage of records must be obeyed. (See Section II of this book.)

In addition to these standards, there are other common considerations. For example, most documentation is done in blue or black ink because often the documents must be copied and other colors of ink do not photocopy well (Borcherding, 2006; Fremgen, 2006). Never document in a permanent medical record using a pencil (it is erasable). Some facilities do not allow practitioners to document using erasable pens. Other facilities require the ink to be waterproof (Borcherding, 2006). Of course, when documentation is done on computer, the default color of ink used by most printers is black.

Another common consideration is that all handwritten documentation needs to be legible (Fremgen, 2006; Kuntavanich, 1987; Ranke, 1998). For some people, this means printing rather than writing in script (Fremgen). Again, if documentation is done on the computer, usually legibility is not a problem unless the printer is running low on ink, as long as the font size is large enough that people with varying visual acuity can read it (10- or 12-point size font).

Finally, all of the considerations in Chapter 5 about documenting with CARE and Section II (ethical and legal considerations) apply. All documentation must be clear, accurate, and relevant, and exceptions must be documented.

▼ ELECTRONIC MEDICAL RECORD ▼

In 2004, President Bush called for the conversion to an electronic medical record for everyone in this country by 2014 (Tieman, 2004). This record would be portable, so it could follow the patient, and contain documentation of the patient's history, including every physician visit, test, and treatment (Tieman). Many, but not all, hospital and health care systems, clinics, and private practitioners have already made the conversion. It's been reported that in the aftermath of Hurricane Katrina, more than a million Gulf Coast residents found themselves without any access to their medical records, including pharmacy records (Rogers, 2005). This made it much more difficult to provide health-related services to the hurricane survivors that were left in the area with little more than the clothes on their backs.

There are many advantages to having an electronic medical record (EMR). In addition to improved access to the records, computerized records are easier to read, take less time to locate, decrease the duplication of information, and help streamline the billing processes (Shamus & Stern, 2004). Used properly, the EMR can reduce the amount of paper used and decrease storage space needed. The data in the EMR can be used to organize data that can be helpful for tracking staff productivity, identifying referral patterns, and marketing management (Shamus & Stern). In large health care systems, with multiple providers entering and retrieving client information, electronic systems can alert providers to duplicate physician orders, potential adverse drug reactions, and conflicting medication prescriptions. Some disadvantages include the high cost in time and money for hardware, software, and training; the need to back up the systems in case of power outages and system crashes; and the use of templates—which may limit the information that is entered into the record (Hesse & Siebens, 2002).

There are two kinds of hardware systems with which occupational therapy practitioners can enter data into the EMR. The first kind is a computer work station, such as a desktop computer or kiosk that may be set up in central locations (Shamus & Stern, 2004). These may include keyboards and monitors, or touch screens. The second kind comprises the handheld systems such as laptop and notebook computers, or personal data applications (PDAs). These hardware systems differ in their portability, memory capability, and ease of data entry (Shamus & Stern).

Just as with paper documentation, the EMR data can be entered onto a blank page (knowledge-based systems) or a form (template-driven systems) (Shamus & Stern, 2004). A template-driven system can be set up so that the occupational therapy practitioner is cued to enter all the necessary data for the type of document being generated; the system can allow for the use of checklists and menus of words/phrases. While a properly developed template-driven system can reduce the amount of time fully trained staff spend on documentation, the system may not allow much flexibility for situations where "normal" documentation is inadequate. A knowledge-based system can be configured to meet the needs of the setting, and is generally more flexible and user-friendly, but takes longer to learn to use.

Using the EMR while in the presence of the client presents some interesting challenges. First, clients have concerns over the privacy of the information being entered into the computer (Baker, Reifstech, & Mann, 2003). This is greatly affected by whether or not the client can see the screen. Second, the practitioner tends to guide the conversation with the client to facilitate ease of data entry, rather than letting the client's responses guide the conversation. Finally, if the clinician has to turn away from the client to enter the data, that reduces the time the clinician spends observing or talking with the client, and could lead to errors and unsafe situations (Baker, et al.).

▼ STRUCTURE OF THIS SECTION OF THE BOOK ▼

Chapter 9 focuses on documentation of the initial contact a clinician has with a client. This includes referrals for intervention, physician's orders, and screenings.

Chapter 10 discusses the ways in which evaluation reports are written. As part of that discussion, the purposes and focus of evaluations, methods of recording evaluation data, interpreting the data, and summarizing the data are presented.

Chapter 11 centers on goal setting. Clinicians may set goals as part of an evaluation report or as part of an intervention plan. Several methods for writing goal statements are offered.

Chapter 12 presents methods for documenting intervention plans. Specific information about documenting progress summaries and intervention methods/strategies are set forth.

Chapter 13 addresses various forms of progress notes. The two most common kinds of progress notes are SOAP and narrative formats. This chapter looks at these and other formats in detail, with practice opportunities for the readers of this text.

Finally, Chapter 14 presents discontinuation (discharge) summaries. It offers information on documenting the plan for discontinuation and for follow-up if needed.

REFERENCES

American Occupational Therapy Association. (2007). *Guidelines for documentation of occupational therapy.* Retrieved June, 16, 2008, from http://www.aota.org/Practitioners/Official/Guidelines/41257.aspx

Baker, L. H., Reifsteck, S. W., & Mann, W. R. (2003). Connected: Communication skills for nurses using the electronic medical record. *Nursing Economics 21,* 85–87.

Borcherding, S. (2006). *Documentation manual for writing SOAP notes in occupational therapy* (2nd ed.). Thorofare, NJ: Slack.

Fremgen, B. F. (2006). *Medical law and ethics* (2nd ed.). Upper Saddle River, NJ: Prentice Hall.

Hesse, K. A. & Siebens, H., (2002). Clinical information systems for primary care: More than just an electronic medical record. *Topics in Stroke Rehabilitation 9*(3), 39–57.

Kuntavanich, A. (1987). *Occupational therapy documentation: A system to capture outcome data for quality assurance and program promotion.* Rockville, MD: American Occupational Therapy Association.

Ranke, B. A. E. (1998). Documentation in the age of litigation. *OT Practice, 3*(3), 20–24.

Rogers, M. (2005). *Hurricanes, health records and you.* Retrieved August 27, 2006, from http://msnbc.msn.com/id/9431650/

Shamus, E. & Stern, D. (2004). *Effective documentation for physical therapy professionals.* New York: McGraw-Hill.

Tieman, J. (2004). Lurching into the future: Bush sets 2014 goal for EMRs, calls for incentives. *Modern Healthcare 34,*(18) 18. Retrieved July 31, 2006 from Infotrac database.

CHAPTER 9

Client Identification: Referral and Screening

INTRODUCTION

There are several different ways in which an occupational therapy practitioner can discover that she or he has a new client. Depending on the setting in which the occupational therapy practitioner works, she or he can find out by phone, fax, a conversation in a hallway, a written note (a prescription-like form or a handwritten order in a chart), or by a computer alert system (electronic health record). This notification usually comes in the form of a referral or an order.

▼ REFERRALS ▼

A referral is a suggestion from someone that a particular client would benefit from occupational therapy services. Occupational therapists can receive referrals from almost anyone. A parent can call up and refer a child for services. A nurse can refer a client who is struggling to stay in his or her home despite failing health. A chiropractor can refer a client who needs work on body mechanics. A dentist can refer a client with severe jaw pain. A physical therapist, teacher, nursing assistant, or any other person working with someone who has or is at risk of having an occupational performance deficit can make a referral for occupational therapy services. There are no rules or regulations preventing an occupational therapist from receiving referrals from anyone. However, third-party payers, such as managed care organizations and governmental reimbursement systems, often will not pay for services provided to a client with only a referral, unless the referral comes from a physician.

▼ ROLE DELINEATION FOR REFERRALS AND ORDERS ▼

The AOTA has established standards for referrals. These can be found in the *Standards of Practice for Occupational Therapy* (2005a) in Appendix C of this book. These standards require that occupational therapists are responsible for receiving and responding to referrals (and orders). *The Standards of Practice* (2005a) also require occupational therapists to refer clients to other practitioners (other occupational therapists with specific expertise or other professionals) when a client needs a provider with expertise beyond his or her own. This is also a standard in the AOTA Code of Ethics (2005b). In order to ensure appropriate referrals or orders, it is incumbent upon both the occupational therapist and the occupational therapy assistant to educate referral sources on the appropriateness of referrals or orders for occupational therapy services (AOTA, 2005a). The AOTA standards do not recommend that occupational therapy assistants receive or respond to referrals or orders (AOTA, 2005a).

An order is a referral written by a physician. It is like a prescription. Just as a pharmacy must fill a prescription written by a licensed physician, an occupational therapist must comply with a physician's order. Many people use the phrase "physician referral" rather than "physician order." The AOTA (2005a) prefers the term "physician referral." If a client is referred to occupational therapy, often an order from a physician (or nurse practitioner, chiropractor, optometrist, or other legally defined health care professional, depending on state and payer regulations) is required in order to get paid for providing services. There is no national requirement that says occupational therapy practitioners need a physician's order or referral before providing services. Some state licensure laws and some payers require a physician's order for an occupational therapist to see a client.

If an occupational therapist receives a referral for occupational therapy services, and talks to the referral source to find out why the referral was made, the occupational therapist can then contact the physician and ask for an order (or referral). When contacting a busy physician, the occupational therapist needs to have a pretty solid idea of why the client would benefit from occupational therapy evaluation and intervention. In fact, whether or not a busy physician is involved, the occupational therapist and occupational therapy assistant need to clearly understand and articulate why occupational therapy services would be beneficial for every client served by occupational therapy. An occupational therapist who observes a client or does a screening and thinks occupational therapy services would benefit the client can initiate an order by contacting the physician (or other legally defined licensed health care professional) and discussing the ways in which occupational therapy services could benefit the physician's client.

It is up to the occupational therapist, using his or her best clinical judgment, to determine if the referral or order for occupational therapy is appropriate. It is also up to the occupational therapist to determine if additional orders are needed. For example, I have seen orders come through to a rehabilitation department (occupational therapy, physical therapy, and speech-language pathology) for physical therapy for ADLs. The physical therapy staff hand the order to the occupational therapy department and have the occupational therapists call the doctor to explain that it is occupational therapy that works on ADLs and request that the doctor change the order. Conversely, I have seen orders come through for occupational therapy to provide diversional activities. Generally speaking, third-party payers do not pay for diversional activities, so it behooves the occupational therapist to discuss the situation with the physician and determine if the client has occupational performance issues. The occupational therapist should also consider whether a referral to recreation therapy might be more appropriate for the client than occupational therapy.

Physician orders (referrals) should contain certain information. The order (referral) should specify the full name of the client, the date, and sometimes the time the order was written, the full name and credentials of the physician (or equivalent according to state law and payer requirements), the reason for the referral (order), and the frequency and the duration of occupational therapy services (AOTA, 1995). Frequency refers to how often the intervention sessions will occur. Duration refers to how long it is expected to take to meet the needs of the client. Some settings also require intensity of intervention to be included in the order. Intensity refers to the length of time for any one session. An order (referral) for occupational therapy services six times a week (frequency) for three weeks (duration) of 30-minute sessions twice a day (intensity) would satisfy this part of the requirements. If any of these factors are missing, and they often are, the occupational therapist is responsible for contacting the physician to clarify the orders. Sometimes, the occupational therapist completes the evaluation, then, on the basis of the results of the evaluation, contacts the physician to clarify the frequency, intensity, and duration. These are called clarification orders.

An ongoing order is often needed for continued payment for services, especially from Medicare. Having the client's physician sign the plan of care (intervention plan) serves as ongoing orders. Medicare identifies this process as certification and recertification (Prabst-Hunt, 2002). Medicare requires this recertification every 90 days for anyone receiving outpatient occupational therapy (Part B), and the physician has the right to make any changes to

Exercise 9.1

Identify the parts of these referrals:

1.

> 7-10-08
> 8:03 a.m.
>
> Gertrude Silverstein
> #SIL439855GE
> Rm 408B
>
> *Occupational therapy to evaluate and treat for (R) hemisphere CVA bid for 1 wk. Focus on ADLs and IADLs. Provide adaptive equipment as needed along with training in the use of it. Anticipated discharge date 7-17-08.*
>
> *Dr. Sara Bellar*
> #5843-392

_____	Date of referral	_____	Name of physician
_____	Name of client	_____	Frequency
_____	Duration	_____	Intensity

_____ Reason for referral

Is this an adequate referral?   yes   no
Why or why not?

2.

> Kyle Beback
> May 31, 2008
>
> Occupational therapy to evaluate and treat for sensory integration
>
> *Dr. Don Touchme*
> #5883-1202

_____	Date of referral	_____	Name of physician
_____	Name of client	_____	Frequency
_____	Duration	_____	Intensity

_____ Reason for referral

Is this an adequate referral?   yes   no
Why or why not?

the care plan that the physician deems necessary (Centers for Medicare and Medicaid Services [CMS], 2008).

▼ SCREENINGS ▼

Often, but not always, a screening occurs at the first meeting of occupational therapist and client. A screening is a brief, hands-off check of a client to see if further evaluation or intervention is warranted. It often is based on observations of a client and chart review without the direct intervention of an occupational therapy practitioner. Screenings are generally not reimbursable, but can be a good way to identify potential clients for reimbursable services. In most situations, a screening can be done without a physician referral or order. If there is an order for occupational therapy, a screening may simply be a quick chart review before beginning the full evaluation of the client.

In some settings, the occupational therapist routinely screens potential clients. This is referred to as a type I screening (Collier, 1991). For example, an occupational therapist working in a nursing home might screen all new admissions to the facility, or an occupational therapist in private practice might screen visitors to a local health fair. Then, if the screening demonstrates a need for occupational therapy services, an order can be obtained.

In other settings or at other times, the occupational therapist may only screen after receiving a referral. This is referred to as a type II screening (Collier). A screening is not a substitute for an evaluation. Chapter 10 explores evaluations more thoroughly. Evaluations are more thorough and specific than screenings and are reimbursable. It may be tempting at times to use a screening as a substitute for a complete evaluation when time is of the essence. Do not do it. A screening is not adequate for accurately determining a client's strengths and need areas, or for developing goals.

As mentioned in Chapter 3, the word "assessment" means screening in some settings, and is used as a synonym for evaluation in other settings. Be sure you know how the word is used at your facility/agency and for the reimbursement system used.

According to Collier (1991), there are several general guidelines for when to do screenings:

- Screenings are done only when you believe that the potential problems you will find in your screening can be positively affected by occupational therapy intervention. You do not want to conduct screenings for problems that are beyond occupational therapy's scope of practice. For example, you do not want to screen for problems with articulation of words; a speech-language pathologist would do that.

- Screenings are best done when they are timely, that is, they are done at a time when intervention would be effective. It sounds obvious, but you would not screen for developmental delays in high schoolers; you would screen for delays in preschoolers.

- There must be a reason to believe that the population you are screening will have some people who demonstrate the problem you are screening for. If you are screening a healthy population, you must expect that at least a small percentage of people will ultimately need your services.

- Occupational therapy intervention must be available to help alleviate the problems you identify. It makes no sense to provide screenings where or when there are no services available to work on the problems found.

- Finally, use screening methods that you believe are valid and reliable. This does not mean they need to be standardized, but that your methods are sensitive to finding persons with the problems you are looking for.

There are four possible outcomes of screenings. The first is that the client may in fact need occupational therapy intervention. The second is that the client does not need intervention right now, but there is enough concern that it would be worth rescreening in a few months (or whatever time period you think is appropriate). Next is the possibility that the client needs a referral to some other professional. Finally, the client may not need any intervention at all.

▼ ROLE DELINEATION FOR SCREENINGS ▼

The AOTA has established standards for screenings, which can be found in the *Standards of Practice for Occupational Therapy* (AOTA, 2005a) in Appendix C of this book. The occupational therapist is responsible for conducting the screening; however, an occupational therapy assistant, under the supervision of an occupational therapist, may contribute to the screening. The occupational therapist is responsible for selecting the proper tools and methods for screening. Either the occupational therapist or an occupational therapy assistant, under the supervision of an occupational therapist, communicates the results of the screening results and recommendations to other members of the care team, or other appropriate persons (AOTA, 2005a).

▼ CONTACT NOTE ▼

A brief note is usually entered into the medical record to acknowledge that the referral/order was received or that the screening took place. This note contains the date and time the referral was received, and when the client is scheduled to begin the evaluation. If you did a screening, the note should also contain the bottom-line results of the screening. Below are two examples of contact notes.

> *5/2/09. 10:35 a.m. Order received for occupational therapy evaluation and intervention. Introduced myself to the client and scheduled her to come to the clinic this afternoon to begin evaluation process. K. Sapp, OTR/L.*

> *5/2/09. 10:35 a.m. Received referral for occupational therapy evaluation and intervention. Results of screening show that client would likely benefit from occupational therapy intervention to improve functional use of both arms and hands. Evaluation scheduled for this afternoon. K. Sapp, OTR/L.*

Contact notes are also used at other points during the occupational therapy process. The AOTA *Guidelines for Documentation of Occupational Therapy* (2007) recommend that all contacts between the occupational therapist or occupational therapy assistant and the client be documented, including telephone contacts and meetings with others. Missed sessions should be documented using a contact note (AOTA; Fremgen, 2002). AOTA guidelines further recommend that the therapist should document client or caregiver training in a contact note, being sure to include the names of those present for the training and the client's response (if present).

In some settings, a contact note is written for each contact with a client, including each intervention session. These notes include specific intervention participation (type of intervention and client response to the intervention), significant communication to or from a client, modifications made to the environment or tasks, and/or any equipment (assistive or adaptive devices) fabricated or modified (AOTA, 2007). Some settings prefer a more complete progress note (SOAP, DAP or narrative format) (see Chapter 13). Some settings use a combination of the two, writing a contact note for every client contact, and a SOAP, DAP, or narrative note on a weekly or biweekly basis to summarize the client's progress.

Exercise 9.2

In which of the following situations would it be appropriate to do a screening?

1. A doctor's order comes to the occupational therapy department in an acute care hospital to evaluate a client.

2. You work in a hand therapy clinic. Your caseload has fallen off recently. There is a health fair coming to the strip mall across the street from your clinic. The health fair coordinator suggests that you offer free grip and pinch strength testing.

---

3. You have a friend who is a building supervisor for a new assisted living facility. She would like you to come once a month to screen all new residents for things like fall prevention and other safety concerns. The facility does not have occupational therapy staff on site. You work in a preschool nearby and have never worked with the elderly before.

4. A nurse asks you to look at a resident of the nursing home at which you work. The resident has been taking longer and longer to eat, and is now the last one to finish even though they serve him first. She asks you to observe the client while he eats lunch and tell her whether you think she should ask the doctor for orders for occupational therapy.

▼ MEDICARE COMPLIANCE ▼

There are hundreds of potential payers for occupational therapy services. Each insurance company, managed care organization, state Medicaid program, or other state-run program sets its own standards for documentation. As a result, there are no clear national standards that meet the requirements of all these payers. Medicare, as a national insurance program, does set national standards for documentation, although the Medicare MACs (Medicare Administrative Contractors) may issue further policies on documentation. Since there are so many payers with individual standards for documentation, and the Medicare standards are often the most stringent of the payer standards, some people recommend using the Medicare standards as the minimum standard for documentation. Certainly in some settings, such as pediatric or some mental health clinics, the Medicare standards may not apply because Medicare is rarely the primary payer. Nonetheless, many payers look to Medicare and follow Medicare's lead for establishing documentation policies.

For the sake of clarity, Medicare defines terms used in its communication with providers. Here are the relevant terms as defined by Medicare (CMS, 2008, pp. 7–9):

> ASSESSMENT is separate from evaluation, and is included in services or procedures (it is not separately payable). The term assessment as used in Medicare manuals related to therapy services is distinguished from language in Current Procedural Terminology (CPT) codes that specify assessment, e.g., 97755, Assistive Technology Assessment, which may be payable). Assessments shall be provided only by clinicians, because assessment requires professional skill to gather data by observation and patient inquiry and may include limited objective testing and measurement to make clinical judgments regarding the patient's condition(s). Assessment determines, for example, changes in the patient's status since the last visit/treatment day and whether the planned procedure or service should be modified. On the basis of these assessment data, the professional may make judgments about progress toward goals and/or determine that a more complete evaluation or reevaluation (see the definitions following this paragraph) is indicated. Routine weekly assessments of expected progression in accordance with the plan are not payable as reevaluations.
>
> EVALUATION is a separately payable comprehensive service provided by a clinician, as defined above, that requires professional skills to make clinical judgments about conditions for which services are indicated based on objective measurements and subjective evaluations of patient performance and functional abilities. Evaluation is warranted, for example, for a new diagnosis or when a condition is treated in a new setting. These evaluative judgments are essential to development of the plan of care, including goals and the selection of interventions.
>
> REEVALUATION provides additional objective information not included in other documentation. Reevaluation is separately payable and is periodically indicated during an episode of care when the professional assessment of a clinician indicates a significant improvement, or decline, or change in the patient's condition or functional status that was not anticipated in the plan of care. Although some state regulations and state practice acts require reevaluation at specific times, for Medicare payment, reevaluations must *also* meet Medicare coverage guidelines. The decision to provide a reevaluation shall be made by a clinician.

The full set of definitions and rules for outpatient occupational therapy documentation can be found at http://www.cms.hhs.gov/transmittals/downloads/R88BP.pdf and excerpts are included in Appendix F of this textbook.

Medicare will only pay for services if there is proper documentation that supports the need for the services and justifies payment for those services (CMS, 2008). According to Medicare, Services are medically necessary if the documentation indicates they meet the requirements for medical necessity, including that they are skilled, rehabilitative services, provided by clinicians (or qualified professionals when appropriate) with the approval of a physician/NPP, safe, and effective (i.e., progress indicates that the care is effective in rehabilitation of function) (CMS, 2008, p.23).

In order for Medicare to pay for a service, such as occupational therapy, the service must meet certain requirements. The three main requirements are:

- The client must be under the care of a physician who certifies the plan of care.
- The services provided must require the skills of an occupational therapist or an occupational therapy assistant under the supervision of an occupational therapist. This means that the assessment, evaluation, and intervention require the knowledge, expertise, clinical judgment, decision making, and abilities of occupational therapy practitioners. A skilled occupational therapy practitioner may also be required out of concern for client safety. If an aide can do it, or a family member can do it, then it no longer requires a skilled occupational therapy practitioner, and Medicare will no longer pay for it.
- The services are the appropriate for the individual needs of the client. This means that the type of service, the frequency, the intensity, and the duration of the services are specific to the client's condition. (CMS, 2008).

Documentation for any Medicare client needs to show how the care provided meets all three of these criteria. A payer should be able to read your documentation and see that your skills are required, that the care is appropriate, and that a physician has certified the plan of care (CMS, 2008). A screening can be done without a physician's order or referral, but an evaluation and ongoing intervention required an order/referral from a physician. An order/referral from a physician is evidence of physician involvement in the care of the client.

SUMMARY

The occupational therapist usually makes contact with a client after an order or referral is received for services. The referral can come from any source, including the client or the client's family, other health, social service, or education professionals or physicians. Most payers require either a referral or an order from a physician.

A screening is often the first contact an occupational therapy practitioner has with the client. Sometimes screenings are routinely done for all new admissions to a program or facility. Other times, screenings are conducted at the request of another health, social service, or education professional. Screenings are brief and are generally based on chart review, interview, and observations. A screening helps determine if a full-blown evaluation would be beneficial. A screening can occur before obtaining an order for occupational therapy services, or it can occur after receiving a referral or order.

A contact note is usually written to verify that the occupational therapist has received the referral or order, a screening was done, and to indicate whether further evaluation and/or intervention will be necessary. In addition, a brief contact note may be written to document every subsequent contact the occupational therapist or occupational therapy assistant has with the client throughout the course of occupational therapy service delivery. The contact note documents communication with the client or client's caregiver as well as a description of the interventions implemented and the client's response to the intervention. Contact notes are also written to document reasons for missed sessions and the content of telephone conversations with the client.

REFERENCES

American Occupational Therapy Association. (1995). Elements of clinical documentation. *American Journal of Occupational Therapy, 49,* 1032–1035.

American Occupational Therapy Association. (2005a). Standards of practice for occupational therapy. *American Journal of Occupational Therapy, 52,* 866–869.

American Occupation Therapy Association. (2005b). Occupational therapy code of ethics—2005. *American Journal of Occupational Therapy, 54,* 614–616.

American Occupational Therapy Association. (2007). *Guidelines for documentation of occupational therapy.* Retrieved June, 16, 2008, from http://www.aota.org/Practitioners/Official/Guidelines/41257.aspx.

AOTA. (2008). Occupational therapy practice framework: Domain and process. *American Journal of Occupational Therapy 62,* 625–683.

Centers for Medicare and Medicaid Services. (2008). *Pub100-02 Medicare benefit policy: Transmittal 88.* Retrieved May 8, 2008, from http://www.cms.hhs.gov/transmittals/downloads/R88BP.pdf.

Collier, T. (1991). The screening process. In W. Dunn (Ed.), *Pediatric occupational therapy: Facilitating effective service provision* (pp. 10–33). Thorofare, NJ: Slack.

Fremgen, B. F. (2002). *Medical law and ethics.* Upper Saddle River, NJ: Prentice Hall.

Moyers, P. A. & Dale, L. M., (2007). *The guide to occupational therapy practice, 2nd ed.* Bethesda, MD: AOTA Press.

Prabst-Hunt, W. (2002). *Occupational therapy administration manual.* Albany, NY: Delmar.

CHAPTER 10

Evaluation Reports

INTRODUCTION

The initial evaluation report is one of the most important documents that you will write. All of the other documents (e.g., progress notes, intervention plans, discontinuation summaries) are dependent on a clear and valid initial evaluation report. Evaluation reports demonstrate the need for occupational therapy services. If a need for your services is not documented, why should anyone pay for them? Without documentation of an evaluation, it is difficult to identify the client's level of function prior to intervention. In other words, a baseline is needed from which you, other team members, and payers can see progress (Moyers & Dale, 2007).

This chapter focuses on the components of a well-written evaluation report. The evaluation report is dependent on the skills of the occupational therapist in collecting and interpreting data. This book does not cover specific instructions for conducting evaluations, nor will it recommend specific assessment tools. There are many resources available to occupational therapist practitioners that describe selecting and administering the proper assessment tool and interpreting the data gathered. This chapter assumes you have the data and now need to write about it.

▼ ROLE DELINEATION IN THE OCCUPATIONAL THERAPY EVALUATION PROCESS ▼

The occupational therapist is responsible for the occupational therapy evaluation process (American Occupational Therapy Association [AOTA], 2005). An occupational therapy assistant, under the supervision of an occupational therapist, may contribute to the process. Either an occupational therapist or an occupational therapy assistant may educate the client and others (as appropriate) about evaluation procedures and the reasons for the evaluation.

The occupational therapist determines the most appropriate assessment tools to use (AOTA, 2005). The occupational therapy practitioner administering the assessment is responsible for following established protocols for administration of standardized tests.

The occupational therapist is responsible for summarizing, analyzing, and interpreting the data (AOTA, 2005). He or she also uses that information to develop an appropriate intervention plan based on the client's current functional status. The occupational therapist follows established guidelines for documentation of evaluation results in a time frame and format accepted by the facility/agency, payer requirements, applicable accreditation agency standards, and state and federal laws and regulations. Occupational therapy practitioners also follow confidentiality standards in communicating the results of the evaluation process to others involved in the care of the client. An occupational therapy assistant, under the supervision of an occupational therapist, may contribute to these processes.

Finally, AOTA (2005) standards state that it is the occupational therapist that makes recommendations for evaluation or intervention by other professionals, based on the occupational therapy evaluation results. In practical terms, this means that the occupational therapist has ultimate responsibility for every stage of the evaluation process. However, an occupational therapy assistant can be a very valuable contributor to the evaluation process. As appropriate to the skill of the occupational therapy assistant and the condition of the client, the occupational therapist can delegate parts of the evaluation process to the occupational therapy assistant. An occupational therapy assistant must demonstrate service competence when administering any part of the evaluation process, including standardized tests. State licensure laws may contain specific language describing criteria for delegation of duties to an occupational therapy assistant as well as the type and amount of supervision required. It is always prudent to check with your state's licensing (or registration or other form of regulation as appropriate) authority for specific requirements.

▼ CORE CONCEPTS OF EVALUATIONS ▼

Polgar (1998) identified three main purposes for doing an evaluation: Evaluations are done (1) to describe a client's current level of performance, (2) to predict future function of that client, and (3) to measure the outcomes of occupational therapy intervention. While there may be times when you conduct an evaluation without providing intervention afterward, often you will need to write your evaluation report with all three purposes in mind. As a result, you will need to describe the unique circumstances of your client's situation, predict future function through goal setting, and establish a baseline from which future performance can be measured and compared.

Occasionally, an evaluation is completed and no intervention is needed. In this case, the evaluation serves as documentation of a client's function at the point in time of the evaluation. If another evaluation is completed at a later date, it can be used to compare to the initial evaluation, to see if functional skills have been gained or lost. If the occupational therapist is functioning in a consultant role, the evaluation may be written with the expectation that others will carry out the intervention. In this case, careful attention to the language of the evaluation report will be needed so that those charged with implementation will understand exactly what needs to be done.

Moyers and Dale (2007) identified the focus of the evaluation process as "the client's engagement in occupations to support participation in the community or in organizations." (p. 22). It would follow, then, that the focus of your evaluation report would be on engagement in occupations rather than on client factors that influence performance. The *Occupational Therapy Practice Framework* (AOTA, 2008) suggests that the evaluation process focuses on finding what the client wants to do, needs to do, used to do, and can do, and on identifying those factors that support or inhibit performance.

Both of these perspectives suggest a "top-down" approach to conducting the evaluation. A top-down approach considers occupational roles and performance first and then discerns the factors that contribute to the occupational performance (Stewart, 2001; Weinstock-Zlotnik & Hinojosa, 2004). The specific tasks that a person will need to do or wants to do are considered first; the specific "foundational skills (performance skills, performance patterns, context, activity demands, and client factors) are considered later" (Weinstock-Zlotnik & Hinojosa, p. 594).

Some models and frames of reference support the top-down approach; however, others support a "bottom-up" approach. In a bottom-up approach, the foundational factors are evaluated first; then occupational performance is addressed (Weinstock-Zlotnik & Hinojosa, 2004). The bottom-up approach calls for an examination of a client's assets and limitations first, under the assumption that, as the limitations are eliminated, reduced, or compensated for, the occupational performance will naturally improve (Weinstock-Zlotnik & Hinojosa). This may be the most reasonable approach to take in some settings, such as in an intensive care unit (ICU) where the patient may not be able to respond verbally, but needs a splint made in order to prevent contractures from developing.

This is why it is so important to base one's evaluation process on a particular model or frame of reference. It gives you a starting point and direction in which to proceed. The model or frame of reference will guide the critical thinking of the occupational therapist in the selection of evaluation methods and assessment tools, as well as the language by which the occupational therapist will describe occupational performance strengths and deficits. Refer to Chapter 4 of this book for further discussion on the influence of models and frames of reference.

Two of the most prominent concepts driving occupational therapy practice today are evidence-based practice and client-centered practice (Law, Baum, & Dunn, 2001). Evidence-based practice means that, to the extent possible, you must be prepared to show that your interpretation of the data collected and plan for intervention are supported by research. This demonstrates to those reading your evaluation reports that you are current in your knowledge of occupational practice and that you know what is effective.

Being client-centered means that the client is a full partner in the evaluation process (Law et al., 2001). As a partner, the client's subjective experiences, as well as the occupational therapist's objective observations and measurements, are both critical to the evaluation process. The establishment of occupational therapy outcomes (goals) is a collaborative effort between the client and occupational therapist. The client's subjective experiences are reflected in the occupational profile, and the objective observations and measurements are reflected in the analysis of occupational performance (AOTA, 2008).

▼ THE EVALUATION PROCESS ▼

The process of evaluation has many steps. These steps are spelled out nicely in the *Guide to Occupational Therapy Practice* by Moyers and Dale (2007) and in the *The Occupational Therapy Practice Framework* (AOTA, 2008). Remember that the term evaluation refers to a process, while the term assessment refers to a tool used to gather information for the evaluation (AOTA, 2005). The process of evaluation includes planning the approach, data gathering, interpreting the data, hypothesizing, setting goals, and planning intervention. Moyers and Dale suggest nine distinct steps in the evaluation process. This is a "top-down" approach. It is important to remember that not every facility or program uses a "top-down" approach. Figure 10.1 illustrates this process.

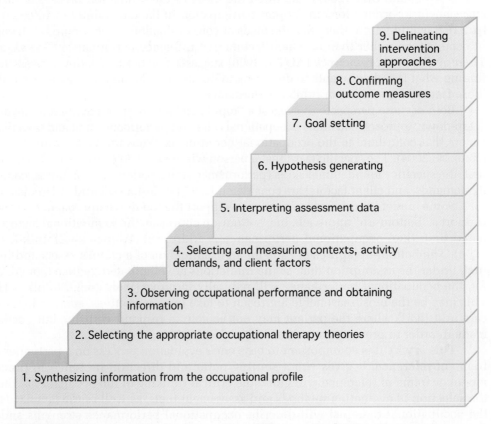

9. Delineating intervention approaches

8. Confirming outcome measures

7. Goal setting

6. Hypothesis generating

5. Interpreting assessment data

4. Selecting and measuring contexts, activity demands, and client factors

3. Observing occupational performance and obtaining information

2. Selecting the appropriate occupational therapy theories

1. Synthesizing information from the occupational profile

FIGURE 10.1 Steps in the Occupational Therapy Evaluation Process. *Source: Moyers & Dale (2007).*

The first step is to synthesize the information that is shared during the occupational profile (Moyers & Dale, 2007; AOTA, 2008). This will allow the occupational therapist to focus on the areas of occupation and the contexts in which the occupations occur for the rest of the evaluation process.

Next, the occupational therapist determines the theoretical approach he or she will employ to guide his or her thinking through the rest of the process (Moyers & Dale, 2007; AOTA, 2008). This requires the occupational therapist to use clinical reasoning skills, and evidence-based practice concepts. The theoretical approach or combination of approaches will shape not only the evaluation process, but the interventions and outcomes of occupational therapy as well.

The third step involves observing and documenting the client's performance in the occupations and activities that are important to the client (Moyers & Dale, 2007; AOTA, 2008). In addition to observing the client while engaged in occupations, this step includes reviewing information provided by the occupational therapy assistant or others who have observed the client's performance. The focus is on the occupation, the effectiveness of the occupational performance, and the client's satisfaction with the effectiveness of the occupational performance. Time will not allow the occupational therapy practitioners to observe the client engage in every possible occupation that might be of concern, so some prioritization is necessary. Target the ones that are of the greatest concern to the client or the client's caregivers (Moyers & Dale; AOTA, 2008).

Next the occupational therapist selects the assessments that will be used (Moyers & Dale, 2008; AOTA, 2008). Either the occupational therapist or occupational therapy assistant, under the supervision of the occupation therapist, then uses the assessments to measure the client factors, contexts, and activity demands. The assessments may be formal tests with specific protocols, or they may be informal, depending on the client's situation and needs.

The fifth step requires the clinical reasoning skills of the occupational therapist. In this step, the assessment data is interpreted so that a clear picture of the supports and barriers to effective occupational performance are identified (Moyers & Dale, 2007; AOTA, 2008). The test manual of a standardized test will provide some guidance for proper interpretation of test results. AOTA (2007) suggests expressing one's confidence in the test results. This can be accomplished by stating whether test scores are consistent with observed behavior. For example, a test may show that a client has poor muscle strength, yet the client is observed using that muscle against gravity during dressing. Or a test could show that a client is not able to follow three-step directions, but during an activity in the occupational therapy room, the client complied perfectly when you asked him to "pick that up, put it on the shelf over there, and then come back and sit in that chair." The results need to be summarized and must relate clearly to the occupational profile (AOTA, 2007).

The next step may blend in with the last one without a clear separation. In this step, the occupational therapist hypothesizes about the client's strengths and weaknesses/need areas in occupational performance (Moyers & Dale, 2008; AOTA, 2008). The weaknesses/need areas will be targeted during intervention planning (next step), and the strengths will be incorporated into the intervention methodology.

In the seventh step, the occupational therapist develops long- and short-term goals for the client to address the weaknesses/needs and the client's desired outcomes (Moyers & Dale, 2008; AOTA, 2008). This happens in collaboration with the client or client's caregivers. The collaboration is a key element in client-centered care.

Next, the outcome measures are confirmed (Moyers & Dale, 2008; AOTA, 2008). The outcome measures are used to determine when therapy will no longer be needed. Outcomes can reflect the client's occupational performance, satisfaction with performance, role competence, adaptation, health and wellness, or quality of life (Moyers & Dale; AOTA, 2008).

Finally, potential intervention approaches are identified (Moyers & Dale, 2008; AOTA, 2008). These will reflect the theoretical approaches embraced by the occupational therapist and shown to be effective for clients with similar needs. The clinician should be prepared to demonstrate that there is evidence to support his or her planned interventions.

▼ COMPONENTS OF AN EVALUATION REPORT ▼

Evaluations vary on many factors. Some are comprehensive; some are problem specific. Some use standardized, formal assessments; some use nonstandardized, informal, activity-based evaluations. There are checklists and self-reporting tools. Remember, evaluation is the process and assessments are the tools (AOTA, 2005). Documentation of evaluation results may be referred to by different terms: assessment summary report, evaluation summary, evaluation report, evaluation note, or assessment report and plan. In this book, the term "evaluation report" is used.

Hinojosa and Kramer (1998) state that an occupational therapist must consider several factors when conducting an evaluation:

1. The development (biological and personal) of the person
2. Contexts
3. The client's relationship with others
4. The client's engagement in occupations
5. The quality of occupational performance
6. The relationship between the client's development (physical and psychosocial) and engagement in occupations.

They go on further to identify beliefs that occupational therapists hold about evaluation (Hinojosa & Kramer, 1998). The first is that the evaluation process is ongoing throughout the service delivery continuum and it is a dynamic and interactive process. Second, we know that assessment tools can have biases, and so can the people who administer them. Assessment tools can have biases in terms of gender, culture, geographic region, educational level, or socioeconomic status of the test taker. Test administrators, including occupational therapists, can carry expectations, personal prejudices, and preconceived notions into the testing situation. Of course, it is hoped that assessment tools that are selected are as free of bias as possible, and that occupational therapists try to not let biases influence the way they administer the test or interpret it. The third belief is that the client's perspective, as well as that of the client's family and caregivers, is incorporated into the evaluation process. Finally, the evaluation report should provide the reader with a comprehensive picture of the client. The report reflects the person's occupational roles, occupational performance, performance skills and patterns, contexts, activity demands, and client factors (AOTA, 2008).

As with all clinical documentation, certain elements must be present in an evaluation report. Besides the usual identification information (client name, date of birth, gender, and diagnoses), the reason for the referral, when the referral was made and who made the referral, and the type/amount of service requested are also included (AOTA, 2007). Assessment tools used in the evaluation process are listed and references are made to other reports, such as the physician's history and physical examination or client intake forms used by the occupational therapist. Precautions and contraindications that could interfere with or cause problems during occupational therapy evaluation and intervention are clearly stated. Examples of precautions and contraindications are that the client could not find his or her own way out of the building in case of a fire, that the client's blood pressure drops dangerously low when seated at a 90° angle, or that the client is combative. Each of these is something any occupational therapy staff member who works with clients or transports them to the clinic needs to know.

Listing the appropriate diagnoses is not as easy as it sounds. You need to identify which condition (there usually is more than one diagnosis, often identified by the referral source) the occupational therapy interventions are being designed to address. If a client has an upper respiratory infection, diabetes, chemical dependency, and a broken hip, which one is the primary condition you are addressing? The term "diagnosis" is used primarily to satisfy third-party payers. In nonmedical settings, a primary concern or occupational deficit may be used instead of a medical diagnosis.

A critical section of the evaluation report is the occupational profile. In this section of the evaluation report, the occupational therapist "describes the client's occupational history and experiences, patterns of daily living, interests, values, and needs" (AOTA, 2008, p. 649). The occupational therapist is trying to understand, from the client's perspective, what the client wants and needs. This requires using a client-centered approach. The occupational therapist needs a solid understanding of the client's past experiences and contexts, current occupational strengths and areas that are problematic, and priorities/desired outcomes (AOTA, 2008, 2007). In addition to gaining valuable insight into the unique situation of your client, discussing the client's situation with him or her helps to build rapport and establish a therapeutic relationship necessary for collaboration with the client throughout the occupational therapy process (AOTA, 2008).

In addition to the occupational profile, an essential part of the evaluation is the analysis of occupational performance (AOTA, 2008). In the analysis of occupational performance, the performance skills, performance patterns, client factors, contexts, and activity demands that affect occupational performance are identified and prioritized. The focus of the analysis of occupational performance is on gathering and interpreting data from assessment tools. It is important to note that the occupational profile and analysis of occupational performance may be performed sequentially or concurrently (AOTA, 2008).

Gathering data for an evaluation occurs primarily in three ways.

1. Observation of occupational performance
2. Interviewing the client and the client's caregivers
3. Selecting and administering assessment tools

Some evaluation reports will also include the initial intervention plan in the form of long- and short-term goals; intervention approaches and methodology; the anticipated frequency, duration, and intensity of occupational therapy services; and recommendations for other services. Goal writing is addressed in Chapter 11, and intervention planning is covered in Chapter 12.

To illustrate the evaluation process, let's pick a client to evaluate.

Case: Jacob Olsen

Jacob "Jake" Olsen is a 20-year-old college basketball star. He is a junior at a major Big Ten school. He has been a starting forward since his freshman year. Since this school has a large athletic department, there are university employees whose only job is to see that the student athletes pass all their courses. Jake loves playing basketball, but not studying for classes, so he appreciates these "tutors." One of the tutors will even write his papers for him since she is paid to type them anyway; she just recycles papers she has typed for other athletes. Jake's other love is computer games. When he is not sleeping, eating, or on the basketball court, he is leaning over his laptop computer (he is a tall man, while the desks are at heights for normal people), playing galactic battle–type games with his joystick. Over time the hours and hours he spent bent over and pressing the button on the top of the joystick have taken their toll on his neck, shoulders, wrist, and thumb. He has pain from his neck to his fingers on his shooting arm. The pain in his thumb has gotten so bad that the trainer advised him to see the team physician. He was diagnosed with "game playing thumb," a combination of tendonitis and osteoarthritis. The physician gives him a thumb support splint to rest the thumb, with strict instructions not to use the thumb for the next couple weeks.

Without basketball or computer games, he is bored. The coach and his fellow teammates are angry with him. He is in constant pain. The pain pills help, but he feels drained of all energy and motivation. His appetite has decreased. The doctor referred him to occupational therapy to use heat/cold to reduce the inflammation and electrical stimulation to assist in pain relief and to "cheer him up," in other words, to keep him motivated.

Using the model of human occupation, the occupational therapist begins collecting data as part of the occupational profile by talking with him. Although she was tempted to give him a lecture on ethics, personal responsibility, and the good of the team, she restrained herself. Instead, she finds out that the areas of occupation that currently concern Jake are that he has nothing to do with his time, no games to play, and writing is impossible (he can't take notes in class now that he has time to go to class and the tutors won't go for him). He wants to get back to his games as soon as possible; he is just itching to do something beside watching TV or going to classes. He wears sweats so dressing is not a problem, and all his meals are prepared for him, so these are not areas of concern.

On the basis of this information, the occupational therapist can select appropriate assessment tools to measure his motor deficits and his play/leisure choices, collect subjective data on his level of pain, and evaluate the ergonomics of his desk and chair. These assessments provide the data for the occupational analysis. She delegates some of the testing to the occupational therapy assistant. On the basis of the data she and the occupational therapy assistant collected, the occupational therapist concludes that the factors affecting his occupational performance are motor skills (poor posture at the computer, repetitive stress on the joints of his thumb), energy (lack of it), dominating habits (computer games dominate his leisure time), and adaptation (anticipating problems, and modifying the environment or his task to accommodate for problems). After she collects and synthesizes this data, she identifies the supports and barriers to his full engagement in the occupations he loves. She identifies his strengths and areas in need of improvement in the analysis of occupational performance. She and Jake then sit down together to write goals and identify a targeted outcome.

▼ WRITING THE REPORT ▼

Evaluation reports can contain objective and subjective information. When reporting subjective findings, record what the client or the client's caregivers said. Objective findings could be test scores, observations, or measurements. It is important to keep the findings separate from your interpretation of those findings.

Descriptive, Interpretive, and Evaluative Statements

In writing, there are descriptive, interpretive, and evaluative statements. Descriptive statements are objective; they describe what you can see, hear, taste, touch, or smell. Interpretive statements are based on observations or data, but draw some inference or conclusion about the observation or data. Evaluative statements pass judgment on something; it is obvious the person making the statement feels good or bad about it, satisfied or dissatisfied, angry or accepting. Table 10.1 gives examples of the different kinds of statements.

Exercise 10.1

Determine whether each statement is a *description* of an event or person, an *interpretation* of an event or person, or an *evaluation* about an event or person.

1. _____ She ate corn flakes for breakfast.
2. _____ She eats corn flakes for breakfast.
3. _____ She could care less what she eats for breakfast.
4. _____ The client's breath smelled like alcohol.
5. _____ Alyah likes to play with blocks.
6. _____ Jake abuses the system of tutors for scholar-athletes.
7. _____ Jake got a high score of 3,203,485 in Galactoids.
8. _____ Jake usually plays computer games 8–10 hours per day.
9. _____ Jake sat with his body forward at 60°, his elbows resting on his knees.
10. _____ Jake's poor posture contributes to his neck, back, and shoulder pain.
11. _____ Avi refused to make eye contact with this clinician during the evaluation process.
12. _____ Avi is stubborn, yet impulsive.

TABLE 10.1 Descriptive, Interpretive, and Evaluative Statements

Type of Statement	Examples
Descriptive	She wore a red dress.
	He sat down on the edge of the bed and took off his shoes.
	He ate everything on the right side of his plate, leaving the food on the left side untouched.
	She looked over her left shoulder and mumbled, "Get away" six times in the half hour she was in the room. No one was standing behind her.
	She said "please" and "thank you" consistently throughout the session.
Interpretive	She usually wears red dresses.
	He had to sit down on the edge of the bed to take off his shoes.
	He did not appear to notice the food on the left side of his plate.
	She seemed to be hallucinating about someone standing too close behind her.
	She demonstrated awareness of her manners.
Evaluative	She wore a beautiful red dress.
	He was too lazy to bend over and take his shoes off.
	He is careless.
	She acted like a crazy person.
	She is a pleasant person.

Reporting Data and Interpreting It

Interpreting data can be tricky. Often people use phrases like "appears" or "seems to." If that is the preferred wording at your facility or program, then use it. Otherwise, stay away from these phrases because they make you sound unsure of yourself. When you are interpreting data/findings, stay away from evaluative statements.

In the evaluation report findings section, you report a summary of the data collected, such as raw scores from tests or specific tasks that the client completed. For example, you could state that the child scored 24 on the Test of Visual Perception. Or you could say that the client completed 5 of the 7 steps of making coffee. In the interpretation section, you

---

Exercise 10.2

Using "R" for report and "I" for interpretation, identify which of the following statements are a report of information and which are an interpretation of information.

1. _____ The client completed her meal in 26 minutes.
2. _____ The client did not complete the task of looking up the phone number for "time and temperature" and making the call.
3. _____ The child is functioning at an age equivalent of 3 years, 6 months.
4. _____ Annette completed all tasks at the 3-year, 6-month level.
5. _____ The client has severely limited range of motion in her left arm.
6. _____ Toby has an attention span of about 3 minutes.
7. _____ Rashad scored 21 on the Beck's Depression Inventory, 2nd edition.
8. _____ Bao bites her wrists when she's angry or frustrated.
9. _____ Savion needed assistance to start each task, but once started, he finished without additional cuing from staff.
10. _____ Juana used the "two bunny ears" method of tying her shoes.

could report the age level of the child's performance, a percentile rank compared to a normal population, or describe client factors that interfere with optimal occupational performance. When you identify a client's needs, you are making an interpretation of the data. For example, when you say that a child needs to work on fine-motor coordination to bring skills up to age level, or needs to improve gross-motor skills to enable him to explore and interact with his environment, you are making an interpretive statement. Reporting data is recording facts; interpreting data gives the data meaning and context.

When you are interpreting the data and paving the way for your plan, it is important to keep the principles of efficiency and effectiveness in mind (Law, et al., 2001). Since the evaluation report may be used by payers to determine if the services will be paid for, you need to make convincing arguments that occupational therapy intervention is necessary to improve the quality of life for your client. Using Jake as an example, one argument could be that poor posture will contribute to lifelong recurring joint injuries and pain. Teaching him ways to arrange his furniture and computer could prevent future injuries. In clinical settings, you often have to show that your services are medically necessary, which may be defined differently by different payers. You can make your arguments more convincing by demonstrating that there is support in the literature for your conclusions (interpretations) and your plan for intervention. You also have to demonstrate that what you plan to do with the client is uniquely based on occupational therapy principles, and not something that could be done through the use of other disciplines in place of occupational therapy.

Exercise 10.3

Given the data provided, write a brief interpretation of that data.

1. *Findings:* Client drooled throughout the meal. He coughed and gagged with water and juice, but not with applesauce, mashed potatoes, or Jell-O. When he chewed, he frequently opened his mouth and protruded his tongue with food on it. Sometimes food fell off his tongue back onto his plate. He was provided with eating utensils, but he did not use them. Client scooped food with both hands, putting large quantities into his mouth at one time. He swallowed five times during the entire meal.
Interpretation:

2. *Findings:* Active range of motion is within normal limits on the right side, but the left shoulder moved 80° in flexion and 70° in abduction (normal is 180° in both directions). Client moved her elbow between 80° flexion and 40° extension (normal is 0–150°). She had no active movement of the forearm, wrist, or fingers. Passive range of motion is within normal limits in all joints and directions.
Interpretation:

3. *Findings:* During the interview, Goran turned away from the interviewer every 1–2 minutes and spoke over his shoulder in unintelligible words, sometimes laughing out loud. He responded to questions with short phrases. He made eye contact with the interviewer for no more than 2 seconds at a time, 3 times during the 10-minute interview. When asked where he lived, he said, "Here." When asked what kind of work he wanted to do, he said, "Guava." He said he "made the Internet" and that "they stole it" from him. His clothes were dirty, his hair uncombed, and his fingernails appeared bitten off, ragged, and dirty. His breath was sour and he gave off a foul body odor.
Interpretation:

Suggested Evaluation Report Format

Figures 10.2 and 10.3 contain sample evaluation report formats. Notice that there are four sections; background information, findings, interpretation, and plan. You can remember these parts with the mnemonic "BiFIP." The first section (Bi) is for background information. It provides the context for the rest of the report. This is where you record the information you gather for the occupational profile (AOTA, 2008). The second section (F) is for reporting the findings. This is where objective data is reported using descriptive language. This is the place to record the analysis of occupational performance (AOTA, 2008). In as few words as possible, explain the client's current level of performance. It is not necessary to list the client's level of function for every possible activity of daily living (ADL) if only a few areas are affected by his or her current condition. Refer back to

---

OCCUPATIONAL THERAPY EVALUATION REPORT AND INITIAL INTERVENTION PLAN

BACKGROUND INFORMATION
Date of report: **Client's name or initials:**
Date of birth &/or age: **Date of referral:**
Primary intervention diagnosis/concern:
Secondary diagnosis/concern:
Precautions/contraindications:
Reason for referral to OT: *(or questions to be answered)*
Therapist: *(Print or type your name, sign, and date the report at the end.)*

Assessments performed: *(Give a brief description of the method(s) used to gather evaluation data; i.e., interview, informal observation, name of formal assessments, etc.)*

FINDINGS
Occupational Profile: *(Describe the client's occupational history and experience, patterns of living, interests, values, and needs that are relevant to the current situation.)*

OCCUPATIONAL ANALYSIS:
    Areas of occupation:
    Performance skills:
    Performance patterns:
    Client factors:
    Activity demands:
    Contexts:

INTERPRETATION
Strengths and areas in need of intervention:
Supports and Hindrances to Occupational Performance:

Prioritization of Need Areas:

PLAN
    Mutually agreed-on long-term goals:
    Mutually agreed-on short-term goals:
    Recommended intervention methods and approaches:
    Expected frequency, duration, and intensity:
    Location of intervention:
    Anticipated D/C environment:

_____
Signature   **Date**

FIGURE 10.2 Occupational Therapy Evaluation Report and Initial Intervention Plan.

OCCUPATIONAL THERAPY PEDIATRIC EVALUATION REPORT

BACKGROUND INFORMATION

Date of report: __/__/20__

Date of birth &/or age: ___

Primary intervention diagnosis/concern:

Secondary diagnosis/concern:

Precautions/contraindications:

Reason for referral to OT: *(or questions to be answered)*

Therapist: *(Print or type your name, sign and date the report at the end.)*

Client's name or initials:

Date of referral: __/__/ 20__

Assessments performed:

☐ Play Observation
☐ Self-care Observation
☐ Parent Interview
☐ Pediatric Evaluation of Disability Inventory (PEDI)
☐ Sensory Profile
☐ Peabody Developmental Motor Scales, 2nd ed. (PDMS-2)
☐ Bruininks-Oseretsky Test of Motor Proficiency, 2nd ed. (BOT-2)
☐ Beery Visual Motor Integration (VMI)
☐ Sensory Integration and Praxis Test (SIPT)
☐ Sensorimotor Performance Analysis (SPA)
☐ Evaluation Tool of Children's Handwriting (ETCH)
☐ Other: _____

FINDINGS

Occupational Profile: *(Describe the client's occupational history and experience, patterns of living, interests, values, and needs that are relevant to the current situation.)*

Occupational Analysis:

Areas of Occupation	Not Tested	Dependent	Max Assist	Mod Assist	Min Assist	Equipment	Independent	Comments
Bathing	☐	☐	☐	☐	☐	☐	☐	
Toileting	☐	☐	☐	☐	☐	☐	☐	
Eating	☐	☐	☐	☐	☐	☐	☐	
Feeding	☐	☐	☐	☐	☐	☐	☐	
Dressing	☐	☐	☐	☐	☐	☐	☐	
Functional mobility	☐	☐	☐	☐	☐	☐	☐	
Grooming	☐	☐	☐	☐	☐	☐	☐	
Safety	☐	☐	☐	☐	☐	☐	☐	
Handwriting	☐	☐	☐	☐	☐	☐	☐	
Meal prep	☐	☐	☐	☐	☐	☐	☐	
Play	☐	☐	☐	☐	☐	☐	☐	
Other (describe)	☐	☐	☐	☐	☐	☐	☐	

FIGURE 10.3 Occupational Therapy Evaluation Report: Quick Form, Pediatrics.

Performance Skills	Not Tested	Absent	Developing	Proficient	Comments
Posture	☐	☐	☐	☐	
Balance	☐	☐	☐	☐	
Fine motor coordination	☐	☐	☐	☐	
Gross motor coordination	☐	☐	☐	☐	
Visual motor integration	☐	☐	☐	☐	
Following directions	☐	☐	☐	☐	
Sensory processing	☐	☐	☐	☐	
Emotional regulation	☐	☐	☐	☐	
Cognitive skills	☐	☐	☐	☐	
Communication and social skills	☐	☐	☐	☐	
Other (describe)		☐	☐	☐	

Performance patterns: Describe the client's

Habits:

Routines:

Roles:

Rituals:

Client factors:

Body Functions	Not Tested	Absent	Impaired	Adequate	Comments
Attention	☐	☐	☐	☐	
Distractibility	☐	☐	☐	☐	
Memory	☐	☐	☐	☐	
Sequencing	☐	☐	☐	☐	
Initiative	☐	☐	☐	☐	
Sight	☐	☐	☐	☐	
Hearing	☐	☐	☐	☐	
Smell	☐	☐	☐	☐	
Taste	☐	☐	☐	☐	
Touch	☐	☐	☐	☐	
Vestibular	☐	☐	☐	☐	
Kinesthetic	☐	☐	☐	☐	
Proprioception	☐	☐	☐	☐	
Temperature	☐	☐	☐	☐	
Pain	☐	☐	☐	☐	
Muscle tone	☐	☐	☐	☐	
Reflexes	☐	☐	☐	☐	
Endurance	☐	☐	☐	☐	
Joint stability	☐	☐	☐	☐	

FIGURE 10.3 (Continued)

Bilateral integration	❑	❑	❑	❑
Praxis	❑	❑	❑	❑
Other (describe)		❑	❑	❑

Body Structure	Deformity	Movement Limitation	Normal	Comments
Head	❑	❑	❑	
Neck	❑	❑	❑	
Shoulders	❑	❑	❑	❑ R ❑L ❑B
Elbows	❑	❑	❑	❑ R ❑L ❑B
Forearms	❑	❑	❑	❑ R ❑L ❑B
Wrists	❑	❑	❑	❑ R ❑L ❑B
Hands	❑	❑	❑	❑ R ❑L ❑B
Trunk	❑	❑	❑	
Hips	❑	❑	❑	❑ R ❑L ❑B
Knees	❑	❑	❑	❑ R ❑L ❑B
Legs	❑	❑	❑	❑ R ❑L ❑B
Ankles	❑	❑	❑	❑ R ❑L ❑B
Feet	❑	❑	❑	❑ R ❑L ❑B
Other (describe)	❑	❑	❑	

Activity demands and contexts: *(describe)*

Specific test results:

Name of Test (subtest)	Raw Score	Standard Score	Percentile Rank	Age Equivalent	Comments

INTERPRETATION

Strengths and areas in need of intervention:

Supports and hindrances to occupational performance:

Prioritization of need areas:

1.

2.

3.

PLAN

Mutually Agreed-on Long-Term Goals	Mutually Agreed-on Short-Term Goals	Recommended Intervention Methods and Approaches	Comments

FIGURE 10.3 (Continued)

Plans for coordination/
communication with school-based team ❏ Phone   **Frequency:**

                                           ❏ Email   **At least __x/mo**

                                           ❏ Conferences   **More often as**
                                                                         needed

Plans for coordination/
communication with family   ❏ Phone   **Frequency:**

                                           ❏ Email   **At least __x/wk**

                                           ❏ Conferences   **More often as**
                                                                         needed

Intervention will be provided ___ x/ week, ____ min sessions, for ___ weeks at
❏ clinic   ❏ home   ❏ other _____

Anticipated D/C environment: ❏ school   ❏ home   ❏ other _____

_____
Signature   **Date**

FIGURE 10.3 (Continued)

Chapter 3 for explanations of each item listed on the format. Next is the interpretation section (I), sometimes referred to as the analysis portion. You want to use interpretive statements in this section to help the reader make sense of your findings. Finally, there is the plan (P) section. This is where you set goals in collaboration with your client, and determine the methodology you will employ to help your client meet those goals. The ultimate goal of occupational therapy intervention, according to AOTA (2008), is "supporting health and participation in life through engagement in occupation" (p. 626). In writing goals, you will need to specifically state which area or areas of occupation the client will participate in. In collaboration with your client, establish concrete, measurable, timely goals. Goal writing will be covered in Chapter 11. Intervention planning will be discussed in Chapter 12.

The BiFIP format is one of several possible formats for writing evaluation reports. A format simply provides a structure for presenting information in an organized fashion. Sections will vary in length according to the amount of information you have to present. Sometimes the structure is invisible; the report is written in a narrative format with a different paragraph for each section.

There are also numerous electronic evaluation report formats for writing evaluation reports on a computer. These usually have space for entering narrative information, some drop-down boxes for common phrases, and some check boxes for routine items. Because each system is different, it is important to get trained on the particular system used in each facility.

Exercise 10.4

Complete the evaluation report on Jake Olsen using the form provided. You may invent test results and other information for this exercise, knowing you would never do such a thing in "real life." The results and additional information you create must be consistent with the case.

OCCUPATIONAL THERAPY EVALUATION REPORT AND INITIAL INTERVENTION PLAN

BACKGROUND INFORMATION
Date of report: 1-15-09 | **Client's name or initials:** Jacob Olsen
Date of birth &/or age: 6-25-84 | **Date of referral:** 1-14-09
Primary intervention diagnosis/concern: Tendonitis of (R) thumb; neck, back, and (R) arm pain
Secondary diagnosis/concern: Depression
Precautions/contraindications: Thumb immobilized until 1-28-09
Reason for referral to OT: Immobilization of thumb interferes with daily life tasks
Therapist: *(use your name with OTS or OTAS as your credential if you are a student)*

Assessments performed: Observation and interview, UMOT interest inventory, ergonomic assessment of dorm room chair and desk, and the Multiple Dimension Hand Assessment.

FINDINGS
Occupational Profile:

Occupational Analysis:
 Areas of occupation:
 Performance skills:
 Performance patterns:
 Client factors:
 Activity demands:
 Contexts:

INTERPRETATION
Strengths and areas in need of intervention:
Supports and Hindrances to Occupational Performance:

Prioritization of Need Areas:

PLAN
 Mutually agreed-on long-term goals:
 Mutually agreed-on short-term goals:
 Recommended intervention methods and approaches:
 Expected frequency, duration, and intensity: 3xlwk for 2 weeks, 45-min. sessions
 Location of intervention:
 Anticipated D/C environment:

_____
Signature   **Date**

Exercise 10.5

For the following case, write an evaluation report. Again, you may make up supplemental information, but the information you add must be consistent with the case.

 Donna is a 23-year-old mother of five, who has been admitted to the locked unit for a 72-hour hold. She was brought in by police. She was found on a bridge over a major river, allegedly throwing her oldest child (6 years old) over the railing and preparing to throw the rest over. She said she planned to jump in after them; none of them could swim. She was despondent and said she did not want to live anymore. The child was rescued by bystanders and all the children were sent to stay with other family members. Tomorrow her case will be heard by a judge, who will hold a commitment hearing.

Donna recently lost her job as a receptionist at a car dealer's, which she had held for 3 months. Prior to that, she had a series of jobs, none of which lasted more than 6 months. She did not graduate from high school, but did complete her GED. Her children are ages 6 (girl), 5 (boy), 3 (boy), 21 months (girl), and 5 months (boy). She is not married. She has a history of chemical dependency, and twice completed inpatient treatment programs. When she was arrested, she tested positive for crack cocaine, and a small amount was found in her coat pocket. She was arrested twice for prostitution and served short (30- to 90-day) sentences.

When you interview her, she does not make eye contact, slurs her speech, gives very short answers, and expresses no interest in returning to independent living. She sees no future for herself. She has not been eating; she has no appetite. She sleeps a little, she says, because they give her "the good stuff." She tears up as she talks about her children. She admits that she has spanked them, sometimes repeatedly, when they "won't leave her alone," but she insists that she loves them with all her heart. She says that it's not her fault that she didn't finish high school, she got pregnant in the summer before sophomore year by a man she met at her cousin's house. He disappeared when he heard she was pregnant, so there was no child support. She stated no man wants to support her or her kids—there are too many of them. She said there are no good jobs for someone like her, so she will never be able to support herself and her kids.

You administer a Beck Depression Inventory, 2nd ed., and she scores a 48, indicating severe depression. You attempt to administer a Kohlman Evaluation of Living Skills, but she says she doesn't feel like doing anything. She tells you that nothing interests her. She says she doesn't do anything with her leisure time except go to bars or watch TV. She does not think she needs help learning child-rearing strategies, nutrition, job-seeking skills, or leisure activities.

▼ REEVALUATION ▼

Evaluation is an ongoing process. While the focus of this chapter has been on documenting an initial evaluation, there is an element of evaluation that occurs throughout the intervention process. At every intervention session, the occupational therapy practitioner makes observations, collects information about changes in the client's circumstances and performance, and sometimes makes adjustments in the intervention methodology. If the intervention is going to occur over several weeks or more, periodic reevaluations are conducted.

Reevaluation may be formal or informal. Informal reevaluation occurs every time the occupational therapist revises the intervention plan (see Chapter 12). A formal reevaluation may involve repeating previous testing so that changes in performance can be measured and documented. Often formal reevaluation occurs when a client is close to being discontinued or at regular intervals, such as yearly for a child with developmental delays.

Nielson (1998) suggests that reevaluation is a three-step process: data collection, reflection, and decision making. Data collection involves gathering subjective and objective information relative to the targeted outcomes identified by the client and clinician. Reflection is a thought process centered on the client's current status, changes in status since the last evaluation, and a judgment on the effectiveness of the current intervention plan. In the decision-making step, the occupational therapist decides whether the current intervention plan is sufficient, whether it should be changed in some way, or whether the client is ready to be discontinued from occupational therapy services.

▼ MEDICARE COMPLIANCE ▼

Medicare requires documentation of an evaluation that demonstrates the necessity for occupational therapy services. The necessity for occupational therapy services is documented through "objective findings and subjective patient self-reporting" (Centers for Medicare and Medicaid Services [CMS], 2008). Under Medicare, only the occupational therapist may conduct the initial evaluation, reevaluation, and ongoing assessment, but may include objective measures or observations made by an occupational therapy assistant. Medicare wants to assure that the occupational therapist is actively involved in the evaluation and ongoing intervention of the client, that he or she does not simply rely on the input of others (CMS, 2008).

In the evaluation report Medicare requires that the clinician document the client's condition and complexities, and the impact these have on the client's prognosis and/or plan of intervention (CMS, 2008). A medical diagnosis established by a physician or a treatment diagnosis identified by the occupational therapist should be part of the evaluation report. For the occupational therapy evaluation, Medicare recommends using the Patient Inquiry by Focus on Therapeutic Outcomes (FOTO) or the Activity Measure—Post Acute Care (AM-PAC) as outcome measures. If one of these two measurement systems is not used, then other commercially available outcome measurement instruments, validated tests and measurements (evidence based), or "other measurable progress towards identified goals for functioning in the home environment at the conclusion of this therapy episode of care" (CMS, 2008, p. 30) may be used. In addition, there should be documentation that supports the illness severity or complexity, identification of other health services the client is receiving for the condition being addressed in the evaluation/intervention plan and/or durable medical equipment needs, the type of medication the client is currently taking, any factors that complicate care or impact severity, and any documentation of medical care prior to the current condition. The occupational therapist must document the client's answer to the question (or why the client cannot answer the question) "At the present time, would you say that your health is excellent, very good, fair, or poor?" (CMS, 2008, p. 28). There also needs to be documentation that indicates the client's social support, such as where the client lives or intends to live at the conclusion of occupational therapy services, who the client lives with or intends to live with, whether this intervention will return the client to the pre-morbid living environment, and whether this intervention will reduce the level of assistance in ADLs or IADLs. The occupational therapist must use his or her clinical judgment to describe the client's current function status. Finally, the occupational therapist must make a determination whether intervention is needed or not needed. If intervention is needed, the occupational therapist must provide an expected time frame and a plan of care (CMS, 2008).

Depending on the setting, the occupational therapist may contribute to the completion of specific forms that are used to determine whether or not the client will continue to qualify for Medicare coverage. For example, in long term care settings, the Minimum Data Set (MDS) 3.0 is used, and in home health, the Outcome and Assessment Information Set (OASIS) is used. The information that occupational therapists contribute to these Medicare documents are informed by data gathered in the evaluation and reevaluation process.

SUMMARY

The evaluation report is a critically important document. When another team member or a payer reads your evaluation report, he or she should have a clear picture of how the client is functioning and what the hope is for change. The report will justify the need for occupational therapy involvement in this case. All the rest of the work you do with that client hinges on an evaluation report that shows a strong need for your services, clearly states where the client is starting from, and establishes a doable plan.

In the evaluation report, describe your findings/data and then interpret them. Without findings, an interpretation is meaningless. The interpretation cannot stand alone; there must be data/findings to back it up. There is a difference between descriptive, interpretive, and evaluative statements. In the findings section, only descriptive statements should be used. In the interpretation sections, interpretive statements are used. Evaluative statements have no place in evaluation reports. Be absolutely sure you distinguish between reporting information and interpreting it. Follow all the guidelines for general documentation as well as professional standards for evaluation reports.

The occupational therapist is responsible for conducting and documenting the evaluation process. An occupational therapy assistant may contribute to the process. The occupational therapist is also responsible for making referrals to other professionals if the client has needs that are better met by another professional.

There are many formats for reporting evaluation results. Medicare has a form that is available in both electronic and paper formats. Other vendors sell documentation systems that include evaluation formats. The format presented in this chapter is a paper-based format called "BiFIP," which stands for background information, findings, interpretation, and plan. The AOTA describes the evaluation process in *The Occupational Therapy Practice Framework* (2008). The evaluation process is client-centered.

Reevaluation occurs periodically throughout the course of occupational therapy service delivery. It may be formal or informal. It should contain subjective input from the client and client's caregivers as well as objective data gathered through observation and testing. The reevaluation helps the occupational therapist determine whether the current intervention plan is sufficient, needs adjustment, or if the client is ready to be discontinued from occupational therapy services.

REFERENCES

American Occupational Therapy Association. (2005). Standards of practice for occupational therapy. *American Journal of Occupational Therapy, 52,* 866–869.

American Occupational Therapy Association. (2007). *Guidelines for documentation of occupational therapy.* Retrieved June, 16, 2008, from http://www.aota.org/Practitioners/Official/Guidelines/41257.aspx

American Occupational Therapy Association. (2008). Occupational therapy practice framework: Domain and process. *American Journal of Occupational Therapy 62,* 625–683.

Centers for Medicare and Medicaid Services. (2008). *Pub100-02 Medicare benefit policy: Transmittal 88.* Retrieved May 8, 2008, from http://www.cms.hhs.gov/transmittals/downloads/R88BP.pdf

Hinojosa, J., & Kramer, P. (1998). Theoretical basis of evaluation. In J. Hinojosa & Kramer (Eds.), *Evaluation: Obtaining and interpreting data.* Bethesda, MD: American Occupational Therapy Association.

Law, M., Baum, C., & Dunn, W. (2001). *Measuring occupational performance: Supporting best practice in occupational therapy.* Thorofare, NJ: Slack.

Moyers, P. A. and Dale, L. M. (2007). *The guide to occupational therapy practice.* Bethesda, MD: American Occupational Therapy Association.

Nielson, C. (1998). Reevaluation. In J. Hinojosa & P. Kramer (Eds.), *Evaluation: Obtaining and interpreting data.* Bethesda, MD: American Occupational Therapy Association.

Polgar, J. M. (1998). Critiquing assessments. In M. E. Neistadt & E. B. Crepeau (Eds.), *Willard & Spackman's occupational therapy* (9th ed., pp. 169–184). Philadelphia: Lippincott.

Stewart, K. B. (2001). Purposes, processes, and methods of evaluation. In J. Case-Smith, (Ed.), *Occupational therapy for children* (4th ed., pp. 190–213). St. Louis, MO: Mosby.

Weinstock-Zlotnik, G. & Hinojosa, J. (2004). Bottom-up or top-down evaluation: Is one better than the other? *American Journal of Occupational Therapy 58,* 594–599.

CHAPTER 11

Goal Writing

INTRODUCTION

Setting appropriate goals, ones that can be measured and are realistic, can help you demonstrate that you did indeed help your client. The trick is to set the goals so that the client can meet them. The goals cannot be so easy that they are not meaningful, yet not so hard that they cannot be accomplished in the time you have to work together. In other words, they have to represent a just-right challenge.

Goal writing is an essential step in both the evaluation and intervention process. Goals are often first established as part of the evaluation process, and then revised as part of the intervention process. Goals guide the direction of interventions. They help occupational therapy practitioners determine the effectiveness of their interventions. If a client is meeting goals, the intervention is likely to be appropriate. If a client is not meeting established goals, perhaps a different approach or intervention method should be tried.

▼ ROLE DELINEATION IN GOAL WRITING ▼

Goals are established in collaboration with the client, or if the client is unable to collaborate, the client's caregiver or guardian (American Occupational Therapy Association [AOTA], 2008). Primary responsibility for the development of intervention plans and goal setting rests with the occupational therapist; however, occupational therapy assistants may contribute to the process (AOTA, 2005). The *AOTA Occupational Therapy Standards of Practice* (2005) further states that "an occupational therapist has overall responsibility for the development, documentation, and implementation of the occupational therapy intervention based on the evaluation, client goals, current best evidence, and clinical reasoning" (AOTA, 2005, Standard III.1).

▼ GOAL DIRECTIONS ▼

The frame(s) of reference you used in determining your evaluation strategies is used to help you frame your goals (see Chapters 4 and 10). The type of setting in which you are working will impact the wording of the goals you write. In writing goal statements, there are a limited number of directions the goals can go. AOTA (2008), in *The Framework,* suggests the ultimate outcome of occupational therapy intervention is "supporting health and participation in life through engagement in occupation" (p. 626). To achieve that outcome, the intervention approaches that you can take with your client are geared toward assisting "the client in reaching a state of physical, mental, and social well-being; to identify and realize aspirations; to satisfy needs; and to change or cope with the environment" (p. 652). *The Framework* further presents the following intervention approaches: create or promote, establish or restore, maintain, modify, or prevent. These intervention approaches can be used to help determine the direction a goal will take. Moyers and Dale (2007), describe six kinds of outcomes: occupational performance, client satisfaction, role competence, adaptation, health and wellness, and quality of life. Based on a synthesis of these two documents, goal directions can be summarized as restorative, habilitative, maintenance, modification, preventive, and health promotion.

Restorative Goals

Restorative goals (rehabilitative or remediative) are used when you have a client who used to be able to do something, but now cannot (AOTA, 2008). This usually happens when there has been an illness or injury. Occupational therapy practitioners working in hospitals, rehabilitation facilities, nursing homes, outpatient clinics, home health, or psychiatric facilities typically write restorative goals. These goals are written to reflect a desired change in function.

Examples of restorative goals include:

- By discharge, client will feed herself three meals a day independently.
- By July 15, 2009, client will state three strengths about herself with no more than one prompt.
- The client will return to work as a carpenter, consistently using good body mechanics, by August 1, 2009.

Habilitative Goals

Goals that teach new skills are often called habilitative goals. Habilitation refers to teaching skills that the client never had, typically because of delayed development. This is different from rehabilitation, which seeks to restore a lost function or to help a client relearn a lost skill. Habilitative goals are often used with children whose development is delayed, or when teaching new skills to adults with developmental disabilities.

Examples of habilitative goals include:

- Eric will write his name legibly on all his school papers by June 10, 2009.
- Pahoa will consistently package the correct number of products, using adaptive jigs if needed, in the sheltered workshop by September 1, 2009.
- Emmalee will demonstrate increased mobility by independently moving from prone on the floor to standing by November 3, 2009.

Maintenance Goals

Maintenance goals seek to keep a client at his or her current level of function despite disease processes that normally would cause deterioration of function (AOTA, 2008). These goals would be written in long-term care or outpatient settings when a client has a progressive or deteriorating condition. Sometimes, maintenance goals are written when the client's condition is so complex that only someone with the specialized knowledge and skills of an occupational therapy practitioner can carry out the intervention. For example, a client with severe contractions may require occupational therapy intervention to open up the hand so that nursing can clean the client's palm and prevent skin breakdown.

One concern about maintenance goals is that many third-party payers will not pay for them. The payers often only want to pay as long as progress is being made. A maintenance goal may be seen as an indication that progress is no longer being made.

Examples of maintenance goals include:

- Client will maintain independence in dressing for the next 3 months.
- Client will actively participate in a current events group eight times in the next 30 days.
- For the next 6 months, client will continue to live in her own home with minimal assistance of home health aide.

Modification Goals

Modification goals (also called compensation or adaptation goals) seek to change the contexts or activity demands rather than change the skills and abilities of the client (AOTA, 2008). In other words, instead of increasing the strength and range of motion of an elderly client, address adapting the environment or tools used to complete the task. These goals are difficult to write in the sense that they can sound prescriptive and limiting. The trick is to be general enough to allow you to experiment and see what products work best, yet specific enough that you have some direction.

Examples of modification goals include:

- By August 12, 2009, Pyter will open boxes, cans, and bags with the use of adaptive equipment as needed so that he can independently prepare meals at home.
- By discharge, client's home will be modified to allow wheelchair access both inside and outside the house.
- In 3 months, the client will return to work with workplace modifications as needed to allow completion of essential functions of the job.

Preventive Goals

Preventive goals are written to assist persons who are at risk of developing occupational performance problems (AOTA, 2008). The person may or may not be completely healthy at the time the goal is written. A preventive goal may be written when the potential exists for a client to get hurt, such as through a repetitive motion injury or self-injurious behavior.

Examples of preventive goals include:

- By discharge, client will demonstrate proper body mechanics while lifting.
- By next session, Reed will list five strategies for removing himself from situations that tempt him to engage in the use of cocaine.
- By next week, Chenyse will identify three friends she can call for help when she begins to feel depressed or overwhelmed.

Health Promotion

Goals that relate to health promotion are written for clients who may not have a disability, but are more about enrichment or enhancement of occupational performance (AOTA, 2008). Health promotion goals may apply to an individual, group, community, or organization. In these settings, there is usually no attempt to correct a performance deficit; rather, the emphasis is on enhancing the contexts and activities to enable maximum participation in life (AOTA, 2008).

Examples of health promotion goals include:

- By the end of this class, parents will demonstrate minimal competency in infant massage.
- Playground surfaces will be replaced to provide a safer play environment for children by May 25, 2010.
- Within the next 3 months, create raised gardens at the community center so that wheelchair-bound gardeners can access their own garden plot.

▼ GOAL SPECIFICS ▼

Goals are also written for varying amounts of time. Long-term goals are overarching goals that guide the intervention to a definite conclusion. Often, long-term goals are the goals that, when met, will determine the time to discontinue therapy. Some facilities call them discharge goals. If a client is expected to receive services for more than one year, then the long-term goal might reflect the progress expected by the end of a year.

Short-term goals are written for specific periods of time, and change from time to time, leading up to the achievement of the long-term goal. In some settings, short-term goals are called objectives (Richardson & Shultz-Krohn, 2001). For example, if the long-term goal is to become independent in dressing, the first short-term goal might address dressing in clothes that have no fasteners, such as sweats. The next short-term goal might include zippers or Velcro. The next might include buttons, snaps, hooks, or ties. The last one might include outerwear (especially in cold climates) such as parkas, mittens, boots, hats, and scarves.

In acute care settings where clients are seen for a short time, the occupational therapy staff may not distinguish between short- and long-term goals. There are just goals. It is not necessary to separate goals by length of time when the occupational therapy practitioner is only going to work with the client for less than a month. Some facilities or programs may not separate long- and short-term goals if the clients are seen for 90 days or less, but some do, so be sure to find out what the facility's standard practice is before you start setting goals.

The way in which you refer to your client in the goal statement will vary by facility or program. In some facilities, the preferred phrase is "the client." In others, it is "the patient," "the resident," or "the participant." Some programs prefer that you use the client's first or last name. The best advice is to either ask your supervisor what his or her preference is, or read the goals written by others in the department.

There are several formats for writing goals, but all of them require the use of action words (verbs). Box 11.1 is a list of some verbs (there are more than those on this list, but these give you an idea) that can be used in goal writing. Of course, a lot depends on how you use the word. For example, when you use the verb *focus* in reference to vision rehab, you can see if the client is focusing on an object. If you use *focus* in reference to thought processes, can you see that?

BOX 11.1   Action Verbs

accomplishes	builds	creates	extends
accommodates	buttons	crochets	facilitates
achieves	buys	crushes	fastens
acquires	calculates	cuts	feeds
acts	calls	dances	finishes
adapts	changes	demonstrates	focuses
adheres	chooses	develops	folds
adjusts	chops	digs	follows
agrees	clasps	diminishes	gains
aligns	cleans	discriminates	gathers
allows	clears	discusses	gazes
applies	closes	displays	generalizes
approaches	collaborates	distributes	gets
arranges	collects	does	gives
asks	comes	doffs	grips
asserts	communicates	dons	grooms
assists	completes	draws	goes
attempts	complies	dresses	handles
attends	conforms	drinks	heeds
avoids	confronts	drives	identifies
bakes	connects	dries	improves
balances	contacts	eats	initiates
bathes	continues	employs	inquires
becomes	contributes	endures	irons
behaves	converses	engages	interacts
bends	cooperates	establishes	jumps
breathes	coordinates	explores	keeps
brushes	corrects	expresses	knits

(continued)

knots	prevents	rinses	stirs
labels	prints	rises	stitches
leads	prioritizes	rolls	stops
leaves	procures	rotates	straightens
lies	promotes	rows	strengthens
lifts	propels	rubs	stretches
lists	provides	runs	succeeds
listens	pulls	says	sucks
locates	punches	scrubs	supports
locks	purchases	secures	sustains
loosens	pursues	seeks	takes
maintains	pushes	selects	talks
makes	puts	sends	taps
manages	questions	sequences	tastes
masters	quits	serves	tends
meets	raises	sets	terminates
modulates	reaches	sews	throws
spreads	reads	shares	tightens
moves	rebuilds	shaves	toilets
obeys	records	shops	touches
obtains	reduces	shows	tracks
opens	reestablishes	showers	transfers
organizes	regards	shuts	transports
navigates	rehearses	signs	tries
notices	rejoins	simulates	types
paces	relates	sings	unwraps
paints	remarks	sits	uses
participates	reminds	skis	utilizes
pauses	removes	sleeps	verifies
pays	repairs	slides	vocalizes
pedals	repeats	snaps	volunteers
performs	requests	socializes	walks
picks	researches	solves	washes
places	responds	sorts	watches
plans	rests	speaks	wears
plays	restores	specifies	wipes
positions	resumes	stabilizes	withdraws
posts	returns	stands	works
practices	reverses	starts	wraps
prepares	reviews	states	writes
presses	revises	stays	zips

Source: Dictionnaire Jeans Anglais Français, Français Anglais (1982).

Verbs that are not action-oriented would rarely, if ever, be used in occupational therapy goals. These are listed in Box 11.2.

Except for maintenance goals, most goals need to describe change, and how that change will be measured. Box 11.3 shows examples of ways to measure change. However, depending on the unique wants, needs, and circumstances of each client, there are many other ways to document change as well. For example, attainment of health status, level of prevention of dysfunction, and client perception of life satisfaction, role performance, or quality of life may be measured qualitatively rather than quantitatively.

BOX 11.2   Verbs to Avoid

commits	feels	loves	resolves
considers	forgives	perceives	respects
contemplates	hears	prefers	sees
decides	imagines	processes	senses
desires	infers	realizes	smells
determines	interprets	recognizes	sympathizes
empathizes	knows	reflects	thinks
enjoys	learns	remembers	wants
expects	likes	represses	

Source: Dictionnaire Jeans Anglais Français, Français Anglais (1982).

BOX 11.3   Ways to Measure Change

Frequency or Consistency

- Percentage (number of successes divided by the number of opportunities for success)
- "x" out of "y" trials
- Consistently

Duration

- Time, such as number of seconds or minutes of sustained activity
- Number of repetitions

Assistance

- Maximum (75% or more of task)
- Moderate (50–74% of task)
- Minimum (25–49% of task)
- Standby
- Setup
- Adaptive equipment
- Verbal cuing/prompts
- Physical cuing
- Independently

Quality of Performance

- Number of errors
- Accuracy
- Amount of aberrant task behavior (i.e., tremors, off-task behavior)
- Amount of pain perceived by client
- Adherence to safety precautions

Level of Complexity

- Amount of instruction
- Number of steps in the process
- Cognitive level
- Multitasking

Participation (may require additional measure)

- Attend
- Engage
- Initiate
- Transition
- Interaction
- Adapt to environmental signals or social cues
- Obtain needed tools and equipment

Other (may require additional measure)

- Express feelings
- Specific task completion
- Variety of environments in which desired behavior will occur
- Level of cooperation
- Complete steps of a task

Source: Moyers & Dale (2007).

▼ FORMATS FOR GOAL WRITING ▼

There are many systems for formulating goals. In this chapter, I share four of these with you. I do not propose that any one system is better than the others; they are all just different. It is good to be familiar with more than one system, as you never know which system your supervisor will prefer.

ABCD

Kettenbach (2004) proposed the "ABCD" method: **A**udience, **B**ehavior, **C**ondition, and **D**egree. The *audience* represents the person who will do the behavior. The *behavior* is what the audience will do. The *condition* describes the circumstances around the behavior. The *degree* describes how well the behavior must be done to meet the goal.

Usually, the *audience* (or actor) is the client (Kettenbach, 2004). Since occupational therapy practice is client centered, this makes sense. Occasionally you might write a goal for a caregiver, but you should never write a goal for what you, the occupational therapist, will do (Kettenbach). What you plan to do, the methodology, belongs in the plan, not in the goal.

A *behavior* is usually something you can see or hear the person doing or saying. Examples of behaviors include reaching, dressing, carrying, demonstrating, expressing, eating, or crocheting. Behaviors represent an action and thus are stated as verbs (Kettenbach, 2004). However, not all verbs represent action. Refer to the word lists earlier in this chapter.

Conditions, circumstances that support the behavior, help to clarify the goal (Kettenbach, 2004). Conditions can represent something in the environment that is necessary for the behavior to occur (Richardson & Schultz-Krohn, 2001). For example, in the goal "The client will independently dress herself in clothes that have no fasteners," *clothes that have no fasteners* is the condition. The client needs access to clothes that do not have fasteners (elastic-waist pants, pull-over tops) in order to meet the goal. Conditions can also be the amount of cuing or assistance needed.

The *degree* is the measurable part of the goal (Kettenbach, 2004). It tells the reader how many, what percent, what degree, or other distinguishing characteristic of the behavior. The degree has to be realistic, functional, and identify a specific time frame. Realistic means that you can reasonably expect the client to achieve the goal in the time frame you establish. Functional means the goal describes an area of occupational performance. The time frame is when you realistically expect the goal to be met. This is dependent on the condition of the client, the frequency and duration of occupational therapy, and your professional knowledge and experience with similar types of clients.

A variation of the ABCD format is ABCDE, which is advocated by Quinn and Gordon (2003). They use the same audience, behavior, condition, and degree as does Kettenbach (2004). The "E" stands for **E**xpected time. The expected time part of a goal is an estimate of the length of time it will take to meet the goal, for example, within a week or within a month (Quinn & Gordon).

Exercise 11.1

Identify the parts of the goal that correspond to the letters ABCD:

1. The client will prepare a complete meal (meat, vegetable, starch, and beverage) independently on three consecutive days. *(Client has osteoarthritis and diabetic neuropathy in her upper extremities.)*

   A:

   B:

   C:

   D:

2. The patient will bathe herself using adaptive equipment, if needed, in less than 15 minutes. *(Client has a right hemiparesis.)*

   A:

   B:

   C:

   D:

3. Bobby will independently retrieve the tools necessary to complete his project in three of the next five sessions. *(Client has chronic schizophrenia and is seen in a day program.)*

   A:

   B:

   C:

   D:

FEAST

Another system for writing goals is FEAST by Borcherding (2005) (see also Borcherding & Kappel, 2002). As with the ABCD method, each letter of the word *FEAST* represents a component of the goal.

F stands for *function*. Functions are the areas of occupational performance that the client hopes to improve or maintain—the focus of the goal. Examples of functions include dressing, eating, shopping, knitting, or navigating the neighborhood.

E stands for *expectation*. In conjunction with the client, you establish what the client will do. Phrases like "the client will" make the expectation clear.

A is for *action*. Actions are expressed as verbs and are often part of the function being addressed, so they may not be a separate part of the goal statement. Examples of action words (verbs) include make, do, reach, carry, write, lift, transfer, and demonstrate.

S stands for *specific conditions*. These are essentially the same as the C in the ABCD model. They identify the level of assistance or other conditions that are necessary for the client to meet the goal. For example, whether the client engages in the activity while sitting or standing, whether the client does it with help or independently, or which body parts will be involved. There may be more than one specific condition listed in the goal.

Finally, the T stands for *timeline*. Good goals give some indication of when you think the goal will be accomplished. This could be stated in terms of the number of intervention sessions, number of weeks, or a specific date.

Exercise 11.2

Identify the parts of the goal that correspond to the letters FEAST:

1. Client will demonstrate safe use of a sharp knife without cuing on three consecutive occupational therapy sessions by June 1, 2009. *(Client had a traumatic brain injury.)*

   F:

   E:

   A:

   S:

   T:

2. Student will consistently write his name with each letter correctly formed by June 15, 2009. *(Client is an 8-year-old child with mental retardation.)*

   F:

   E:

   A:

   S:

   T:

3. Client will retrieve her mail from the mailbox at the end of her driveway on three consecutive days by 4-17-10. *(Client is a middle-aged woman with agoraphobia.)*

   F:

   E:

   A:

   S:

   T:

RHUMBA (Rumba)

A third method for writing goals is RHUMBA (College of St. Catherine [CSC], 2001) or RUMBA (McClain, 1991; Perinchief, 1998). According to Perinchief (1998), the American Occupational Therapy Association (AOTA) developed RUMBA in the 1970s. A *rhumba* (also spelled *rumba*) is an Afro-Cuban folk dance that is especially rhythmic (*The New Encyclopedia Britannica*, 1985). In goal setting, the client represents the music, the goals must "dance" to the client's tune, and each of the parts of the goal must "rhumba" with each other (CSC, 2001). As with the other systems for goal writing, each letter in the word "rhumba" stands for something.

Relevant/**R**elates: *The goal/outcome must relate to something, be relevant.*
How Long: *Specify when the goal/outcome will be met.*
Understandable: *Anyone reading it must know what it means.*
Measurable: *There must be a way to know when the goal is met.*
Behavioral: *The goal/outcome must be something that is seen or heard.*
Achievable: *It must be realistic and doable.* (CSC, 2001, p. 1).

Let's examine each of these in more detail.

The "R" can stand for **relevant** (McClain, 1991; Perinchief, 1998). If a goal is relevant, it answers the question "So what?" Does achieving this goal really matter? Will it make a difference in the client's life? Think about what matters more, that the client can bend her elbow 40° farther or that she can now feed herself? Here are some examples of meaningless goals adapted from CSC's *Goal Writing: Documenting Outcomes* (2001):

1. I will take 94E to 90S, averaging 70 mph and 30 mpg, on Saturday, driving for approximately 7 hours, in my red '02 MX6, by myself, taking enough luggage for 3 days and food for the trip, stopping no more than 3 times.

   So what? What is the point of all of this? Where are you going? Is how you do it more important than getting there? What needs to be stated is the expected outcome, not the method for getting there.

2. Patient will count coins of varying denominations and combinations of up to $.77 with 65% accuracy on 3 of 5 tries each day for 7 of 10 days within 30 days.

   So what? How will this make a significant difference in a client's life? What happens if the patient counts $.77 with 60% accuracy on 4 of 5 tries for 6 of the next 10 days? Is the goal met? Will the next goal be $.78? How will you keep track of all this data? I do not understand this goal; it is too complicated.

The "R" can also mean *relates* (CSC, 2001). The long- and short-term goals must relate to an area of occupation (keep it functional); they must relate to each other, and they must relate to identified wants and needs of the client (the client's music) (CSC, 2001). In other words there must be a clear relationship between the areas of occupation identified during the evaluation process as being in need of intervention, the goal statements themselves, and the intervention strategies used to help meet the goals. For example, if in your evaluation you determine that the client needs to learn to hold a crayon using a three-point grasp, then the goals need to say something about holding a crayon, and the intervention needs to involve crayons. It would be inappropriate to identify the need to hold a crayon, set a goal to improve hand use (too vague), and then suggest intervention strategies using jungle gyms, large balls, and finger painting.

How long is a realistic estimate of the time you expect it will take to reach the goal (CSC, 2001). For long-term goals, it usually means when the client will be discontinued, which may be a specific date or an estimate such as 6 months or a year. For short-term goals, it could be a number of visits, a specific date, or, if you write a new intervention plan, every 30 days, you can assume the short-term goals are meant to be met in 30 days. Since how you state the time frame will vary by the setting in which you are working, always check with your supervisor to see what the standard is in that setting. I have seen some goals that simply state that a client will do something on 3 consecutive days, and then the goal will be met. Well, that is not really putting a time limit on a goal. The client could do the task on 3 consecutive days next week, or 6 months from now. If I am paying for occupational therapy services, I want to know whether to expect the client to meet the goal in 2 weeks or 2 months. If a client needs to do something 3 days in a row, that may be OK as a measurement, but it does not tell me when to expect the goal to be met.

Understandable involves several dimensions. In order for the reader to understand the goal, it first has to be legible (McClain, 1991; Perinchief, 1998). Then it has to make sense to the reader, which means using easily understood, grammatically correct, accurately spelled language free from jargon and using only acceptable abbreviations. Use an active voice rather than a passive voice. This means you say that the client will do something rather than that something will be done; that is, "The client will change her socks," rather than "The socks will be changed by the client." Again, check a grammar guide for more information on active voice. Finally, consider avoiding noncommittal language. Examples of noncommittal language include phrases like "will appear" or "will be able to."

You want the client to do something, not just look like she can do it. There is a difference between actually doing something and being able to do something. If you say the client will be able to feed himself, it does not necessarily mean he will do it. Maybe the nurse does it for him, even though he could do it if they let him. If you say the client will feed himself, it means he will do it himself. The goal has to be so clearly stated that anyone stepping in for you if you are sick will know, beyond a shadow of a doubt, what your plan was for providing services to a client.

If you look at the two goals on page 117 you will see that, in addition to not being relevant, they are also not understandable. The goals contain so many clauses and conditions that it is impossible to know what the focus of the goal really is. I can't even tell how to measure the second example.

Measurable is usually expressed as a quantitative statement that identifies how you will know when the goal is met (CSC, 2001). A goal is not met just because the time frame has elapsed. There has to be a measurement of function. You can measure progress as well as maintenance of function. Examples of measurements include frequency, accuracy, level of efficiency, consistency, grade, degree, speed, level of independence, or duration (CSC; McClain, 1991; Perinchief, 1998).

The *behavioral* component is the same as it was in the ABCD system. The behavior has to be observed, not inferred. It can be reflected as an action verb (see lists earlier in the chapter). By observed, I mean something you can see the client do or hear the client say (Perinchief, 1998). Since you cannot see or hear how a client feels or knows something, these would not be behaviors you would include in goal statements. You can hear a client express his feelings, but you can never be completely sure that because someone says he feels something he actually feels it. You can see if a client can demonstrate a behavior, but that may or may not mean she understands it.

Achievable means that the goal is reasonable and likely to be met in the time frame established (CSC, 2001; McClain, 1991; Perinchief, 1998). It is reasonable given the condition of the client, the frequency and duration of projected occupational therapy sessions, and the contexts of the client and the environment. It is not overly ambitious or too easy.

Exercise 11.3

Identify the parts of the goal that correspond to the letters RHUMBA:

1. By January 2, 2010, the client will accurately cut and paste eight individual letters using the mouse with his left hand in 5 minutes or less. *(Client had a stroke affecting his dominant*

(right) hand and wants to become proficient at using a mouse with his nondominant (left) hand.)

R:

H:

U:

M:

B:

A: *You do not have enough information to answer this, but I assure you it is achievable.*

2. By June 26, 2009, the client will consistently catch himself each time he begins to make self-defeating/self-derogatory statements. *(Client is experiencing major depression and has committed himself to an inpatient psychiatric program following a failed suicide attempt.)*

R:

H:

U:

M:

B:

A: *You do not have enough information to answer this, but it seems achievable.*

3. By the end of the year, Kylie will independently maintain a sitting position without support for 10 minutes, so that she can participate more actively in the world around her. *(Client is a 9-month-old near-SIDS baby seen in her home.)*

R:

H:

U:

M:

B:

A: *You do not have enough information to answer this, but it is achievable.*

SMART

The last system for goal writing is writing SMART goals. There are many versions of SMART goals as well. Angier (1995) says SMART goals mean goals that are specific, measurable, action-oriented, realistic, and timely. The University of Victoria Counseling Services (1996) uses SMART as an acronym for specific, measurable, acceptable, realistic, and time frame. Paul J. Meyer (2002) describes SMART as standing for specific, measurable, attainable, realistic, and tangible. In this book, SMART stands for significant (and simple), measurable, achievable, related, and time-limited.

Significant means that achieving this goal will make a significant difference in this person's life. This implies that you know your client's strengths and need areas so well that you know what will matter most to her (or him); in fact, your goals would ideally be developed in collaboration with her (or him), ensuring significance. By remembering to keep it simple you are more likely to achieve the goal, and it will be easier to understand.

Measurable, as in RHUMBA, means that you have a clear target to aim for, and that you will know when the client gets there (CSC, 2001). The client will dress herself with no more than one verbal cue. The client will feed himself a whole meal in less than 30 minutes. Timothy will check his daily schedule every hour. These are incomplete goals, but I mention them here to emphasize the measurement component of goal writing. One common error I have seen in goal writing is goals that say the client will improve at something without stating how big the improvement must be. For example, the client will improve her accuracy at measuring dry ingredients. How much improvement is enough to say that goal was met?

Achievable also has the same meaning as it does in RHUMBA. It must be reasonable that the client could achieve this goal in the time allotted for it (CSC, 2001). Realistically, not every client will achieve every goal. When you first start out writing goals, you may have to guess a little at how much the client can achieve in your time frame. As you gain experience, your guesses will become more accurate.

Related, in SMART as in RHUMBA, means that the goal clearly has a connection to the client's occupational needs as stated in the evaluation report (CSC, 2001). Long- and short-term goals relate to each other.

Finally, *time-limited* means the goal has a chronological end point (CSC, 2001). You know when to evaluate whether the goal is met. If the long-term goal is met, then it is time to discontinue services. If the short-term goal is met, then it is time to set a new short-term goal that gets the client closer to the long-term goal. If the short-term goal is not met at the designated time, then perhaps that goal needs to be either modified or continued.

Exercise 11.4

Identify the parts of the goal that correspond to the letters SMART:

1. By next week, client will demonstrate proper lifting techniques on 80% of opportunities for lifting boxes weighing 10 lbs. or more. *(Client had a back injury and is now being seen in a work-hardening program.)*

   S:

   M:

   A: *Seems achievable given what we know.*

   R:

   T:

2. By April 22, 2010, Nellie will feed herself with a fork or spoon, spilling two or fewer times per meal. *(Nellie is in a long-term care facility with diagnoses of rheumatoid arthritis, COPD, and macular degeneration.)*

   S:

   M:

   A: *I think it is achievable in the time frame given.*

R:

T:

3. Mandy will cut out basic shapes with scissors within 1/4" of the line consistently by the end of the school year. *(Mandy is in first grade and has fine motor deficits that make her stand out from her classmates.)*

S:

M:

A: *It is achievable.*

R:

T:

Exercise 11.5

Write a goal statement for the following cases using the format listed.

1. **ABCD:** This client has recently had tendon transfer surgery on his dominant hand. The surgeon wants you to make a splint and teach the client how to don and doff the splint. The hand will be immobilized for a week.

2. **FEAST:** This client was admitted yesterday after an episode of mania in which she got little sleep, shopped till she dropped, and then engaged in wild parties involving sex, drugs, and rock 'n' roll. She is loud, often saying and doing things that embarrass other clients, and is in constant motion. Her husband admitted her to get her back on an appropriate medication routine.

3. **RHUMBA:** This client is 6 years old. She has cerebral palsy. She is in occupational therapy to learn to use a new electric wheelchair.

4. **SMART:** This client was badly burned in a house fire. She has had numerous skin grafts. She is past the extreme pain phase, and now rates her pain level as very bad. In occupational therapy, she is working on increasing her reach and grasp with both arms while wearing compression garments.

5. **ABCDE:** This elderly client was recently discharged from the hospital following surgery to remove a brain tumor. She is being seen in her home to increase her endurance and begin to do her own self-cares.

6. **FEAST:** This homeless man needs to work on skills related to budgeting. He has a full-time minimum wage job.

7. **RHUMBA:** This man has schizophrenia and lives in a group home in the community. He is receiving occupational therapy at a sheltered workshop for organizing his work space and staying on task.

8. **SMART:** This 4-year-old child was recently diagnosed with autism. He will only wear soft clothes, avoids certain textures of food, bumps into objects and people, and bites his wrist when he becomes excited.

Exercise 11.6

What is wrong with each goal? Tell which criteria you used to answer this question (ABCD, FEAST, RHUMBA, or SMART).

1. Tiffany will be evaluated for a new wheelchair within the next 30 days.

2. By next week, Dylan will feed himself with minimal assist, 3x/d, for 50% of the meal, using adaptive utensils, with extra time allowed, and a pureed diet.

3. Darnell will complete his resume and send it to 3 potential employers.

4. Hector will bring his memory book to therapy every day for the next week.

5. Hui will express satisfaction with the quality of her work at least 3 times.

SUMMARY

Goal writing is tricky business. You have to think about what the client wants or needs, what is a reasonable amount of time needed to meet the goal, how you will measure it, and assorted other conditions, depending on the format you use for goal writing. Four separate formats for goal writing were presented: ABCD, FEAST, RHUMBA, and SMART. While there are subtle differences between them, they all result in well-written goals.

Goal writing is a collaborative process involving the occupational therapist and the client or client's surrogate (i.e., parent or guardian). An occupational therapy assistant contributes to this process.

Goals are written to help a client improve occupational performance, learn to do a new task, maintain function, modify or adapt contexts to enable performance, prevent occupational performance problems, or promote health (AOTA, 2008). The verbs used to show theaction of the goal will vary by the direction of the goal, but all verbs used should be active rather than passive in nature. Word selection is also important in describing change and the measurement of change.

The ultimate goal in occupational therapy is "*supporting health and participation in life through engagement in occupation*" (AOTA, 2008, p. 626). For each client, the occupations the client wants or needs to engage in will be different. Long-term goals are written to describe the final outcome of occupational therapy intervention and are sometimes called discharge or discontinuation goals. Short-term goals are usually written for a specific period of time, often monthly, but may be written for a week, biweekly, or bimonthly. Long-term goals generally stay the same throughout occupational therapy service delivery, unless the client's life circumstances change. Short-term goals change or are revised often.

Goal writing is an essential part of both the evaluation and intervention processes. Goals give you a yardstick by which you can measure the effectiveness of the intervention approaches and methods used with a given client.

REFERENCES

American Occupational Therapy Association. (2005). Occupational therapy standards of practice. *American Journal of Occupational Therapy, 59*, 663–665.

American Occupational Therapy Association. (2008). Occupational therapy practice framework: Domain and process. *American Journal of Occupational Therapy, 62*, 626–683.

Angier, M. (1995). *Setting S-M-A-R-T goals.* Retrieved December 20, 2002, from http://www.positiveath.net/ideasMA20_p.htm

Borcherding, S. (2005). *Documentation manual for writing SOAP notes in occupational therapy,* 2nd ed. Thorofare, NJ: Slack.

Borcherding, S., & Kappel C. (2002). The OTA's guide is writing SOAP notes. Thorofare, NJ: Slack.

College of St. Catherine. (2001). *Goal writing: Documenting outcomes* [Handout]. St. Paul, MN: Author.

Jeans Anglais Français, Français Anglais. (1982). Dictionnaire. Berlin and Munich: Langenscheidt.

Kettenbach, G. (2004). *Writing S.O.A.P. notes,* 3rd ed. Philadelphia: F. A. Davis.

McClain, L. H. (1991). Documentation. In W. Dunn (Ed.), *Pediatric occupational therapy* (pp. 213–244). Thorofare, NJ: Slack.

Meyer, P. J. (2002). *Creating S.M.A.R.T goals.* Retrieved December 20, 2002, from http://achievement.com/smart.html

Moyers, P. A., & Dale, L. M. (2007). *The guide to occupational therapy practice,* 2nd ed. Bethesda, MD: American Occupational Therapy Association.

Perinchief, J. M. (1998). Management of occupational therapy services. In M. E. Neistadt & E. B. Crepeau (Eds.), *Willard and Spackman's occupational therapy* (9th ed., pp. 772–790). Philadelphia: Lippincott.

Quinn, L. & Gordon, J. (2003). *Functional outcomes: Documentation for rehabilitation.* St. Louis, MO: Elsevier.

Richardson, P. K., & Schultz-Krohn, W. (2001). Planning and implementing services. In J. Case-Smith (Ed.), *Occupational therapy for children* (4th ed., pp. 246–264). St. Louis, MO: Mosby.

University of Victoria Counseling Services. (1996). *Learning skills program: Smart goals.* Retrieved December 20, 2002, from http://www.coun.uvic.ca/learn/program/hndouts/smartgoals.html

CHAPTER 12

Intervention Plans

INTRODUCTION

The intervention plan is where the occupational therapist articulates the expected outcomes and how they will be achieved. It is based on the results of the evaluation and the wants and needs of the client or surrogate (i.e., parent or guardian) (American Occupation Therapy Association [AOTA], 2005a). The development and revision of the intervention plan are a collaborative effort between the occupational therapist, the occupational therapy assistant, and the client (AOTA, 2005a). Medicare uses the term *plan of care* rather than intervention plan (Centers for Medicare and Medicaid Services [CMS], 2008). You may also hear the terms *care plan, treatment plan,* or *plan of treatment* used interchangeably with intervention plan. Regardless of what you call it, the intervention plan tells the occupational therapy practitioners what they are going to do to help the client.

Establishing goals and determining intervention strategies that will be effective, and that third-party payers will pay for, is critical to the ongoing viability of your practice in occupational therapy. If you do not get paid for what you do, you will not be able to make a living at being an occupational therapy practitioner. To be paid for your services, you have to show that the intervention made a difference in your client's life. That is what motivates us to become occupational therapy professionals in the first place—we want to help make people's lives better.

▼ ROLE DELINEATION IN INTERVENTION PLANNING ▼

The occupational therapist is responsible for developing and documenting the intervention plan, and complying with the time frames, formats, and standards required by the facility/agency, accrediting bodies, and payers (AOTA, 2005a). An occupational therapy assistant under the supervision of an occupational therapist may contribute to the intervention plan. The intervention plan includes the frequency, scope, and duration of occupational therapy services. The occupational therapist or occupational therapy assistant under the supervision of the occupational therapist reviews the intervention plan, the rationale for the plan, and the risks and benefits of the plan with the client and appropriate others (AOTA, 2005a). When necessary, the occupational therapist revises the plan of care and documents the revised goals, changes in the client's condition or situation, and the client's performance; the occupational therapy assistant may contribute to the revised intervention plan (AOTA, 2005a).

The intervention planning process makes the client an active partner in the process. As in the evaluation process, it is client-centered. It also requires close interaction between the occupational therapist and the occupational therapy assistant. In some settings, the occupational therapy assistant is the professional who is at the facility day in and day out, while the occupational therapist makes periodic supervision visits to the facility to conduct evaluations, develop and revise intervention plans, and prepare discontinuation (discharge) plans and summaries. This is most likely to occur in settings where the clients are fairly stable, and the occupational therapy assistant is experienced and has demonstrated service competence in a wide variety of clinical skills. In situations like this, the occupational therapy assistant has more regular contact with the clients and can provide extremely valuable input to the occupational therapist regarding the skills and abilities of the client as they relate to occupational performance.

▼ MEDICARE COMPLIANCE ▼

Medicare requires that all services are delivered under a plan of care (CMS, 2008). In addition, Medicare requires certification and recertification of the need for treatment by a physician or nonphysician practitioner (NPP). An NPP is a physician assistant, clinical nurse specialist, or nurse practitioner who is authorized by state law to certify or supervise therapy services. Medicare does not allow chiropractors or dentists to order, certify, recertify, or supervise therapy (CMS).

The plan of care must be established before any occupational therapy services can be provided (CMS, 2008, AOTA, 2008b). The word *established* implies that it is written or dictated by either a physician or NPP, or the occupational therapist who will provide the services. Medicare allows the interventions to begin before the plan is written only if the occupational therapist who established the plan is providing or supervising the occupational therapy interventions. This means that the evaluation and initial intervention can occur on the same day (CMS). As stated earlier in this book, the closer to the actual event (evaluation or intervention) that the documentation of it occurs, the more accurate and trustworthy it will be. In other words, even though Medicare allows interventions to begin before the plan is written, it is crucial to get the plan in writing as soon as possible.

According to Medicare, the plan of care needs to include at least the client's diagnoses; long-term treatment goals; and the type, amount, duration, and frequency of the occupational therapy services (CMS, 2008). The plan needs to reflect the results of the evaluation. Medicare wants the plan to be the most efficient and effective means of treating the client's needs. Occupational therapy is considered reasonable and necessary when it is expected that the therapy will result in significant improvement in the patient's level of function within a reasonable time (AOTA, 2008b). The long-term goals are written for the entire episode of care (number of calendar days from the start of care to the end of care) in that setting. Unless otherwise specified in the plan of care, Medicare assumes that interventions will be provided one time per day (CMS).

Optional, but recommended elements of a Medicare plan of care include short-term goals and specific treatment interventions, procedures, modalities, or techniques (CMS, 2008). Brennan and Robinson (2006) stress that these should always be included because they show why the specialized skills of an occupational therapist or occupational therapy assistant under the supervision of an occupational therapist are needed.

Certification and recertification indicate that the client is under the care of a physician or NPP, and that the physician or NPP approves the plan of care (CMS, 2008). A physician or NPP must certify the occupational therapy plan of care in order for Medicare to pay for the occupational therapy services delivered to a specific client. The certification/recertification occurs when the physician or NPP signs the plan of care, writes a physician's progress note or orders occupational therapy interventions. After initial physician or NPP certification, a recertification is required at least every 90 days, or sooner if there is a need to change the plan of care (CMS).

Brennan & Robinson (2006) identify common pitfalls in documenting the plan of care that could lead to payment denials by Medicare. If the intervention does not have a sufficient level of complexity to justify the intervention by an occupational therapy practitioner, payment can be denied for the services provided. Medicare expects that the intervention plan will change to reflect changes in the client's level of function; if the plan does not change or the client's level of function does not change, that could be grounds for a Medicare denial of coverage. The outcome goals have to be based on some kind of baseline measure; failure to do so could result in a Medicare denial. Finally, while standardized test scores are helpful in determining outcomes, outcomes tied to a specific test score are meaningless because a test score is not the same as functional performance in an area of occupation (Brennan & Robinson).

In each publication, find the information that pertains to the documentation of the delivery of occupational therapy services. What limits does Medicare set?

▼ CONCEPTS FOR INTERVENTION PLANNING ▼

To help your client make progress toward his or her desired outcomes, you must select intervention strategies that will lead your client in the same direction as the mutually agreed-upon goal(s). This requires knowledge of both the skills and abilities of your client and the qualities of the activities (occupations) so that there is a match between what the activity has to offer and what the client needs. For example, if a client has difficulty with problem solving, you need an activity that requires some problem solving, but at a level that is just a bit above where the client is currently functioning. In this case, perhaps problems that require abstract thought, such as story problems in math or exercises of the "2-minute mysteries" type, would be too hard. Instead, an activity that involves real-life situations with rules to follow, such as getting from one place to another within the building or using a substitutions list at the back of a cookbook, would be a better place to start.

An intervention plan is not engraved in stone; it is subject to change as the client's condition and contexts change. If the occupational therapist believes that a change in the goals or intervention strategies, including the frequency, intensity, or duration of intervention sessions, is needed, he or she writes up a new intervention plan. If the client is a Medicare Part B (outpatient) recipient, the Medicare forms require a physician signature every 90 days, so changing the frequency or duration on that form carries the weight of a doctor's order (CMS, 2008). Factors to consider when changing the frequency or duration include the client's potential to benefit from services, the degree of dysfunction, outcomes research on clients with similar conditions and interventions, potential for caregiver follow-through, and possible complications that could change the client's rate of progress (Moyers & Dale, 2007).

Intervention plans are established as soon as the occupational therapist determines that the client needs intervention and may be reviewed every 30 days, 60 days, quarterly, or semiannually (twice a year), depending on the setting, the needs of the client, and the demands of the payer.

The intervention plan must consider not only the client's goals, skills, abilities, and deficits, but also the client's values, beliefs, current and desired state of health and well-being, contexts and environments of the client and the setting in which the intervention will occur, and activity demands (AOTA, 2008a). In addition, the occupational therapist must use the best available evidence in determining the best course of action for the interventions.

▼ PARTS OF AN INTERVENTION PLAN ▼

The BiFIP format that was used in Chapter 10 can also be used to format an intervention plan. The background information, findings, interpretation, and plan sections may contain similar, yet different, content from an evaluation report.

The first intervention plan you write for any one client might be part of the evaluation report, or it may be a stand-alone document, depending on the policies of the facility at which you work. If it is part of the evaluation report, then there is no need to repeat identification/ background information. However, if it is a stand-alone document, then you will need to include the same kind of identification information that you included on your evaluation report (AOTA, 2007):

- Client name, gender, and date of birth
- Date of the document (may be part of the signature) and the type of document; name of agency/facility and department
- Intervention diagnosis/condition and other diagnoses/conditions
- Precautions and contraindications

An electronic health record system may automatically insert this information once the client's name or client ID number is entered.

The next section of an ongoing intervention plan is findings. On an intervention plan the findings section is for reporting a brief summary of progress since the last intervention plan was written, within the client's current context. Then describe progress or lack thereof using the language of the *Occupational Therapy Practice Framework* (AOTA, 2008a), addressing the client's performance in areas of occupation, and the performance patterns and skills, contexts, client factors, and activity demands that impact the client's occupational performance. Remember that in this section, you are reporting data, not interpreting it.

There is a difference between reporting on the current status of a client and reporting the progress made by that client (McQuire, 1997). According to McQuire, a status report tells what a person can do now with no comparison to prior performance, while a progress report contains some comparative statements. If you want to convince a payer or a referral source that you have provided a worthwhile service, you must choose your words carefully so they show progress. (There will be more information on this in the next section of this chapter.)

The third section of an intervention plan is for recording your interpretation of the findings. This is where you record any barriers or challenges to attaining the short- and long-term goals, and identify the client's current strengths and supports.

The fourth section of the intervention plan is for spelling out what you hope to accomplish in the next review period, adjustments to the short-term goals, intervention strategies, or the duration, frequency, and intensity of intervention sessions can be made. AOTA (2007) specifically states that the short-term goals must be "related to the client's ability and need to engage in desired occupations" (p. 4).

Along with revising goals, you must determine appropriate intervention strategies and methods given the client's current condition and contexts (AOTA, 2007). For example, you will determine if a particular client is a good candidate for using adaptive equipment, or whether teaching the client an adaptive technique would be better. In the course of your occupational therapy education, you will learn many strategies for interventions.

AOTA (2007, 2008a) distinguishes between intervention approaches and types of intervention. The intervention approaches are (AOTA, 2007, 2008a):

- Create or promote
- Establish or restore
- Maintain
- Modify
- Prevent

Types of intervention are the "consultation process, education process, advocacy, therapeutic use of occupations or activities, and therapeutic use of self" (AOTA, 2007, p. 3).

The people reading your intervention plans (other facility staff, physicians, third-party payers, quality management personnel, lawyers, etc.) must be able to see the logical thinking that went into your plan. They have to see that if you set a long-term goal to improve someone's dressing skills, then the short-term goals and methods of intervention must also directly relate to dressing. Not everyone who reads your intervention plan will understand the link between improving dexterity and improving dressing, so if your intervention plan calls for stringing 14-inch beads, it will not make logical sense. If, however, your intervention plan calls for learning to don and doff certain articles of clothing with certain types of fasteners, it will make logical sense. (More about this later in this chapter.)

AOTA (2007) also requires that the service delivery mechanisms and plan for discharge be included in this section. Service delivery mechanisms include such details as who will provide the services, where the services will be provided, and the frequency and duration of services. The plan for discharge includes criteria for discontinuing occupational therapy services, discharge disposition (where the client will be discharged to), and the need for follow-up care.

The last part of the plan section is the outcome statement. In the outcome statement, you state the desired outcome of occupational therapy. Examples of outcomes include (AOTA, 2007, p. 3):

- improved occupational performance
- adaptation
- role competence
- improved health and wellness
- prevention of further difficulties
- improved quality of life
- self-advocacy
- occupational justice

The last part of the intervention plan is for signatures. Every intervention plan needs to be signed by an occupational therapist. The *AOTA Guidelines for Documentation of Occupational Therapy Practice* (2007) suggests including the name and position of each person responsible for overseeing the implementation of the plan. Each time you sign a document, always include the date it was written in the signature line.

▼ SUMMARIZING PROGRESS ▼

Generally, you will write an intervention plan for a client every 30–90 days. Between intervention plan revisions, you will write progress notes (see Chapter 13). On your initial intervention plan, you will not be able to summarize progress, but on subsequent intervention plans you will. It is helpful to go back over the progress notes written over the last month (or whatever the interval between plans is in your setting) while you summarize changes since the last intervention plan was written.

It is important to give the reader an accurate picture of progress. Inaccurately reporting progress so that it appears faster or slower than reality is fraud (see Chapter 7). Do not do it. As stated in the AOTA *Code of Ethics*, "Occupational therapy personnel shall refrain from using or participating in the use of any form of communication that contains false, fraudulent, deceptive, or unfair statements or claims" (2005b, Principle 6.C). It is further elaborated in the AOTA *Guidelines to the Code of Ethics*, "All documentation must accurately reflect the nature and quantity of services provided" (AOTA, 2006, 1.5) and, even more explicitly, "Occupational therapy personnel do not fabricate data, falsify information, or plagiarize" (2006, 2.8).

So how do you describe progress accurately? Choose your words carefully. Understand how others interpret words. Some words are "loaded," that is, some readers will twist them in ways you never intended (see Chapter 2). When you write, "Continues to have difficulty with _____," a payer might interpret it as "not making progress." In reality, the client has made progress, but not as fast as you had hoped. Think about the difference between these words:

Attends	Participates
Understands	Complies or demonstrates
Approachable	Sociable

In each of these pairs, the word on the right is more active. If you write that a client attended occupational therapy sessions, a reader could interpret that as the client came into the room, but did not do anything. If you write that the client participated in the occupational therapy session, it does imply that the client engaged in the process. Someone can nod and say she understands, but unless you see them do it, are you sure she can do it? *Approachable* implies that you can go up to this person and initiate conversation. *Sociable* implies that this person is equally comfortable approaching others and being approached by others. Box 12.1 contains a list of words that convey progress or change.

When you summarize progress over time, the focus needs to be on function. Describe the new occupations the client does now that he or she could not do last month (or whatever your time frame is). The World Health Organization's ICF document (see Chapter 3) contains a comprehensive list of activities that might be helpful to you as you think about function (WHO, 2002). Focusing on function means making sure you address what the client does, not the underlying skills and abilities. For example, if a client is now able to reach to the top shelf in

---

BOX 12.1   Descriptive Words for Progress Notes

Describing Physical Behavior		Describing Social Behavior	
Adapts	Hesitantly	Acceptable	Curious
Against gravity	Holds	Adapts	Decides
Assistance	Imitates	Aggressive	Demanding
Athetoid	Inconsistent	Agitated	Demands
Awkward	Independent	Alert	Demonstrates
Barely	Jerky/jerkily	Angry	Dependable
Bouncy	Less	Antagonistic	Destructive
Careful	Limits	Anxious	Diligent
Clumsy	Maintains	Apathetic	Distractible
Compensate	Minimum	Approachable	Drowsy
Complains	Mildly	Appropriate	Easily upset
Completely	Moderate	Argumentative	Elated
Consistent	Modifies	Argues	Empathetic
Coordinated	More	Asks	Encouraging
Crooked	Precise	Attentive	Engaging
Creates	Rapid	Aware	Enjoys
Crepitus	Regressed	Behaves	Enthusiastic
Delayed	Rigid	Boisterous	Establishes
Deliberately	Roughly	Bored	Euphoric
Dependent	Shaky	Careful	Evasive
Difficulty	Slow	Changeable	Even disposition
Easily	Smoothly	Cheerful	Excessive
Effort	Softly	Childish	Excitable
Effortless	Spastic	Complacent	Explores
Endurance	Steady	Complains	Explodes
Energetically	Stimulating	Complies	Expresses
Even	Strength	Confident	Fearful
Exertion	Swiftly	Confused	Flat affect
Gently	Tentative	Consistent	Flexible
Gracefully	Thoroughly	Contributes	Flexibility
Guarded	Tires	Consults	Follows
Haphazardly	Uneven	Converses	Friendly
Heavily	Violently	Cooperative	Fussy
	Withdraws		Gathers
	With ease		Giddy
	Writhe		Guarded

(continued)

Hostile
Hyperactive
Immature
Impolite
Impulsive
Inappropriate
  touching
Inappropriate
  laughter
Inattentive
Incessantly
Inconsistent
Initiates
Intrusive
Involved
Irritable
Lethargic
Limits
Listens
Manipulative
Moody
Narcissistic
Observes
Obsessive
Overdependent
Pacing
Passive–
  aggressive
Permissive
Pleasant
Polite
Preoccupied
Proud
Quarrelsome
Receptive
Reliable
Reserved
Respectful
Responsible
Responsible
Restless
Reticent
Rigid
Satisfied
Seductive
Self-confidence
Sensitive
Shallow
Shy
Sluggish
Sociable
Socialize
Suspicious
Tenacious
Tense
Terse

Tolerant
Trepidation
Unaffected
Unassuming
Uncomfortable
Unpopular
Unrealistic
Vacillates
Volunteers
Withdrawn

Describing Cognition

Adapts
Alert
Attentive
Aware
Clarifies
Concentrates
Conscious
Consults
Decisive
Demonstrates
Determines
Distinguishes
Distractible
Explores
Fidgety
Follows
Follows routine
Follows rules
Forgetful
Formulates
Identifies
Impatient
Inattentive
Inquisitive
Intellectually
  curious
Interprets
Knowledgeable
Is Realistic
Learns from
  mistakes
Needs reminders
Obtains
Organizes
Perseverate
Prefectionistic
Prepares
Prioritizes
Problem-solves
Reads
Refuses
Relaxed
Reliable

Retains
Seclusive
Selects
Thoughtful
Thoughtless
Writes

Describing Participation

Attends
Contributes
Conversation
Diligent
Engages
Expresses
Eye contact
Industrious
Initiates
Participates
Quiet
Reserved
Responds
Responsive
Sociable
Solitary
Talkative
Team player
Terminates

Describing Appearance and Touch

Appropriate
Ashen
Bewildered
Blush
Body odor
Bored
Clean
Clenches
  teeth
Colors clash
Concerned
Damp
Dirty
Disheveled
Disordered
Disrepair
Drooling
Ecstatic
Erect posture
Excessive
  layers
Eyes get big
Fastidious
Flushed

Furrowed
  brows
Fussy
Glared
Goosebumps
Grimaces
Hot (temperature)
Ill-fitting
Mannerism
Monotone
Neat
Pale
Poised
Presents
Puffy
Raises eyebrow
Scarred
Shiny
Shivered
Sloppy
Slouched
  posture
Smiles
Sneer
Sweaty
Teary
Tired
Torn clothes
Unaware
Uncombed
Unkempt
Worn out

Describing Speech

Babbles
Clear
Disarticulates
Echolalia
Expresses
Expressive
Flat
Gibberish
Grunts
Lisps
Mispronounces
Monotonous
Mumbles
Pressured
Rambles
Rapid
Repetitive
Slow
Slurred
Word
  substitutions

the kitchen and bring down what she needs from that shelf without assistance, that is focusing on function. If, instead, you report that the client has increased range of motion to 170° in shoulder flexion, you are not reporting on function. Reporting increased range of motion is nicely measurable, but just because someone can move his arm farther does not necessarily mean he uses it to do anything that his functional performance has improved. Another example would be describing ways a client demonstrates improved self-esteem rather than stating the client scores 26% higher on a test of self-esteem. Perhaps the client is now checking her appearance in the mirror before leaving her room, or she is expressing confidence in her skills.

How do you demonstrate progress? By choosing words that show change as much as possible while still being honest. On an intervention plan, it is not necessary to describe everything the client did over the past month; hit only the highlights, only ones that directly relate to the goals you set last month. To do otherwise would result in a lengthier document than you want to write and than anyone wants to read. Evaluation reports can be long, but intervention plans usually have limited space for recording progress.

What do you write if there has not been the progress you had hoped for? Explain what barriers to progress were encountered. There is probably a reasonable explanation for the lack of expected progress; maybe there was a medical complication or change in life circumstance that got in the way. Whatever the explanation, keep it simple and short. Explain how you will modify your intervention plan to encourage greater progress.

In some places, the payers allow maintenance therapy. In maintenance therapy, a client has a condition that is likely to cause functional deterioration. Occupational therapy intervention can delay or prevent this deterioration. If this is the case, showing progress is not expected; maintaining function is good. Do not try to describe progress when maintenance is the goal.

▼ DOCUMENTING INTERVENTION STRATEGIES ▼

Once you and the client have reviewed progress to date and revised short-term goals toward which to work (the outcome or long-term goal is not likely to change, although under some circumstances it might), your thoughts can turn toward intervention strategies to use to help the client meet those goals. The section of the intervention plan where the intervention strategies are listed may be called "interventions," "strategies," "approaches," "methods," or some combination of these words. This is the section where you have to tell the reader what you plan to do to help the client meet his or her goals. To distinguish this from the intervention approaches described earlier, the term "strategies" will be used here.

Strategies can include specific techniques for intervention that are suggested by the model or frame of reference you are using (see Chapter 4), the manner in which you approach the client, general principles for intervention, types of adaptive aids/assistive technology, or task/environmental modifications that will be tried (AOTA, 2007). It also includes whether the client would be best served in an individual or group session (Moyers & Dale, 2007).

As you develop intervention plans, remember that problem identification (evaluation results), goal setting, and intervention strategies all have to relate directly to each other. One way to ensure this interrelationship is to use a frame of reference to guide your thinking. Specific intervention techniques are usually explained by the frame of reference you are using. If you refer back to Chapter 4, you can see how knowledge of a frame of reference can direct your thinking about how to approach the client and the problem. For example, if you were using a biomechanical approach with a client who has had a stroke, your strategies would reflect splinting and range of motion exercises. If instead you were using a contemporary task-oriented approach, you would have the client practice functional activities that are meaningful to the client. If you were using a cognitive disabilities or cognition and activity approach, you would focus on ways to adapt techniques or the environment to enable task performance.

The way you approach the client should be specified in your intervention strategies section. This can have several meanings. It could mean that you identify whether you approach the client at eye level, whether you approach the client like you are the expert or a partner in recovery, or whether you approach the client at bedside or in the clinic. Will you follow the client's suggestions or will you be making suggestions? Will you be firm or flexible? Some of this will depend not only on the frame of reference, but also on the age and condition of the client and the philosophy of the program that is serving the client. For example, the program philosophy may emphasize clients taking an active role in their recovery, and all staff need to actively listen to what the client is saying, letting the client direct the activities he or she tries. Another program may have rigid rules to follow, and the client must obey staff directions.

Other information to record in the strategies section of the intervention plan includes the types of assistive technology, adaptive equipment, or task/environmental modifications the client will try and what home programs or training will be provided to the client or client's caregivers. Since your strategies are simply descriptions of what you will try during the plan period, you can suggest many options. If you put the specific type of equipment in the goal statement, you get locked into using that equipment. If the goal says that the client will do something with or without adaptive equipment, you are freer to experiment. Then in the strategy section, you can list several possibilities for different types of equipment or different techniques.

In addition to establishing goals and intervention strategies, the plan section includes the occupational therapist's recommendations on the frequency, duration, and intensity of occupational therapy intervention sessions (AOTA, 2007). Along with this information, intervention plans specify the location of intervention sessions (e.g., bedside, clinic, client's home) and the anticipated environment to which the client will be discharged (AOTA, 2007).

When you first start out writing intervention plans and client goals, it is not uncommon for your professor or supervisor to ask that you specifically state your rationale for the goals you set and the intervention strategies you suggest. This is actually a good way to start out because it forces you to articulate why you made the choices you did. In most clinical settings, your rationale will be implied; there will not be time or space to spell out your rationale on every intervention plan. To help you think about your rationale, consider the following questions:

- Why did you choose the goals you wrote down?
- How do they relate to the client's needs?
- How do your intervention strategies relate to each goal?
- What frame of reference (or model of practice) guided your thinking?
- Were there goals or strategies that you considered, but chose not to record? If so, why?

Exercise 12.2

For the following goals, suggest three activities that the client could engage in to help reach his or her goals, and then state your rationale for the suggested activities.

1. Client: 2-year-old female with Down syndrome whose lack of coordination and low muscle tone interfere with her ability to engage in age-appropriate play activities.

   Goal: The client will successfully participate in three age-appropriate play activities by 6 months from now.

   Three suggested activities:

   Rationale:

2. Client: 54-year-old man with a traumatic amputation of his right arm just below the elbow.

   Goal: In the next 30 days, Mr. Smith will spontaneously begin to use artificial arm with hook to pick up solid objects.

Three suggested activities:

Rationale:

3. Client: 72-year-old woman with a total hip replacement.

   Goal: Ellie will dress herself independently, with or without the use of adaptive equipment, by April 10, 2009.

   Three suggested activities:

   Rationale:

4. Client: 28-year-old woman with postpartum depression.

   Goal: Naomi will initiate conversations with three people outside her family in the next 2 weeks.

   Three suggested activities:

   Rationale:

▼ SAMPLE INTERVENTION PLANS ▼

Figure 12.1 shows a sample intervention plan format. Sample intervention forms are also provided in Appendix G. Figure 12.2 contains three sample intervention plans (based on plans developed by occupational therapy students at the College of St. Catherine). They have been modified and simplified, with only one long-term goal and two short-term goals listed, whereas in reality there may be more goals than that. However, I will caution you to avoid setting too many goals in one plan. I have seen plans with eight or more goals that the practitioner expects client to accomplish in a month or two. While the client may have lots of areas that need work, it would be better to focus on a few and do well with them than try to work on too many goals and not do as well.

▼ REVISING INTERVENTION PLANS ▼

The longer you work with a particular client, the more likely it is that you will need to revise your intervention plan. This is not necessarily a sign that your plan is not working, but it just means that it takes time to effect significant changes in a person. Intervention plans are usually revised on a regular schedule, such as every 30 or 90 days, often depending on the requirements of the third-party payer and/or the condition of the client.

Revising the intervention plan allows you to step back from day-to-day intervention and really evaluate whether the plan is working or not. If it is working, then maybe the time is right to take things to the next level. If it is not working, then this is a good time to figure out what you could do differently. Maybe you were too ambitious in your goal setting and need to set smaller goals. Maybe you were not ambitious enough and you need to set higher goals. Maybe you need to consider taking the interventions in a whole new direction. It is up to the occupational therapist to evaluate the effectiveness of the intervention plan. Any changes in the plan should be made in consultation with the client and/or client's caregiver (AOTA, 2007).

OCCUPATIONAL THERAPY INTERVENTION PLAN.

BACKGROUND INFORMATION
Date of report: Client's name or initials:
Date of birth &/or age: Date of referral: M   F
Primary intervention diagnosis/concern:
Secondary diagnosis/concern:
Precautions/contraindications:
Reason for referral to OT: *(or questions to be answered)*
Therapist: *(Print or type your name and credential; you will sign and date the report at the end.)*

FINDINGS
Occupational Profile: *(Describe the client's occupational history and experience, patterns of living, interests, values, and needs from the client's perspective that are relevant to the current situation.)*

Progress *(Progress toward goals so far; reasons for progress or lack thereof.)*
    Areas of occupation:
    Performance skills:
    Performance patterns:
    Activity demands:
    Client factors:
    Contexts:

Equipment/orthotics issued:

Home programs/training:

INTERPRETATION
 Analysis of occupational performance: *(Describe the barriers and challenges, supports and strengths.)*

PLAN

Long-term Goal	Short-term Goal	Methods/Approaches

Expected frequency, duration, and intensity:
Location of intervention:
Anticipated discontinuation environment:

_____
Signature   Date

FIGURE 12.1   Sample Occupational Therapy Intervention Plan.

```
                              OT Intervention Plan
                              Functional Rehab, Inc

Name: Jamie Shooter      DOB: May 18, 1960        Date of Report: Nov. 3, 2009
Precautions/Contraindications: Non-weight bearing for six weeks
Reason for referral: Increase mobility for independence in self-care

Occupational Profile: Jamie was working as a human cannonball for the circus when he was seriously injured in a freak
accident 3 days ago. He has multiple fractures of his lower extremities, a dislocated (R) shoulder, and numerous contusions, cuts,
and scrapes all over his body. He had a severe concussion with loss of consciousness for 10 minutes following the incident. Prior
to the injury he was healthy and physically fit.

Analysis of Occupational Performance: Client is in a great deal of pain and resists moving quickly or through his
entire range. He is totally dependent in transfers and dressing. He requires moderate assist for grooming and hygiene and
minimal assist for feeding. Jamie expressed frustration with his condition, saying he is not used to lying around and has
always been active. He thinks boredom will be one of his biggest challenges because he knows he can recover from the
physical injuries, but the recovery will not come as quickly as he would like. He loves his job and hopes to return to circus
work, although he thinks the doctor is unlikely to recommend a return to being shot out of a cannon. He says he loves the
rush he feels flying through the air, so if he can't do that, then maybe he will consider the trapeze.

Problems prioritized:      #1 Needs to increase mobility for self-care skills
                           #2 Needs to decrease dependence on others for self-care skills
                           #3 Needs to stay occupied

Long-term goal:
Client will transfer independently from bed to wheelchair by Dec. 15, 2009.
```

Short-term goals for Problem #1	Intervention approaches/methods for #1
By November 20, client will transfer from the mat table to the wheelchair with moderate assist on three consecutive tries.	Strengthening activities Instruction in safe techniques Practice pushing up on arms to bear weight on his arms without moving to another surface
By Dec. 1, client will transfer from the mat table to the wheelchair with stand-by assist and verbal cues as needed on three consecutive tries.	Strengthening activities Activities involving weight bearing on arms

```
Frequency of OT sessions: 2x/day
Duration of OT sessions: 30 min
Expected length of OT services: 6 weeks


_____  Date:_____
Signature(s)
```

FIGURE 12.2   Sample Intervention Plans.

OT Intervention Plan
Functional Rehab, Inc

Name: _Loretta Mojo_   **DOB:** _4-28-05_   **Date of Report:** _Nov. 3, 2009_
Precautions/Contraindications: _Strong aversion to any touch_
Reason for referral: _Aversion to touch is interfering with everyday life_

Occupational Profile: _Loretta is a 4-year-old girl with autism. She developed normally until she was 18 months old when she seemed to regress to earlier developmental stages. She has strong aversive responses to any form of touch. General health has been good, with only a few ear infections._

Analysis of Occupational Performance: _According to Loretta's mom, Loretta has become increasingly aversive to almost any touch. She is removing her clothes because they appear to irritate her, making it difficult for Loretta to go out in public. She screams when anyone touches her. She fights her bath, especially getting her hair washed. She walks on tiptoes so that her whole feet do not have to touch the floor. Loretta's mom reports that Loretta is a very picky eater and will not let them hug her. This last point seemed to be of the greatest concern to her mom as evidenced by her tears at this point in the interview. Results of sensory integration testing confirm aversion to touch, and deficits in processing both tactile and proprioceptive input._

Problems prioritized: #1 _Needs to tolerate touch so that she can be hugged and give hugs_
                               #2 _Needs to tolerate touch so that she can wear clothes of varying textures and get her hair washed calmly_
                               #3 _Needs to increase the variety of foods she will eat_

Long-term goal:
Loretta will share hugs with parents and loved ones within 1 year.

Short-term goals for Problem #1	Intervention approaches/methods for #1
Loretta will receive one hug without withdrawal during three consecutive OT sessions within 3 months.	_Sensory integrative techniques for tactile processing that will gradually increase in duration and intensity._ _Begin with her applying the stimuli and moving toward the OT applying them._
Loretta will initiate a hug with a parent following OT sessions on four out of five opportunities within 5 months.	_Progressive touching activities such as handshaking, putting her arm around an object or person, and then to a hug._

Frequency of OT sessions: _2x/week_
Duration of OT sessions: _45 min_
Expected length of OT services: _1 year_

_____ **Date:**_____
Signature(s)

FIGURE 12.2   (Continued)

OT Intervention Plan
Functional Rehab, Inc

Name: _Yolanda Odor_   **DOB:** _Jan. 18, 1963_   **Date of Report:** _Nov. 3, 2009_
Precautions/Contraindications: _None_
Reason for referral: _Needs to improve personal hygiene_

Occupational Profile: _Yolanda is a 46-year-old woman with schizophrenia. She has been living in community housing; however, recent complaints of poor hygiene resulting in strong body odor has resulted in increasingly angry exchanges with housemates. According to Yolanda, she would bathe if she needed to, but she sees no need to. She also does not think that her bathing habits are anyone's business but her own. She also says she had been faithful in taking her medications, but has stopped taking them because she feels she no longer needs them._

Analysis of Occupational Performance: _Client has a very strong body odor; stringy, greasy hair, and has not shaved her legs or armpits in quite some time (judging by the length of the hair). During observation, she did not wash her hands no matter how soiled they became. She did not wash her hands after going to the bathroom. Client reports not using toothpaste, soap, or deodorant in weeks. She also says she does not notice any particular odor about her. Her clothes had multiple spots where food had landed on them._

Problems prioritized: #1 _Needs to improve personal hygiene skills_
                                #2 _Needs to improve personal grooming skills_

Long-term goal:
Within 1 month, Yolanda will independently complete all personal hygiene tasks.

Short-term goals for Problem #1	Intervention approaches/methods for #1
Within 1 week, Yolanda will wash her hands with soap and water after each time she uses the toilet.	_Visual reminders in the bathroom_ _Coaching and verbal reminders_
Within 3 weeks, Yolanda will independently initiate showering at least 4 days per week.	_Adaptive equipment and instruction in the safe use of this equipment as needed_ _Calendar to keep track of showers_ _Coaching and feedback_

Frequency of OT sessions: _3x/week_
Duration of OT sessions: _60 min_
Expected length of OT services: _6 weeks_

_____   **Date:** _____
Signature(s)

FIGURE 12.2   (Continued)

Exercise 12.3

This exercise is called "Create-a-Client." In this exercise, you will create an imaginary client and develop a mini-intervention plan for this client. I suggest that you create a memorable client, someone you think would be fun to work with. You can create a serious case that is simple or complex, or you can create a bizarre and unique client. Use the following format to write about your client.

First, establish background information on your client. Create a memorable name for your client. Determine the client's age, diagnoses, and occupational profile. Then summarize the occupational needs of the client. Determine what performance skills, performance patterns, contexts, activity demands, or client factors contribute to the problems. Next, prioritize occupational needs and establish goals for this client. Finally, suggest intervention strategies.

Create-a-Client
I. Background Information
Name: _____ **Age:** _____
Diagnoses: _____

II. Findings:
    Occupational Profile:
    Summary of Progress (since last intervention plan):

III. Interpretation:
    Strengths and Need Areas:
    Prioritize Occupational Needs:
    1.
    2.
    3.

IV. Plan:
    One long-term and two short-term goals for top priority:
    LTG:

    STG:

    STG:

    Possible interventions:
    Frequency, Intensity, Duration:

_____ **Date:** _____
Signature

Exercise 12.4

Write an intervention plan based on the following cases:

1. Butch is a 46-year-old man with autism, seizures, and sensory processing disorder. He lives in a shared apartment and works at a sheltered workshop 5 days a week. At the sheltered workshop, he packages craft kits that will be sold at a chain of craft stores nationally. Butch shares his apartment with 2 other men; all are autistic, and there is a staff person available from 4 p.m. to 9 a.m., Monday to Friday, and 24 hours a day on weekends. With setup by staff, Butch dresses himself, and he assists with cooking and cleaning. For leisure activities, Butch does jigsaw puzzles, rides the exercise bike, goes for walks, and watches TV. Over the last 2 months, the staff at the workshop and at his home have noticed an increase in Butch's self-stimulatory and noncompliant behaviors. He has increased the frequency and intensity of his rocking and mumbling to himself, and hand-flapping. He is saying "no" when he is asked or told to do something, refusing to comply with instructions about 50% of the time. In the last week, he has started to refuse to shower and has gotten pickier about his food. He has not had any medication changes. At the workshop, about 2 months ago, he was moved into a different room, but the task remained the same. He is now in a room with higher functioning clients. At home, last month, the carpeting was replaced with a laminate floor in the living room, and the walls were painted blue. One of his roommates has been having more visitors lately. The staff at the apartment called for an occupational therapy consultation to evaluate and plan a new sensory diet and environmental adaptations as necessary in an effort to restore Butch to his prior level of function.

2. Marcus is a 3-year-old born with Fragile X syndrome. He is nonverbal. His mother completed a Sensory Profile on him, and he appears to have oversensitivity to noise, but undersensitivity to touch. He bites his wrists. He walks independently, but has problems with balance and motor planning. He is a very picky eater, he drinks out of a sippy cup, and does not chew his food well. Sometimes the food falls out of his mouth. Marcus does not dress himself and he is not potty trained. Bathing him and washing his hair are extremely challenging as he is very resistive; he screams and hits, trying to stop the process. His mom reports that it takes two people to give him a bath or wash his hair, and he is inconsolable when it is over. His pediatrician referred him to a pediatric clinic that specializes in sensory integrative evaluation and interventions.

3. Mariah is an 87-year-old woman with mild congestive heart failure, who fell while walking her dog and broke her right hip. She is cognitively very sharp. She was a college professor (English) who kept teaching into her early seventies. Prior to her fall, she lived independently with her husband (age 89), and wire-haired fox terrier, Scarlett. They live in a small house in the city. They both gave up driving 2 years ago. Mariah had surgery to repair her hip 3 days ago and was transferred from the hospital to a subacute unit in the long-term care facility near her home. She has two daughters and six grandchildren who live within 10 miles of this facility. She hopes to return home in 2 weeks. While in the subacute unit, she will receive both occupational and physical therapy twice a day.

SUMMARY

In this chapter you have learned about writing intervention plans. The intervention plan is a vital document that is used by payers to determine whether continued intervention is needed, by coworkers to communicate the client's current status and progress, and by the occupational therapy personnel to evaluate the effectiveness of intervention programs.

Generally speaking, a client receiving ongoing intervention from occupational therapy will have an intervention plan developed immediately after the evaluation, and then periodically until services are discontinued. Except when the client is working on maintenance goals, each successive intervention plan should show progress in the client's areas of occupation. If progress is not made, an explanation for the lack of progress must be given.

The occupational therapist is responsible for writing, revising, and communicating the intervention plan. An occupational therapy assistant contributes to the intervention planning process. It is a client-centered process.

In addition to necessary client identification information, intervention plans usually contain a brief summary of progress, revised goals, and intervention strategies. Intervention strategies include frequency and duration of services, manner of service delivery, place of service delivery, types of adaptive equipment/environmental adaptations, task modifications, home programs, and training for the client and the client's caregivers. While intervention plans are written in ink, they are not engraved in stone. They are expected to change as the client's circumstances and condition changes.

REFERENCES

American Occupational Therapy Association. (2005a). Standards of practice for occupational therapy. *American Journal of Occupational Therapy, 59*, 663–665.

American Occupation Therapy Association. (2005b). Occupational therapy code of ethics—2005. *American Journal of Occupational Therapy, 59*, 639–642.

American Occupational Therapy Association. (2006). *Guidelines to the code of ethics. American Journal of Occupational Therapy, 60*, 652–658.

American Occupational Therapy Association. (2007). Guidelines for documentation of occupational therapy. Retrieved June, 16, 2008, from http://www.aota.org/Practitioners/Official/Guidelines/41257.aspx

American Occupational Therapy Association. (2008a). Occupational therapy practice framework: Domain and process. *American Journal of Occupational Therapy, 62*, 625–683.

American Occupational Therapy Association. (2008b). Medicare Basics. Retrieved August 8, 2008, from http://www.aota.org/Practitioners/Reimb/Pay/Medicare/FactSheets/37788.aspx

Brennan, C., & Robinson, M. (2006). Documentation: Getting it right to avoid Medicare denials. *OT Practice, 11* (14) 10–16.

Centers for Medicare and Medicaid Services. (2008). *Pub100-02 Medicare benefit policy: Transmittal 88.* Retrieved May 8, 2008, from http://www.cms.hhs.gov/transmittals/downloads/R88BP.pdf

McQuire, M. J. (1997). Excellence and efficiency in documentation. *OT Practice, 2*(12), 36–41.

Moyers, P. A., & Dale, L. M. (2007). *The guide to occupational therapy practice* (2nd ed.). Bethesda, MD: American Occupational Therapy Association.

World Health Organization. (2002). *International classification of function.* Geneva, Switzerland: Author. Retrieved May 22, 2002, from http://www3.who.int/icf

CHAPTER 13

SOAP and Other Methods of Documenting Ongoing Intervention

INTRODUCTION

Written documentation of ongoing intervention comes in different sizes and formats, but all are intended to provide a record of intervention sessions. In most cases, they are written following each intervention session; however, in some cases, they may be written weekly or other time interval. These notes may be called progress notes, progress reports, encounter notes, daily notes, or similar names, but will be called progress notes in this text. Typically, a progress note covers a longer time interval than a daily, contact, or encounter note (Brennan & Robinson, 2006).

Progress notes should be more than simply a listing of the types of activities in which a client has engaged. They are called progress notes because they are supposed to show progress. Therefore, the notes need to include information about the client's response to interventions and how current performance is different from previous performance (American Occupational Therapy Association [AOTA], 2008; Brennan & Robinson, 2006). Any unusual or significant event, assistive or adaptive equipment issued or tried, and any client/caregiver instruction also need to be documented (AOTA, 2008). Ultimately, a progress note or progress report has to show that the skills of an occupational therapy practitioner contributed to the progress a client has made toward the goals established in the intervention plan; how the client is different as a result of occupational therapy interventions (Brennan & Robinson).

Contact notes, are intended to be shorter, and reflect the client's response to intervention during that day or that intervention session (Brennan & Robinson, 2006). A contact note may be in any of the formats described in the following sections, or may be in the form of a log or flow sheet. Since this note reflects one session or one day's sessions, the emphasis is not on progress, but on what services were provided and how the client responded to that intervention, including adaptive equipment issues, and any client or caregiver education provided (AOTA, 2005; Brennan & Robinson, 2006).

There are three main kinds of progress notes: narrative, SOAP, and DAP (FIP). Narrative notes are notes that are written in paragraph form. SOAP and DAP (FIP) notes have specific labeled sections. All three types of notes are discussed in this chapter. In addition, ways to document progress in checklist or graphic forms, such as progress flow sheets and attendance logs, are discussed.

▼ ROLE DELINEATION FOR PROGRESS REPORTING ▼

The occupational therapist, with contributions from the occupational therapy assistant, performs reevaluation during the ongoing intervention process (AOTA, 2005, 2008). He or she documents changes in the client's occupational performance, short-term goals, and anticipated discharge environment (AOTA, 2005). The occupational therapist is responsible for modifying the interventions as the client's contexts, wants, needs, and responses to interventions change. The occupational therapy assistant, under the supervision of an occupational therapist, offers suggestions for modifying intervention methods. Progress notes may be written by either the occupational therapist or occupational therapy assistant. Notes written by an occupational therapy assistant are usually reviewed and cosigned by the occupational therapist when required by statute, regulation, accrediting agency, payer, or facility/agency policy (AOTA, 2005).

Documentation of intervention requires that the occupational therapist and occupational therapy assistant work closely together. As mentioned in Chapter 12, in some settings, the occupational therapy assistant works without on-site supervision by an occupational therapist. Depending on state licensure or registration laws, the stability of the clients, and the service competency of the occupational therapy assistant, an occupational therapist may provide on-site supervision a couple days a week, once a week, or once every couple weeks. When the occupational therapist does not see the client on a daily basis, he or she relies heavily on the occupational therapy assistant to report changes in the client's condition and client's performance in areas of occupation. The occupational therapist uses this information along with his or her own observations, interviews, and data gathering to recommend any modifications to the ongoing implementation of intervention. These modifications are documented in progress notes and revised intervention plans.

▼ SOAP NOTES ▼

SOAP notes are another of medicine's acronyms. SOAP stands for **S**ubjective, **O**bjective, **A**ssessment, **P**lan, which are the component parts of this type of progress note. One of the advantages of this type of note is that it is quite common and the reader knows just what kind of information to find in what part of the note. Professionals from all health care disciplines write them. The SOAP format can also be adapted for use as an evaluation report or discontinuation summary (Borcherding, 2005; Borcherding & Kappel, 2002).

Dr. Lawrence Weed is credited with developing SOAP notes in the 1960s as part of his efforts to make client charting more client-centered (Borcherding, 2005; Borcherding & Kappel, 2002; Kettenback, 2004). He reorganized a client's medical record so that there would be a master list of the client's problems from the perspective of all the disciplines working with the client, and then a section for progress notes that all disciplines could write in (as opposed to separate sections of the chart for each discipline). Weed named this system the Problem Oriented Medical Record (POMR). The SOAP note format has become so popular that today, even if facilities do not use POMR, the SOAP note is still the preferred format for note writing (Borcherding, 2005).

Here are some sample progress notes written in SOAP format.

Case 1: Helen, Alzheimer's client in day care setting

S: "Where do I go? What do I do?"

O: Upon entering the building, Helen waited for her daughter to tell her which way to turn. Once in the room, she helped herself to a cup of coffee. Then she sat down and sipped her coffee until she received further instructions. She imitated the exercises that the group leader demonstrated. Halfway through the exercise group, she stood up, put her coffee cup in the garbage, and thanked everyone for a pleasant experience. She started to leave the room. She blushed and hid her face when told that the group was not over yet.

A: Helen appears to be dependent on the verbal cues of others in her environment to direct her behavior. In the absence of verbal cues, she gets confused.

P: Pair verbal and visual cues for Helen, or use verbal cues alone. Continue to encourage participation in small-group activities. Provide a structured environment with a consistent, posted schedule. Continue monthly occupational therapy consultation.

Bobbi Babinski, OTR/L 11-1-09

S: "I used to be able to do this without thinking about it. Now I have to concentrate so hard on it I wonder if it's worth it."

O: Client participated in a 30-minute occupational therapy session to work on functional activities with his unaffected (nondominant) hand. Bob attempted to use a computer mouse with his left hand by playing a game of solitaire. He moved quickly to the general area that he wants the mouse to be. He moved slowly and hesitantly to the precise spot he needed; however, he often overshot the mark. Bob clicked the mouse with his index finger easily; however, he had minimal success holding the mouse button down while dragging the mouse. It took 20 minutes to complete one game of solitaire.

A: Bob has not yet achieved adequate coordination with either hand to allow him to perform mouse activities to his satisfaction.

P: Try a touchpad mouse. Encourage moving slowly and carefully. Practice using left hand for other activities during the day. Continue twice-daily occupational therapy as per plan of care.

Carrie Ingwater, COTA/L 3-2-09

Bobbi Babinski, OTR/L 3-2-09

Subjective

The subjective part of the SOAP note usually refers to the client's subjective comments about problems, complaints, life circumstances, goals, current performance, limitations, or other comments that are relevant to the services you are providing (Borcherding, 2005; Borcherding & Kappel, 2002; Kettenbach, 2004; Kuntavanish, 1988; Quinn & Gordon, 2003). You may directly quote the client or paraphrase, but direct quotes must be marked as such with quotation marks. A direct quote can be very effective at illustrating the client's attitude, use of language, denial, or loss of memory. However, simply writing "I feel icky" does not really tell the reader much (Borcherding & Kappel, 2002; "Tips on Medical Progress Notes," 2002). If a client says that, ask him or her for clarification, then write down the client's description of his or her aches, pains and feelings. "I feel tired and my chest and shoulder hurt" conveys more specific information. A relative or caretaker may also say something that is significant, and these comments can also be recorded in the subjective section of the SOAP note. Sometimes a client is nonverbal. If that is the case, you can document nonverbal communication such as smiles, nods, and gestures as appropriate.

Exercise 13.1

Which of these statements belong in the subjective section of the SOAP note?

1. _____ Ndebe appeared tired and listless.
2. _____ Client said she is hearing voices telling her to cut her hair.
3. _____ Raësa got dressed by herself today.
4. _____ Cyndee's mother said that Cyndee has not been sleeping well the past 3 nights.
5. _____ "I am fat and ugly."
6. _____ Client is resistant to all suggestions.
7. _____ "Where am I?"
8. _____ Client made several lewd comments throughout the session, accompanied by sexually suggestive hand gestures.
9. _____ Saji's shirt was misbuttoned, untucked, and stained.
10. _____ Tamara came to the clinic with brown smudges around her mouth and on her hands. She said, "I ate cake for breakfast."

Some people advocate using statements like "Client denies feeling suicidal" ("Sample Medical SOAP Notes," 2002). I think the word "denies" sounds like you do not believe the client; it sounds judgmental. I prefer wording such as "Client reports she is not having suicidal thoughts."

Pick your "S" carefully. Make sure it is relevant to the intervention addressed in your note. For example, if you are writing a SOAP note about the client's functional skills in meal preparation, an "S" about what the client watched on TV last night is not relevant. If there is nothing relevant to report in the "S" section, you can draw a circle with a line through it (Ø) to indicate that you thought about it but there was nothing relevant to write about. Leaving it blank might look like you forgot to write something there.

Objective

The objective section is the place for recording observations, data collected, and other facts (Borcherding, 2005; Borcherding & Kappel, 2002; Kettenbach, 2004; Kuntavanish, 1988; Quinn & Gordon, 2003). The emphasis of this section should be on the client's performance, not simply a listing of activities the client engaged in. The information you record in this section should be the indisputable truth. It is harder than it looks to keep your interpretations out of this section. Remember the Description, Interpretation, Evaluation (DIE) discussion in Chapter 10? This would be a good time to review that material.

If the client made an attempt to open a carton of milk, but gave up before getting it open, would you say "The client was unsuccessful at opening a milk carton" or "The client is dependent in opening milk cartons"? Both sentences are probably true and accurate statements. The first sentence is descriptive of a particular event. The second is a generalization; it makes the claim that the client would be unlikely to open any milk carton. This makes the second sentence an interpretive statement that belongs in the "A" section rather than the "O" section.

Another consideration when writing the "O" section is that in some settings, the preference is to document only what the client can do, not what the client cannot do. In other settings, it is expected that both strengths and limitations will be documented. However, the "O" section should not read like a list of the client's failings.

The actual intervention is not as important as how the client responded to the intervention (Borcherding & Kappel, 2002). Your powers of observation are essential in writing good progress notes. Record the client's reaction to the intervention. Here are some possible "O" statements:

- Client pulled away from contact with the shaving cream.
- Client was dressed in plaid pants and a striped shirt.
- Jalele made fleeting eye contact with other members of the group.
- Client stacked the plates eight high on the bottom shelf of the overhead cabinet.
- Client was instructed in use of stocking aid; she demonstrated proper use of it.
- Client dressed herself independently, except for minimal assist for shoes and socks.
- Selena entered the room and went straight to the coffee pot.
- Client spontaneously used his right hand to pick up his coffee cup.

Exercise 13.2

Which of the following statements belong in the "O" section of the SOAP note?

1. _____ The client's eyes were red and watery.
2. _____ Bob seemed to be frustrated.
3. _____ He pushed away from the table and left the room.
4. _____ She spit out the strawberries.
5. _____ Pevitra wants to be recognized for good behavior.
6. _____ Esai ate all of one food before eating the next food on his plate.

---

7. _____ The client appears bewildered when others get annoyed with him for invading their personal space.

8. _____ The client has a habit of twisting her ring around her finger during personal conversations.

Borcherding (2005) and Borcherding and Kappel (2002) suggest that the "O" section begin with a statement of where and why the client was seen. Some settings and payers also expect the note to contain the amount of time the client was in occupational therapy since the last progress note. For example, the section might start with this sentence: "Demitri participated in two 45-minute occupational therapy clinic sessions this week to develop age-appropriate social skills." Or "Etta received occupational therapy today for 60 minutes in her home to work on meal preparation and housekeeping skills."

The "O" section can be organized chronologically, that is, describing events in the order in which they happened (Borcherding, 2005; Borcherding & Kappel, 2002). This gives the reader a good idea of exactly what transpired during occupational therapy intervention sessions. If you are working with a client such as a child with sensory integration dysfunction where the sequence of interventions is important, then this is the best format.

Some authors (Borcherding, 2005, Borcherding & Kappel, 2002; and Kettenbach, 2004) suggest that objective data can be categorized to make the note appear more organized. Headings can be used to clearly identify separate topics such as test results, functional activities, or body parts. When reporting range of motion or strength data for multiple joints, a chart can be used to display the information. A chart is easier to read and refer back to than a long sentence with multiple measurements.

Exercise 13.3

Practice organizing the "O" section for the following cases.

Case 1: You are working with a client who has severe rheumatoid arthritis, resulting in joint deformities of the fingers of both hands. He wants to be able to keyboard so he can email his son. On his right hand, the thumb IP joint can flex to 40°. Thumb abduction is 55°. The MCP joint can flex to 30°. The index finger has DIP, PIP, and MCP flexion of 45°, 85°, and 50°, respectively, with 35° of hyperextension at the DIP and 35° of MCP extension. There is ulnar drift of index, middle, ring, little fingers of 30°, 30°, 35°, and 40°, respectively. Both the middle and ring finger had 50° of DIP flexion. The little finger has no movement at the DIP joint. The PIP joint of the middle, ring, and little finger are 50°, 40°, and 30°, respectively. There is 30° of flexion and extension for the MCP joints. On his left hand, the thumb IP joint can flex to 40°. Thumb abduction is 55°. The MCP joint can flex to 70°. The index finger has DIP, PIP, and MCP flexion of 50°, 60°, and 50°, respectively. The index finger has 40° of hyperextension at the DIP joint and 40° of MCP extension. There is ulnar drift of index, middle, ring, little fingers of 20°, 30°, 30°, and 40°. Both the middle and ring finger had 30° of DIP flexion. The little finger has no movement at the DIP joint. The PIP joints of the middle, ring, and little finger flex to 60°, 50°, and 45°, respectively. There is 35° of flexion and 40° of extension for the MCP joints.

Fill in each of the following tables using the data in the previous paragraph.

L	Thumb	R
_____	IP flexion	_____
_____	MCP flexion	_____
_____	Abduction	_____

	Index finger	
_____	DIP flexion	_____
_____	DIP extension	_____

```
_____    PIP flexion          _____
_____    MCP flexion          _____
_____    MCP extension        _____
```

Middle finger
```
_____    DIP flexion          _____
_____    PIP flexion          _____
_____    MCP flexion          _____
_____    MCP extension        _____
```

Ring finger
```
_____    DIP flexion          _____
_____    PIP flexion          _____
_____    MCP flexion          _____
_____    MCP extension        _____
```

Little finger
```
_____    DIP flexion          _____
_____    PIP flexion          _____
_____    MCP flexion          _____
_____    MCP extension        _____
```

Ulnar Drift
```
_____    Index                _____
_____    Middle               _____
_____    Ring                 _____
_____    Little               _____
```

Finger	DIP flexion	DIP extension	PIP flexion	MCP flexion	MCP extension	Abduction	Ulnar drift
R thumb							
L thumb							
R index							
L index							
R middle							
L middle							
R ring							
L ring							
R little							
L little							

Next, answer the following questions:

1. Of the three methods of presenting information (narrative, list, and table), which do you think is the easiest to read and understand?

2. Can you think of another way to organize this information?

Assessment

The assessment or "A" portion of the SOAP note is where you explain what all this data (the subjective and objective) means (Borcherding, 2005; Borcherding & Kappel, 2002; Kettenbach, 2004; Kuntavanish, 1988; Quinn & Morgan, 2003). This is where your professional judgment and skills come into play.

The assessment section is where data recorded in the "S" and "O" sections is analyzed, summarized, and prioritized. No new information should be added in the "A" section that is not supported by information recorded in the "S" and "O" sections. In some facilities, the "A" section begins with a problem list (Borcherding, 2005). By listing the problems in order of importance to the client you let the readers (which often includes payers) know why occupational therapy is involved in this case. There is no need to use complete sentences in the problem list. Examples of problems could be:

- Impaired self-care skills
- Decreased hand function
- Decreased job skills
- Low self-esteem
- Limited access to services in his community
- Difficulty feeding herself
- Limited attention to tasks

Typically, in those facilities where the "A" section includes a problem list, the "A" section also includes both long- and short-term goals and a summary. The summary explains to readers the correlations between the "S," "O," and "P" sections, justifies your recommendations, clarifies progress made, explains any difficulties in obtaining information, and makes suggestions for further testing.

Here is an "A" section using this type of format:

A: Problem list: Limited ROM in Ⓡ shoulder, impaired dressing, grooming, and hygiene skills.

Long-term goal: By discharge, return to independence in dressing, grooming, and hygiene.

Short-term goals: In two sessions, pt. will grasp objects at shoulder height without moving his trunk.

In three sessions, pt. will use both hands to shampoo his hair.

In three sessions, pt. will use both hands to dry and style his hair.

Summary: Pt. is using trunk rotation to substitute for Ⓡ shoulder flexion. He has improved since last visit in that he now is using his Ⓡ arm for some tasks. Would benefit from continued occupational therapy.

In other facilities, the "A" will be presented in a more narrative way without listing problems or setting goals. In this method, the "A" would consist of wording similar to what one would write in the summary sections of the "A" part of the preceding note.

Examples of "A" statements would be:

- Client is independent in dressing.
- Laleh needs verbal cues to stay on task.
- She is ready to go on a home visit.
- He has difficulty with impulse control.
- Client is dependent in toilet transfers.
- Client is able to manage her own medication routine.
- The client has demonstrated gains in using fasteners since last report. She now can button and unbutton buttons ½ inch in diameter without assistance.

It might seem unnecessary to remind you that what you write in the "A" section must directly relate to what you write in the "S" and "O" sections, but this has consistently been one of the hardest things for students to learn to do. Often what happens is that students write great "A" statements, but when you look at the "O" section, there is nothing supporting the conclusions drawn in the "A" section. For example:

S: Client reported pain in his shoulder every time he moves in any direction
O: Client twisted his trunk and extended his Ⓡ elbow to reach objects in front of him rather than flexing his shoulder. Once positioned, he grasped various objects including a cup, a glass, a fork, a scissors, and a pen.
A: He writes legibly with his right hand.
P: Continue OT sessions 3x/wk to improve functional use of RUE.

While the "O" does mention that he grasped a pen, there are no observations related to actually using the pen. The "A" is a big leap of thinking and it is unsupported by anything in the "O" or "S" sections. A better "A" for this note would be, "He is protecting his shoulder by substituting trunk and elbow movement for shoulder movement. However, this is an improvement over last session when he refused to use the hand/arm at all." The "A" section is not the place to bring in new information (Borcherding, 2005). Everything you write in "A" has to be supported with evidence in the "S" and "O" sections.

One technique that can be helpful in writing "A" sections that connect to "S" and "O" sections is to go through the first two sections sentence by sentence and ask yourself what it means for the client (Borcherding, 2005; Borcherding & Kappel, 2002). Ask yourself what it is about what the client said or did that is important enough to write down. What does it tell you about the client's performance in areas of occupation? What does it tell you about performance skills, patterns, or client factors? You may find a difference between what the client said and what the client did. You may notice whether or not there has been an improvement in function.

Exercise 13.4

Which of these make good "A" statements on SOAP notes?

1. _____ She has to be told to come out of her room.
2. _____ Client tried to use the TV remote control to call home.
3. _____ Client completed 75% of the task without assistance.
4. _____ Usha does not interact with peers.
5. _____ He used public transportation independently.
6. _____ Ashton can tolerate a moderately noisy environment for up to 10 minutes.
7. _____ Client's statements are inappropriate to the situation.
8. _____ Benjamin refused to taste the meal.
9. _____ Willow is making good progress.
10. _____ Paula cooked the entire meal one handed.

In addition to the interpretation of data, justification of the goals, inconsistencies, progress, difficulty in obtaining information, and suggestions for further intervention (Borcherding, 2005; Borcherding & Kappel, 2002; Kettenbach, 2004), you can also include information on the client's strengths, deficits, and motivation (Kuntavanish, 1988). The keys are to not restate the "O" in "A," and be sure that every statement in "A" is supported by evidence in "O."

Plan

The plan section is where you very clearly spell out what your plan is for helping the client achieve his or her goals. It often states the frequency, duration, and intensity of occupational therapy and suggestions for intervention. It can also include the location of the intervention

Exercise 13.5

1. Write an "A" for the data presented in Exercise 13.3.

2. Write an "A" for the following cases ("S" and "O" provided).

Case 1: 3-year-old boy with muscular incoordination and autism

S: "Keep that away from me!" (response to presentation of plate of shaving cream)

O: Deshaun received 45 minutes of occupational therapy intervention for sensory and motor skill development. He ran away when a plate of shaving cream was brought toward him. He tipped over his chair in his attempt to run away. As each new sensory activity was introduced, Deshaun started flapping his hands. At least five times during the 1-hour session, he bent over forward, placed his head on the floor, and rocked back and forth. He refused to go down a 3-foot long slide, or through a 5-foot long plastic tunnel. When held upside down by his ankles and swung gently, he repeatedly asked to do it again. He also asked to have the weighted blanket put on him three times during the session.

A:

Case 2: 78-year-old man who had a stroke 1 month ago, resulting in left-sided hemiparesis and visual neglect (hemianopsia).

S: "I don't see why I can't drive myself to the golf course for a round of golf, I'm fine. They wouldn't have let me home from the hospital if there was anything really wrong. I can use the golf club for a cane on the course." Client says he has no problem with his left side and all this talk about "left side neglect" is just "garbage."

O: When client attempted to putt using a golf club, he put the club in his left hand and then grasped it with his right. His left hand consistently fell off the club during the back swing. When a plate with chips on the right side and dip on the left was placed in front of him, he ate only the chips, never the dip.

A:

sessions (i.e., bedside, clinic, or home) and equipment issued to the client (Kettenbach, 2004). The "P" section should be written with sufficient clarity that if you get sick and cannot come to work the next time the client is supposed to be seen, a substitute occupational therapy practitioner could step in and do what you would have done.

Examples of the "P" statements include:

- Continue OT 3x/wk for self-care skills development. Try adaptive feeding equipment such as a plate guard and large-handled utensils.
- Continue OT bid, 5x/wk for brain injury retraining program. See in room in a.m. for dressing, grooming, and hygiene, and in clinic in the afternoon for meal prep, safety, and problem solving.
- As per plan of care, client will be seen 5x/wk for 30-minute sessions for the next 2 weeks. Will work on toilet transfers and manipulation of clothes necessary for toileting next visit. Caregiver instruction will be included.
- Client will participate in activity group and assertiveness group daily.

It is not uncommon to see the "P" section written with differing levels of specificity depending on the writer. Generally, the more specific the better.

Figures 13.1 and 13.2 show some sample progress notes. Read through them and see what you think about the quality of the notes. Consider how useful and informative the information is. Review the criteria for Documenting with CARE (Chapter 5).

All the SOAP notes in Figure 13.1 technically have subjective information in the subjective space, objective information in the objective space, and so on; however, the notes

Exercise 13.6

Which of these make good "P" statements?

1. _____ Practice writing his name three times per day.
2. _____ Engage client in conversations about child care.
3. _____ She should be more careful in the kitchen.
4. _____ Increase repetitions as tolerated.
5. _____ Instruct in splint care and maintenance.
6. _____ Client needs to spend more time on leisure occupations.
7. _____ Client will work on chewing food at least 10 times before swallowing.
8. _____ Client should do this more often.
9. _____ Continue OT 2x/wk.
10. _____ Talk with caregivers about follow-through on the unit.

The client, Susie, is a 4-year-old girl with cerebral palsy, who is seen in an outpatient rehabilitation center. Although only a few notes are shown here, assume that the notes follow a similar pattern twice a week for several months.

Jan. 4, 2009
    S: No new complaints today.
    O: Today we worked on fine motor skills using blocks and pegs.
    A: Susie tolerated everything fairly well today.
    P: Continue OT 2x/wk per plan of care.

Jan. 6, 2009
    S: No new complaints today.
    O: Today we worked on functional activities for fine motor development including large and small pegs, using hand over hand assistance as needed.
    A: Susie tolerated everything fairly well today.
    P: Continue OT 2x/wk per plan of care.

Feb. 11, 2009
    S: No new complaints today.
    O: Today we worked on:
        1) Grasp and release using small pegs and a pegboard
        2) Gross motor coordination using adaptive scissors
        3) Spatial relationships by stacking measuring cups
        4) Writing
    A: Susie tolerated everything fairly well today.
    P: Continue per POC 2x/wk.

March 17, 2009
    S: No new complaints today.
    O: Today we worked on PNF diagonal patterns by reaching for things while sitting on a large ball, weight-bearing by rocking back and forth while on all fours, throwing beanbags to work on grasp/release, and turning pages of a book.
    A: Susie tolerated everything fairly well today.
    P: Continue OT 2x/wk per plan of care.

FIGURE 13.1   Bad Example of SOAP Notes (#1).

lack any really useful information. Figure 13.2 shows two SOAP notes where the objective and assessment sections contain information that belongs in the other section or have assessment statements that are not supported by objective information.

The client, Susie, is a 4-year-old girl with cerebral palsy, who is seen in an outpatient rehabilitation center. Although only a few notes are shown here, assume that the notes follow a similar pattern twice a week for several months.

Jan. 4, 2009
    S: "No"
    O: Today we worked on fine motor skills using blocks and pegs. She cannot seem to get a stack of more than three 1" cubes without knocking it down in the process of adding the fourth block. She lacks coordination to stack them higher. Using a whole hand grip on large pegs, she placed six in a row before she refused to do anymore.
    A: Susie did fairly well today. She was less resistive to fine motor tasks.
    P: Continue OT 2x/wk per plan of care.

Jan. 6, 2009
    S: "No"
    O: Today we worked on functional activities for fine motor development including large and small pegs. She needed hand-over-hand assistance with the small pegs. She could pick them up between her thumb and index finger, but could not get them to stand up in the holes.
    A: Susie needs to continue to work on fine motor tasks. She was unable to stack four or more 1" blocks.
    P: Continue OT 2x/wk per plan of care.

Feb. 11, 2009
    S: Ø
    O: Today we worked on:
            1) Grasp and release using small pegs and a pegboard to make a big square shape. She didn't seem to understand the concept of alternating colors to make a pattern.
            2) Fine motor coordination using adaptive scissors. She made a few snips on a piece of paper, but threw the scissors down when the OT tried to guide her to cut along a line.
            3) Spatial relationships by nesting measuring cups. She nested three cups (1/4 c., 1/2 c., 1 c.). She liked this activity, nesting and unnesting them repeatedly.
            4) Writing. She scribbled with a large crayon. She refused to make an S.
    A: Susie did fairly well today. She seems to be getting used to working with the occupational therapist.
    P: Continue per POC 2x/wk.

March 17, 2009
    S: "OK"
    O: Today we worked on PNF diagonal patterns by reaching for things while sitting on a large ball. She pulled plastic figures off a shelf and dropped them in a bucket. We worked on weight-bearing by rocking back and forth while on all fours. Once she got started rocking she didn't want to stop; she appeared overstimulated and excited. We worked on throwing beanbags to work on grasp/release, as well as turning the pages of a book. She is doing better at quickly releasing objects.
    A: Susie had a great day! She was happy throughout the session.
    P: Continue OT 2x/wk per plan of care.

FIGURE 13.2   Bad Example of SOAP Notes (#2).

Exercise 13.7

Write the P section for each of the three cases in Exercise 13.5.

        Case 1: Client with severe arthritis
            P:

Case 2: Client with sensory defensiveness
P:

Case 3: Client with left-side neglect
P:

Exercise 13.8

Label the following statements according to where they would best belong in a SOAP note. Use "S" for subjective, "O" for objective, "A" for assessment, and "P" for plan. Then use these statements to write one coherent SOAP note. You may add transitional phrases to make the note flow better.

1. _____ The client sat on the side of the bed waiting for dressing direction.
2. _____ The client is unable to initiate dressing.
3. _____ She walks to the kitchen when dressed carrying her purse, ready to go to day care.
4. _____ When told what clothes to put on she gets dressed.
5. _____ What am I supposed to wear?
6. _____ The buttons on her blouse are not lined up.
7. _____ While sitting there, she removes her nightclothes.
8. _____ Clothing will be carefully placed in proper sequence and laid out the night before, so the client can see the clothes on the chair when she gets up.
9. _____ When given cues, can dress herself with minor errors.
10. _____ She puts her anklets on under her TED stockings.

S:

O:

A:

P:

Exercise 13.9

Analyze the following SOAP notes. Tell what is good about them and what needs improvement.

Case 1: Client is a 78-year-old woman who had a stroke affecting her left side 3 months ago. Her left arm has been in a sling with only a little active range of motion in her elbow and shoulder. Then 3 days ago, she fell outside on the sidewalk, breaking her right arm. It is now in a cast. She is now attending an intensive program to facilitate movement in her left arm (constraint induced movement therapy [CIMT]).

S: "I felt so helpless with two useless arms. I can't believe I was able to feed myself with my left arm."

O: Client participated in 6 hours of outpatient occupational therapy today. Fitted with a universal cuff, she was able to feed herself using a spoon, with minimal spillage. It required her to use both elbow flexion and trunk movements to get the applesauce scooped up and into her mouth. It was the first time she had fed herself since breaking her arm.

A: Client is making progress in the functional use of her left arm. She was not able to get the spoon to her mouth yesterday.

P: Continue participation in CIMT program 6 days per week as established in plan of care. Provide adaptive equipment as needed.

Case 2: Client is a 19-year-old man who lost his left arm in a farm accident (he is right-handed) 3 weeks ago.

S: "I still can't believe my arm is gone. It's unreal. There are times I swear I can still feel it, like a fly crawling on it, but when I look there's nothing there. Nothing."

O: Withdraws from light touch within 1.5 inches of wound. He demonstrated proper stump wrapping technique. Instructed on how to massage area in preparation for artificial arm.

A: Stump is healing well, and he is on track for getting an artificial arm. He is ready to be fitted with a temporary arm.

P: OT bid, 6 days per week, to reduce sensitivity of stump, prepare stump for artificial arm, and begin training in the use of an artificial arm.

▼ DAP NOTES ▼

DAP notes are very similar to SOAP notes in that each letter stands for one section of the note: **D**escription, **A**ssessment, and **P**lan. This format is less common than either the narrative or SOAP note. They can also be called FIP notes, as in **F**indings, **I**nterpretation, and **P**lan.

The description (findings) section is much like a combination of the "S" and "O" section of a SOAP note. In this section, you describe what you see and hear during the occupational therapy session. It can include quotes, paraphrases, observations, measurements, or test results. This is where you provide evidence that you are making progress. Be sure that everything in this section is fact based, and not a conclusion or inference on your part.

The "A" and "P" ("I" and "P" for FIP notes) sections are exactly like those in SOAP.

Figures 13.3 and 13.4 show examples of DAP notes.

Note 1: Helen, Alzheimer's client in day care setting

D: Upon entering the building, Helen waited for her daughter to tell her which way to turn. "Where do I go? What do I do?" Once in the room, she helped herself to a cup of coffee. Then she sat down and sipped her coffee until she received further instructions. She imitated the exercises that the group leader demonstrated. Halfway through the exercise group, she stood up, put her coffee cup in the garbage, and thanked everyone for a pleasant experience. She started to leave the room. She blushed and hid her face when told that the group was not over yet.

A: Helen appears to be dependent on the verbal cues of others in her environment to direct her behavior. In the absence of verbal cues, she gets confused.

P: Pair verbal and visual cues for Helen, or use verbal cues alone. Continue to encourage participation in small-group activities. Provide a structured environment with a consistent, posted schedule.

Bobbi Babinski, OTR/L 11/2/2009

FIGURE 13.3 Example of DAP Notes (#1).

FIGURE 13.4   Example of DAP Notes (#2).

Exercise 13.10

Write concise SOAP notes and DAP notes for the following cases.

Case 1: Toddler boy with seizure disorder and sensory processing disorder (sensory hyper-sensitivity)

Tommy was brought to the therapy clinic today by his father. Although Tommy has been here twice a week for the last 3 months, and has always seen the same occupational therapist, he was resistant to separating from his father and coming with the OT. He held on to his father and refused to let go. His father described breakfast this morning as very difficult. Tommy threw his sippy cup, refusing to drink from it. He spit out his oatmeal and pushed the spoon away. He asked for his bottle, and after a while dad gave up and gave Tommy his bottle. Tommy refused to sit in a chair in the clinic, so Tommy's dad held him in his lap at the table. Cheerios® and Cheetos® were placed on the table. Tommy picked up a piece of the cereal and put it in his mouth. He held it in his mouth while putting two more pieces in. He gagged on them. Next he tried Cheetos®. He smiled when he tasted it, but spit it out rather than swallow it once it softened in his mouth. He saw the orange residue on his hand and started flapping his hand and screaming. He allowed his father to wipe it off with a damp cloth. He took three sips of milk from a covered cup. He withdrew when his father tried to wipe his chin with the same cloth. His father then sat Tommy on the floor (carpeted), but Tommy immediately stood up and started bouncing up and down. The OT tried to engage Tommy in playing with toy cars made of smooth plastic. He held on to one for 5 seconds, another for 3 seconds. He watched the whole minute the OT played with the cars, but did not make any attempt to reach out and grab any cars. When presented with a toy tree that was bristly, Tommy refused to touch it. He kept two fingers (usually his left hand, but occasionally his right) in his mouth throughout most of the session. He cried and tried to jump off a low platform swing. Next Tommy was brought by his dad over to the water table. Tommy watched for a minute or two, but refused to put his own hands in, no matter how the OT or his dad begged him to try it. Tommy rolled a ball between himself, the OT, and his dad for a couple minutes. Although the OT and his dad sat on the floor, Tommy remained standing. He did allow his dad to put him on the floor with his legs spread like the OT and dad, but he only stayed like that for about 10 seconds. This is longer than he has ever stayed on the floor before in the clinic. At about halfway through the session, he left dad and held the OT's hand as they walked over to the easel. Dad stayed by the door. After about 2 minutes, Tommy stopped scribbling and began to

---

look for dad, dropped everything, and ran to hug dad around the knees. They sat back down at the table again and tried the Cheetos® again. This time the OT held one while Tommy licked the orange coating. He said it tasted good. The OT asked Tommy to copy her while she demonstrated chewing without food in her mouth. Tommy moved his lower jaw up and down. Then she demonstrated taking a small bite of Cheetos®, chewing and swallowing it. Tommy imitated her, and swallowed a small piece. He did this three times before starting to gag. OT discussed with dad the possibility of trying the copying game at home at mealtime. Also discussed trying to engage Tommy in games where he sits on the floor. First try it with long pants on, then in shorts. Since some progress was observed today, I recommend continuing services twice a week.

S:

O:

A:

P:

D:

A:

P:

Case 2: 82-year-old woman who fractured the head of her left femur and then had a heart attack trying to crawl to a phone in her bedroom. She has been in the hospital for 10 days and is transferring to a transitional care facility in 2 days.

Mrs. Anderssen was seen today in her room for work on toilet transfers and dressing. She transfers from bed to wheelchair with minimal assist using a transfer belt and a pivot transfer. This is an improvement, since she was requiring moderate assist 2 days ago. She propelled herself to the bathroom and washed her face and upper body with a washcloth independently. The toilet seat is raised to same height as wheelchair seat. Toilet also has handrails. Client locked the wheelchair at a right angle to the toilet, put both hands on the arms of her wheelchair, and using both arms and her right leg raised herself to standing. She moved her right hand to the toilet rail, pivoted on her right leg, and sat down on the toilet with stand-by assistance. She independently obtained and used toilet paper. She reached behind her and flushed the toilet while still sitting. Then she again used her arms and right leg to stand and then used a pivot transfer with minimal assist to get back to the wheelchair. She reports that except when OT is in her room, the nurses give her a lot of assist with toilet transfers. She has not yet tried toileting independently while wearing street clothes, which would require her to worry about adjusting her clothing. We will attempt to do it this afternoon.

She propelled herself into her room and in front of her closet. From her closet she used a long-handled reacher to get a hanger down from the hanging rod. She removed a sweat suit and replaced the hanger, again using the reacher. Then she got her bra and panties out of a drawer. She removed her gown and put on her bra (using the hook in front, then twisting it around and pulling up the straps) and sweatshirt without assistance. Next she used a sock aid to put on anklets. It took three tries and some verbal cues, but she did do it without physical assist. Then she used the dressing stick to put her panties and pants on and pull them just over her knees. This was a slow process and she expressed some frustration at how tired and slow she felt. Until she fell, she was a very active woman and participated in a local mall-walking club. It is probably because she was in good condition for her age that she has made the progress that she has. She slid her feet into Velcro sneakers with a long shoehorn. She pushed herself up to standing, pausing for a couple seconds to make sure her balance was good. She steadied herself with her left hand on the bed. Finally, she pulled her panties and pants the rest of the way up and then sat back down in her chair. The entire process of washing, toileting, and dressing took 35 minutes. She reports that it used to take her 10 minutes to do all that, although she didn't have to use all that extra equipment. She is progressing as planned. OTR left instructions for undressing with both Mrs. Anderssen and the nursing staff.

S:

O:

A:

P:

D:

A:

P:

▼ NARRATIVE NOTES ▼

If the narrative progress note is written directly in the client's medical record, it is usually done in a section of the medical record set aside for that purpose. Notes are entered as close to the time of intervention as possible since the notes are expected to be in chronological order. Therefore, narrative notes written directly in the medical record need to be dated, and often the time the note was written is also recorded (Fremgen, 2006; Ranke, 1998). Since the pages of the progress note section of a client's medical record already contain the client's identifying information, there is no need to repeat it in the note. The length of time of the intervention session is usually recorded.

How do you show that your client is making progress? The easy way would be to write "The client is making progress." However, this would be woefully inadequate. Why should anyone reading the record take your word for it? You have to show that the client is doing something now that he or she could not do before; you have to show a change in the client's occupational performance.

Figure 13.5, shows three examples of narrative notes.

Narrative format is often used to write a contact note. This is a note written to document contact with a client, usually, but not necessarily, during a therapy session. For example, a contact note may be written when you instruct a caregiver in proper transfer techniques or splint care. A contact note could be written to document the reason for a missed intervention session. A contact note might also be used to document that you met the client and scheduled the client to come to the occupational therapy room to begin the evaluation (or

Note 1: Helen is an 84 y.o. female with Alzheimer's disease.
She receives OT on a monthly consultative basis.

Helen attended her day program for people with Alzheimer's 5 days a week for the past month. She received social and recreational programming, one congregate meal, a short rest period each day, and occupational therapy consultation. In addition to Alzheimer's, the client has high blood pressure and circulatory problems in her left leg. She wears a TED stocking. Her medications are stable. She is a widow of 2 years.

Helen helped herself to coffee without asking for permission or directions. She stayed with the morning exercise group for about 20 minutes (it is a 45-minute group) each day. At about that time, she typically got up to throw her coffee cup away, and tried to continue on out of the room. Helen allowed the group leader to redirect her back to the group, and then she continued to participate in the exercises until she was told that the group is over. Then she asked what was next. When asked the name of the program, she said she was not sure she ever knew the name of it.

Helen has been consistent in her behavior for the last month. According to staff, she is less agitated since moving into small-group activities instead of the large group she was in 2 months ago. She is dependent on verbal cues for the completion of most activities. She expresses her confusion with frequent questions.

Helen will continue to attend the 5x/wk Alzheimer's program. Staff will provide her with a highly structured, small-group experience. The client will continue to ask many questions, and these will be responded to in short, simple sentences. Staff will post a daily schedule near the clock.

Bobbi Babinski, OTR/L Nov. 1, 2009

Note 2: 27 y.o. with LCVA (Bob)

Bob participated in a 30-minute session to work on functional activities with his unaffected (non-dominant) hand. Bob attempted to use a computer mouse with his left hand by playing a game of solitaire. He moved quickly to the general area that he wants the mouse to be. He moved slowly and hesitantly to the precise spot he needed; however, he often overshot the mark. Bob clicked the mouse with his index finger easily; however, he had minimal success holding the mouse button down while dragging the mouse, such as when he wanted to move a card to a different pile. He expressed concern about how much more he had to concentrate on the movements than he had to when he used his right hand. It took 20 minutes to complete one game of solitaire.

Carrie Ingwater, COTA/L 3/2/09

Bobbi Babinski, OTR/L 3/2/2009

Note 3: 9-month-old infant who was found blue
(not breathing) in her crib 2 weeks ago

Rina was seen today for a 30-minute session. She did not make eye contact with the occupational therapist, but she did respond to sound and to touch. She did not try to locate a toy by sight, but when a rattle was touched to her fingertips or the back of her hand, she turned her hand to grasp the rattle and shake it. From a prone position, she rolled to the right and to the left in response to noise. She rolled in a straight line to her right but was slower and less direct rolling to her left. Mild ATNR present, stronger when her head is turned to the left. Rina supported her weight on her right arm when prone on elbows with a toy in her left hand. After three attempts, she was not able to support her weight on her left arm when prone on elbows with a toy in her right hand. While she is able to use both arms to reach and grasp for toys, she is showing greater strength and endurance on her right side. Her vision continues to appear impaired. The plan is to continue to see Rina twice a day for the duration of her hospitalization to work on movement and play skills and to monitor for any sign of returning vision.

Stephanie Smith, OTR/L 7/02/09

FIGURE 13.5 Examples of Narrative Notes.

for you to come to the client's room and begin the evaluation there if that is the plan). In a case like this, the contact note might look like this:

> Saw Mrs. Smith in her room today. Explained what occupational therapy is and that she was referred to occupational therapy to work on her self-care skills. She said she understood her doctor's concern, but that she was sure that her left side was not affected by the stroke and that she really did not want to waste my time when I could be helping someone who really needs my help. She agreed to humor me and come to the occupational therapy clinic this afternoon at 1:30. I told her I would send an aide to come and bring her to the clinic. Britta Farver, OTR/L, 9-23-09

or

> Went to client's room to bring her to the clinic. She said she felt really nauseous today, and a bit light-headed and would prefer to skip this afternoon's session. Checked with the nurse who was aware of the situation and concurred that she should not participate in occupational therapy this afternoon. Mika Vica, OTR/L, 9-23-09

Exercise 13.11

Write a narrative progress note based on the following cases:

Case 1: Kiki is a 6-year-old receiving occupational therapy following a car accident. She had a severe head injury. Last week she visually tracked a toy while supine over a 60° horizontal arc. She did not reach for the toy. During passive ROM to her upper extremities, she cried out with each movement. She was dependent in all her ADLs. This week, she tracked the toy while sitting over a 90° arc horizontally and 40° vertically. She cried out during shoulder passive ROM, but not during elbow, wrist, or hand PROM. Showing about 10° active ROM in Ⓡ elbow spontaneously, but not on command. She remains dependent in all her ADLs. She received occupational therapy twice a day, 5 days this week, and once on Saturday.

Note:

Case 2: 88-year-old woman with osteoarthritis in her knees, COPD, and diabetic neuropathy, who received home-based occupational therapy following hospitalization for pneumonia, resulting in diminished strength and endurance. She received occupational therapy twice a week, and you write a note after each visit. Her goals are to prepare light meals for breakfast and dinner (Meals on Wheels for lunch), dress and undress herself without fatigue, and safe showers. In addition, the client wants to be able to take care of her houseplants and play solitaire, even though holding things in her hands is difficult. During this 45-minute visit, occupational therapy worked on using a kitchen stool to sit on while preparing a meal, shower transfers using the bath bench you brought for her to try, and trying adaptive equipment for dressing and card playing. (*Write the narrative note, using an educated guess on how much progress she has made since you saw her 3 days ago.*)

Note:

▼ PROGRESS FLOW SHEETS ▼

Flow sheets can show the progress a client is making on specific activities in a very concise way. Flow sheets are typically tables or graphs where measurements can be recorded at regular intervals, generally after each intervention session. It makes it easy for the reader to see at a glance whether progress is being made in a particular area of need for a client. For example, you could chart the length of time it takes for your client to complete a meal, the number of dishes the client unloaded from a dishwasher and put away in a cabinet, or the degrees of active range of motion of a client's wrist. When progress flow sheets are used, then the narrative, SOAP, or DAP note may be written weekly or biweekly rather than after every intervention session.

There are several advantages of using flow sheets to track progress. One is that they are easier to read than lengthy progress notes. The data recorded is kept to a minimum, and is organized in an easy-to-follow format. Second, instead of relying on someone saying a client has made progress, you have solid, objective data that shows the progress. Another advantage is a flow sheet contains a lot of data but uses minimal space, so it conserves paper. Using a flow chart keeps the clinician focused on interventions that are specific to the client's goals, and less chance to go off on tangents. It makes it easy for a substitute clinician to know what to expect a client to do in the next occupational therapy session. Third, flow charts provide reliable data that can be used to write progress summaries. In those settings where progress notes are written weekly or biweekly, a clinician who can reflect that data off the flow sheet will have written a more reliable note than one who writes from memory alone. This is particularly helpful if the client's medical record is ever called into court.

There are also disadvantages to using flow sheets. Often, there is space enough to record a number or other objective measurement, but not room for descriptions of performance. There is no place to record the client's reaction to the intervention. There may be a place to record new interventions, but there may not be, depending on the form used.

Figure 13.6 is a sample progress flow sheet for an adult with mental retardation being seen in a sheltered workshop. In this case, only brief objective data is recorded.

Intervention \ Date	6-4-09	6-6-09	6-8-09	6-11-09	6-13-09	6-15-09	6-18-09	6-20-09	6-22-09	6-24-09	6-26-09
Number of correct packets assembled independently	6	6	7	6	7	7	7	8	7	8	
Number of times in a 30-min period client needed redirection	8	9	8	8	7	6	8	6	6	5	
Degree of assist needed in lunch line (dep = 5, max = 4, mod = 3, min = 2, indep = 1, P = physical, V = verbal)	3P 4V	3P 4V	3P 3V	3P 3V	2P 3V	3P 3V	3P 4V	2P 3V	2P 3V	2P 3V	
Number of times during lunch client engages in self-stimulatory behavior	6	7	6	6	6	6	5	6	5	5	
Initials	KC TC	KC	KC	KC	KC	KC	KC TC	KC	KC	KC	

Signatures:		
Initials:	Name:	Credentials
KC	Katie Clapsaddle	OTS
TC	Thomas Carter	OTD

FIGURE 13.6 Sample Progress Flow Sheet (A).

Goal area	Date: 7-20-09	Date: 7-22-09	Date: 7-24-09	Date:
Dresses self in 15 min or less with no more than 2 cues Feed self meal w/o spilling	21 min 2 v cues 1 phys prompt Breakfast: Used fork; no spilling when stabbing meat, but did spill 3x when scooping eggs	21 min 1 v cue 1 phys prompt Breakfast: Used fork for eggs, fingers for meat; eggs fell off 2x	19 min 1 v cue 1 phys prompt Breakfast: Used spoon for oatmeal; no spilling	
Actively participate in one group activity per day	Attended bingo game when aide escorted her, but did not play	Attended current events group, made 1 comment in 30-min session	Attended current events group, made 2 comments in 30-min session	
Develop a repertoire of individual activities (6) in which to engage	Discussed former hobbies; used to enjoy crocheting, knitting, reading magazines and novels, cooking, walking, and dog grooming.	Showed her where magazines are kept for resident use and provided library cart schedule. Provided a large crochet hook and her choice of yarns.	Resident has 6 inches of a scarf crocheted. Reports that her hands hurt after a while. Told her about a program to crochet afghans for kids at homeless shelter.	
Provider name	Mo Chu Yan, COTA/L	Mo Chu Yan, COTA/L	Mo Chu Yan, COTA/L	

FIGURE 13.7 Sample Progress Flow Sheet (B).

Figure 13.7 is a sample of a progress flow sheet for a woman in a nursing home. The therapist records objective data in the appropriate box. It does allow for observations to be recorded as well as number of cues, number of repetitions, time to complete task, or whatever measure is included in the goal. Some forms use short-term goals rather than a problem statement.

In some settings, there may be a separate flow sheet for each goal area. If this is the case, you can graph progress. For example, if you were working on having a client with schizophrenia and attention deficit disorder (ADD) increase attention to task, you could graph the amount of time the client worked on a task before his first redirection, or the number of redirections in a 1-hour session. The graphs might look like Figure 13.8. You can see at a glance that progress is being made, even before you read the data. Figure 13.9 shows a type of bar graph, but you could use a line graph where you connect the dots plotted like this as well.

Flow sheets must be signed at the bottom of the page, but each entry is usually simply initialed. There can be a key at the bottom that looks like the one on the bottom of Figure 13.8. This lets readers know who worked with the client on what day.

Progress flow sheets cannot entirely replace progress notes. They may decrease the frequency with which progress notes are written from daily to weekly or biweekly in some settings. Not every setting uses progress flow sheets.

▼ ATTENDANCE LOGS ▼

Attendance logs, at minimum, identify when the client had therapy. Many also identify which occupational therapy personnel worked with the client that day, and how long the therapy session was. Some also identify which type of intervention happened during which

Maximum uninterrupted time attending to task:										
15 min										
14 min										
13 min										
12 min										
11 min										
10 min										
9 min										
8 min										
7 min										
6 min										
5 min										
4 min										
3 min										
2 min										
1 min										
Task	1	1	1	2	2	2	3	3	3	3
Date 2009	9-8	9-9	9-10	9-11	9-14	9-15	9-16	9-17	9-18	9-21
Initials	KS	KS	KS	KS	CJ	KS	KS	KS	KS	KS

Tasks: 1 = wipe tables   2 = put chairs on tables   3 = vacuum

Signatures:

Initials:	Name:
KS	Katrina Sanchez, MA, OTR/L
CJ	Cecilia Jorgenson, COTA/L

FIGURE 13.8   Sample Progress Graph.

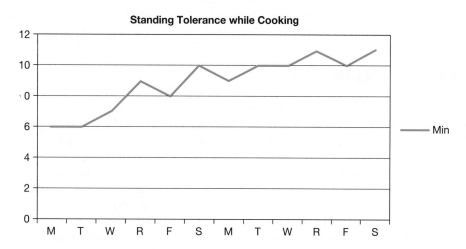

Dates: August 17–29, 2009

FIGURE 13.9   Progress Graph.

intervention session. An attendance log can be used for billing therapy services if it is designed to be compatible with the billing system used at that facility.

Most commonly, I have seen attendance logs on a clipboard in the department with a separate page for each client. When the client is discontinued, the attendance log may go in the client's permanent record, the department file, or the billing office, depending on facility policy.

Attendance logs can be set up much like the first example of a flow chart, with dates across the top and interventions listed along one side. If the attendance log is used for billing, then the interventions are labeled so that they coincide with billing codes. In the box that correlates to the date and intervention, the clinician records the number of billable units of that intervention, or the number of minutes of that intervention. The biggest difference between the attendance log and the flow sheet is the attendance log does not include any data on the client's performance, only that a particular intervention was worked on.

▼ PHOTOGRAPHIC AND VIDEO DOCUMENTATION ▼

It is often said that a picture is worth a thousand words. If that is the case, then it would seem logical that visual evidence of a client's performance would strengthen the documentation. With the availability of digital cameras, visual documentation is getting easier and less cumbersome.

There are several ways in which visual evidence can be used. Still pictures of proper positioning of a client can be used both as an educational aid for clients and/or caregivers and as evidence of the caregiver/client education in the medical record. Before-and-after intervention pictures of resting hand position, posture, range of motion, sensory tolerance, or other intervention provide eloquent evidence of the effect of intervention.

Video can be used to show how a client functions in a particular environment to aid in the evaluation process (Kashman, Mora, & Glaser, 2000). A video camera can be less intrusive than adding a person into an environment for the purpose of observing behavior. The video can capture antecedents to behavior, such as with a child with autism. By using video, an occupational therapist can replay the event to look for details in both the environment and client to help in understanding behavior (Kashman et al.). A video can also be used to document the client carrying out an activity, as proof that the client understood the instructions.

Using video or photographic documentation raises issues of privacy and confidentiality. Many facilities have policies and procedures to govern the use of video or photographic documentation which must be followed very carefully. Some require a separate release form before photos or video can be taken, some include it in the general release form signed by the client or responsible party upon admission. Always check to see what the facility policy and procedure are before taking any pictures.

▼ MEDICARE COMPLIANCE ▼

Medicare requires a progress report (progress note) at least every 10 treatment days or once every 30 calendar days, whichever is less (Centers for Medicare and Medicaid Services [CMS], 2008). The progress report must be signed by the occupational therapist providing the interventions or supervising the occupational therapy assistant who is providing the interventions. The progress report should contain a description of progress; plans for continuation or discontinuation of treatment; plans to change long- or short-term goals; and statements of the client's rehabilitation potential—that "maximum improvement is yet to be attained" (CMS, p. 35) and that the expected improvement is likely to occur in a "reasonable and generally predictable period of time" (CMS, p. 36). If you are using a SOAP format for your progress note, these items belong in the "A" section, and clear, objective data to support the "A" belong in the "O" section.

Medicare also requires documentation of "all treatments and skilled interventions" (CMS, 2008, p. 36) in a treatment note. The treatment note is written for every treatment session, and will be used to compare to billing statements as verification that the services billed for were delivered (CMS). If your treatment note contains the information required in a progress report, you do not need to write additional progress reports. Each treatment note should contain the date of service, the specific interventions provided and billed, the total time the client received treatment during that session, the total of the "timed code treatment minutes" (CMS, p. 37), and the signature of the occupational therapy practitioner who provided the service (and cosignature of the occupational therapist if the service was provided by an occupational therapy assistant). Medicare says that optional information that can be included in the treatment note includes patient self-report (the "S" of your note), any adverse reactions to an intervention, any "significant, unusual or unexpected changes in clinical status" (CMS, p. 38), equipment provided to the client, communication you have with another provider of services about your client, and anything else you think is important to document (CMS).

SUMMARY

In this chapter we explored documentation of intervention, including three types of progress notes. The narrative note is written in paragraph form, and often reads as if one is telling a story, which is in fact what one is doing. SOAP (subjective, objective, assessment, plan) and DAP (description, assessment, plan) perform the same function as narrative notes, but do it in a prescribed fashion. Progress notes do not simply list activities, but describe what progress has been made, how the client reacted to the interventions, and what functional skills the client has demonstrated.

SOAP notes are used by many health care disciplines in many settings. The "S" part of the note is where subjective information, such as the client's perspective on the problem, is recorded. The "O" is for objective data, the information about what the client did without judgment or interpretation. In the "A" section, you make sense out of the information in the "S" and "O" sections by interpreting it and assessing it. Finally, in the "P" section, you state what you plan to do with the client so that the client can achieve his or her goals.

DAP notes are also sometimes called FIP (findings, interpretation, plan) notes. They are very similar to SOAP notes. In the "D" section, you combine the subjective and objective information that would normally be recorded in separate sections in a SOAP note. In the "A" section you assess the meaning of the information in the "D" section, and in the "P" section you record the plan.

Narrative notes contain the same information as SOAP and DAP but the information is not labeled as such; rather, it is written in paragraph format. Narrative notes may be written in great detail, or may only hit the high points. A specific kind of narrative note, a contact note, may be written to document contact with a client or client's caregiver (as part of an occupational therapy session or outside of regular sessions) or to document the reason for a missed intervention session.

Progress flow sheets and attendance logs were also discussed in this chapter. These documents provide information on when a client received intervention and, to a limited extent, what was worked on. These documents can supplement, but not replace, writing progress summaries.

The occupational therapist is responsible for ensuring that progress reports get written in accordance with standards and regulations for timeliness and content and are communicated to the client or other involved party (in accordance with privacy regulations). Occupational therapy assistants, under the supervision of an occupational therapist, contribute to the process. Either the occupational therapist or the occupational therapy assistant may write the progress report. In most situations, as part of routine supervision, the occupational therapist will cosign notes written by the occupational therapy assistant.

REFERENCES

American Occupational Therapy Association. (2005). Standards of practice for occupational therapy. *American Journal of Occupational Therapy, 59,* 663–665.

American Occupational Therapy Association. (2008). Guidelines for documentation of occupational therapy. *American Journal of Occupational Therapy 62,* 684–690.

Brennan, C, & Robinson, M. (2006). Documentation: Getting it right to avoid Medicare denials. *OT Practice, 11*(14) 10–15.

Borcherding, S. (2005). *Documentation manual for writing SOAP notes in occupational therapy* (2nd ed.). Thorofare, NJ: Slack.

Borcherding, S., & Kappel, C. (2002). *The OTA's guide to writing SOAP notes.* Thorofare, NJ: Slack.

Centers for Medicare and Medicaid Services. (2008). *Pub100-02 Medicare benefit policy: Transmittal 88.* Retrieved May 8, 2008, from http://www.cms.hhs.gov/transmittals/downloads/R88BP.pdf

Fremgen, B. F. (2006). *Medical law and ethics* (2nd ed.). Upper Saddle River, NJ: Prentice Hall.

Kashman, N., Mora, J., & Glaser, T. (July 3, 2000). *Using video tapes to evaluate children with autism.* Retrieved on October 3, 2008, from http://www.aota.org/Pubs/OTP/1997-2007/Features/2000/37217.aspx

Kettenbach, G. (2004). *Writing SOAP notes* (3rd ed.). Philadelphia: F. A. Davis.

Kuntavanish, A. A. (1988). *Occupational therapy documentation: A system to capture outcome data for quality assurance and program promotion.* Rockville, MD: American Occupational Therapy Association.

Quinn, L. & Gordon, J. (2003). *Functional outcomes: Documentation for rehabilitation.* St. Louis, MO: Saunders.

Ranke, B. A. E. (1998). Documentation in the age of litigation. *OT Practice, 3*(3), 20–24.

Sample Medical SOAP Note. (2002). Retrieved September 5, 2002, from http://cpmcnet.Columbia.edu/dept/ps/2002/SOAPmed.html

Tips on Medical Progress Notes. (2002). Retrieved September 5, 2002, from http://cpmcnet.Columbia.edu/dept/ps/2002/SOAPmed.html

CHAPTER 14

Discontinuation Summaries

INTRODUCTION

When the client achieves all of his or her goals, moves out of the facility, refuses to continue in the program, or achieves maximum benefit from occupational therapy, a discontinuation summary must be written (American Occupational Therapy Association [AOTA], 2005). This summary, also called a discharge summary or discharge report, needs to show the client's progress from the beginning of occupational therapy services to the end. It is the final justification of your services.

The terms "discontinuation" and "discharge" are distinct but overlapping terms. Discontinuation occurs when a client stops, or discontinues, services from a particular provider. The term "discontinuation" is used in *The Framework* (AOTA, 2008). The term "discharge" is often used to describe what happens when a client leaves a facility or clinic. The *Guidelines for Documentation of Occupational Therapy* (2007) uses the term discharge to describe the end of service delivery. Since services are often discontinued when a client is discharged, the words are often used interchangeably. In this book, the document that is written when a client stops receiving occupational therapy services is referred to as a discontinuation summary.

▼ ROLE DELINEATION IN DISCONTINUATION ▼

The occupational therapist determines when a client is ready to discontinue services (AOTA, 2005). The occupational therapy assistant may recommend discontinuing services to a client. The occupational therapist prepares, implements, and documents the discontinuation plan, including appropriate follow-up resources and reevaluation needs. The occupational therapy assistant contributes to the process of implementing the discontinuation plan and in documenting the changes in the client's engagement in occupations (AOTA, 2005, 2007).

▼ MEDICARE COMPLIANCE ▼

Medicare Part B (outpatient) requires a discontinuation summary (discharge summary) at the end of each episode of care (Centers for Medicare and Medicaid Services [CMS], 2008). If a comprehensive discharge summary is written by the physician, Medicare does not require the occupational therapist to write a separate discontinuation summary. When the occupational therapist writes the discharge summary, it covers the time period since the last progress report, ending on the day of discharge. If the discharge was "unanticipated in the plan or previous Progress Report, the clinician may base any judgments required to write the report on the Treatment Notes and verbal reports of the assistant or qualified personnel" (CMS, 2008, p. 33). Medicare Part A (inpatient) discontinuation follows the facility's policies for documenting discontinuation.

▼ COMPONENTS OF A DISCONTINUATION
SUMMARY ▼

In some facilities the discontinuation summary is an interdisciplinary effort. At a rehabilitation facility or rehabilitation unit of a hospital, members of the rehabilitation team may dictate their part of the summary, and have a secretary type up one report in a narrative format that includes information from occupational therapy, physical therapy, speech-language pathology, nursing, social work, psychology, and other represented disciplines. While dictation can save the clinical staff some time (you can talk faster than you can write), it requires a certain amount of skill. First, you have to speak clearly and spell out any terms that you think the secretary may not be familiar with. You have to identify the punctuation marks so the secretary knows when to include them. Be aware that every word or sound gets transcribed, so side conversations and "ums" and other "filler" words could show up in print. Long pauses waste time for the transcriber. You have to proofread the document for errors before you sign it. The advantage of the interdisciplinary format is that it gives a very complete picture of the client.

At other facilities there may be a paper or electronic form or format to follow for discontinuation summaries. Generally, no matter whether you dictate, fill out a form, or write the report electronically, the same basic information is provided. First, there is, as always, identifying information. Next is a summary of the occupational therapy services provided and the client's response to the intervention (AOTA, 2007). The *Guidelines for Documentation of Occupational Therapy* lists the following items that should be found in this part of the document (AOTA, 2007):

- Starting and ending dates of service
- Frequency/number of session
- Summary of the interventions provided
- Summary of the client's progress in occupational therapy goals
- Occupational therapy outcomes (engagement in occupations)
  - Initial status of client
  - Ending status of client
  - "Client's assessment of efficacy of occupational therapy" (AOTA, 2007, III.A.2.c.)
- Recommendations, including adaptive equipment, home programs, home adaptations, and specialized instructions

Finally, any follow-up plans or referrals to other professionals are documented. Of course, the occupational therapist signs and dates the document.

It is important to be comprehensive, yet concise when reporting on progress toward goals and occupational therapy outcomes. If a client has been receiving occupational therapy intervention for several months or more, you may want to focus more on the long-term goals than on each and every adjustment to short-term goals. However, if a client was seen for a few days to a few weeks, you may address each short-term goal.

When addressing the initial and ending status of the client in relation to engagement in occupations, the emphasis will clearly be on occupations rather than on changes in client factors, activity demands, or even contexts. However, contexts, especially those related to the client's discharge disposition, are very important. The client's discharge disposition is the place the client is being discharged to; it could be to the client's home, extended care facility, assisted living facility, home care, outpatient program, or other community-based service (Moyers, 1999). Your evaluation of the client's ending status is dependent on the discharge disposition.

In order to make appropriate recommendations for follow-up or referrals in the discontinuation summary, the discharge disposition is also essential (Moyers, 1999). If a client is being discharged to another facility, you need to know what services are available at that facility in order to make an appropriate referral. If the client will be receiving occupational therapy intervention at the new facility, it is helpful if the occupational therapists can talk with each other. However, in order to do that, permission to discuss the client's status must be obtained from the client or client's legal guardian in order to comply with confidentiality regulations (i.e., HIPAA;

see Chapter 6). If a client is being discharged to his or her home, community-based services can be recommended, but the occupational therapist has to know what kinds of services are available in the area. This is where working as a team with a social worker can be a real help. For example, you might recommend that a client participate in a community-based 12-step program (i.e., Alcoholics Anonymous), join a health club or community-based exercise program, or seek further help from a vocational rehab program (Moyers, 1999; Moyers & Dale, 2007).

You may recommend that the client come back in a few months for a recheck because you expect the client will progress or regress on his or her own and may need more occupational therapy at that time, or the client may have some medical interventions planned (e.g., surgery, botox injection) that will result in a change of functional status (Moyers, 1999). Orthotic devices or adaptive equipment may need to be checked periodically for wear and fit. For any of these reasons or others, recommending the client come back in three months for a recheck may be a good idea. However, if you make such a recommendation, be sure it is documented in the discharge summary.

Figure 14.1 shows a sample format for a discontinuation summary report. 14.2 shows a sample completed discontinuation summary report.

Occupational Therapy Discontinuation Report

Date of report: Name:
Date of birth &/or age: Date of initial referral: M   F
Primary intervention diagnosis/concern:
Secondary diagnosis/concern:
Precautions/contraindications:
Reason for referral to OT:
Reason for OT discontinuation:

Therapist: *(Print or type your name and credential; you will sign and date the report at the end.)*

Description of OT intervention: *(Include service delivery model, duration/frequency of interventions, # of intervention sessions or beginning and end dates of interventions, location of interventions, and types of interventions provided.)*

Brief summary of progress toward goals: *(Statements of progress toward or achievement of long-term goals or reasons why goals were not met.)*

Occupational therapy outcomes:
    Initial performance in areas of occupation:
    (Concise summary of the client's initial performance in the areas of activities of daily living, instrumental activities of daily living, education, work, play, leisure, and social participation.)

    Current level of performance in areas of occupation:
    (Concise summary of current performance and expectations for performance within the contexts of the client's anticipated environments following discontinuation.)

Contextual aspects related to discontinuation:
(Concise summary of the cultural, physical, social, personal, spiritual, temporal, and/or virtual contexts.)

Discontinuation recommendations:
(Concise description of discontinuation plans, other referrals, follow-up, home program suggestions, support systems, and caregiver suggestions.)

_____   _____
Signature   Date

FIGURE 14.1   Sample Discontinuation Summary Report Format.

Occupational Therapy Discontinuation Report

Date of report: Sept. 30, 2009   **Client's name:** Sadie Clapsaddle
Date of birth/age: March 26, 1980   **Date of initial referral:** Sept. 23, 2009   M   (F)
Primary intervention diagnosis/concern: Depression with suicide attempt
Secondary intervention diagnoses/concerns: History of cutting
Precautions/contraindications: Do not allow to use sharp instruments without close supervision. Count sharps at end of session.
Reason for referral to OT: Evaluate and treat for depression. Increase self-esteem.
Reason for discontinuation of OT: Completed 7-day inpatient program.

Therapist: Carla McShane, OTR/L

Description of OT intervention:
Sadie was seen in the occupational therapy clinic twice a day for 6 of the 7 days she was here. Provided with unconditional support and encouragement. Participated in self-esteem and assertiveness group as well as task group.

Brief summary of progress toward goals:
Sadie's initial goal for herself was to begin to get involved in activities that interested her in the past. She used to paint, but stopped painting when her children were little. Her children are now teenagers. She also wanted to learn to say "no" to members of her family who demanded that she do things for them, without feeling guilty and changing her mind because of it. She met both goals.

Occupational therapy outcomes:
Initial performance in areas of occupation:
Sadie initially sat with her head down; she did not initiate conversation or activities. She was compliant with all therapist requests. She said nothing interested her anymore. Sadie did not initiate any interactions with peers or staff. She did not comb her hair unless she was told to do it. She reported that prior to her hospitalization she just sat at home doing nothing. She was not interested in painting, a hobby she gave up 14 years ago when she had her first child.

Current level of performance in areas of occupation:
During her week here, she rehearsed saying "no" during role-playing exercises with the therapist. By the end of the week, when the therapist would ask Sadie for favors like "Could you clean up the sink?" Sadie said "no" and stuck with that answer. If the therapist asked for volunteers to do something, Sadie literally sat on her hands to keep from volunteering. With the help of the occupational therapist, Sadie signed up for a painting class through Sadie's local community education program. Sadie reports that she is excited about taking a painting class. She said she liked the paintings she made in occupational therapy. She met with her husband and children and told them that they had to start doing some things for themselves when she came home. They agreed to take on some of the work she usually does. Sadie said she was amazed that her family was so unaware of her feelings. She made a commitment to express her feelings on a more regular basis, and they agreed not to "blow her off." Sadie is returning to her home with twice-a-week outpatient visits with a counselor.

Contextual aspects related to discontinuation:
Home has been a stressful place for Sadie, but she and her family say they are committed to making things less stressful by sharing Sadie's load.

Discontinuation recommendations:
Sadie will participate in counseling sessions twice a week. She will attend a painting class through community education.

Carla McShane, OTR/L   _Sept. 30, 2009_
Signature   Date

FIGURE 14.2   Sample Discontinuation Report.

▼ SOAP FORMAT ▼

Some facilities use the SOAP format for their discontinuation summaries (Borcherding, 2005; Borcherding & Kappel, 2002; Kettenbach, 2004). In a discontinuation note, the "S" would describe something the client said about her progress, or the client's subjective description of current function. The "O" would report objective data regarding performance in areas of occupation. This can include both initial and ending data. The "A" would articulate your assessment or interpretation of the data in "O." You would summarize those areas where significant progress occurred and identify areas where progress was not made. The "P" would be where you indicate home program instructions, follow-up recommendations, and referrals to other professionals. Figure 14.3 shows a sample format for a SOAP-based discontinuation summary. Figure 14.4 shows a SOAP-based discontinuation summary for the same client as in Figure 14.2.

Occupational Therapy Discontinuation Report

Date of report: Name:
Date of birth &/or age: Date of initial referral: M   F
Primary intervention diagnosis/concern:
Secondary diagnosis/concern:
Precautions/contraindications:
Reason for referral to OT:
Reason for OT discontinuation:

Therapist: *(Print or type your name and credential; you will sign and date the report at the end.)*

S: *(Client's subjective description of progress or occupational performance)*

O: *(Description of occupational therapy services)*

Long-term Goal	Short-term Goal	Methods/Approaches

A: *(Your assessment [interpretation] of progress)*

P: *(Home programs, follow-up recommendations, and referrals to other professionals)*

_____   _____
Signature   Date

FIGURE 14.3   Sample Discontinuation Report, SOAP Format.

Occupational Therapy Discontinuation Report

Date of report: Sept. 30, 2009   **Client's name:** Sadie Clapsaddle

Date of birth/age: March 26, 1980   **Date of initial referral:** Sept. 23, 2009   M   F

Primary intervention diagnosis/concern: Depression with suicide attempt

Secondary intervention diagnoses/concerns: History of cutting

Precautions/contraindications: Do not allow to use sharp instruments without close supervision. Count sharps at end of session.

Reason for referral to OT: Evaluate and treat for depression. Increase self-esteem.

Reason for discontinuation of OT: Completed 7-day inpatient program.

Therapist: Carla McShane, OTR/L

S: "I am looking forward to the painting class. It will be like taking a 'mini-vacation' twice a week."

O: Sadie was seen in the occupational therapy clinic twice a day for 6 of the 7 days she was here. Provided with unconditional support and encouragement. Participated in self-esteem and assertiveness group as well as task group.

Long-term goals	Initial performance	Ending performance
Sadie will say "no" and stick to that answer.	Client complied with all requests of the occupational therapist.	Client said "no" to three requests on last 2 days of OT, did not change her answer.
Look people in the eye, maintain eye contact for 10 seconds.	Client looked down, did not make eye contact.	Maintained eye contact with therapist and peer for 10 seconds on six occasions in last 2 days of OT.
Engage in painting with watercolors.	Started painting after several prompts.	Independently initiated painting upon entering OT clinic. Signed up to take painting class through community education.

A: Client made good progress. She achieved all of her goals. She is taking steps to take charge of her life, such as taking a painting class, talking with her family and negotiating shared workloads, and not backing down once she says "no"?

P: Sadie will participate in counseling sessions twice a week. She will attend a painting class through community education.

Carla McShane, OTR/L   _Sept. 30, 2009_

Signature   **Date**

FIGURE 14.4   Sample SOAP Discontinuation Report.

SUMMARY

The discontinuation of services brings closure to a case. It provides the final justification for the services that were provided. In this document, you provide an overview of the client's progress and plans for the future. Because it is a summary, it does not need to be a session-by-session recap of what happened. Rather, it hits the highlights and reflects progress toward occupational therapy outcomes.

A discontinuation summary may be written in narrative or SOAP format. Either way, the discontinuation summary must contain specific information about the client's change in status and recommendations for follow-up and referral to other services. Knowing the client's discharge disposition is essential for making accurate statements about the client's status at discharge and what services can be recommended after discontinuation of occupational therapy services.

REFERENCES

American Occupational Therapy Association. (2005). Occupational therapy standards of practice. *American Journal of Occupational Therapy, 59*, 663–665.

American Occupational Therapy Association. (2007). *Guidelines for documentation of occupational therapy.* Retrieved June, 16, 2008, from http://www.aota.org/Practitioners/ Official/Guidelines/41257.aspx

American Occupational Therapy Association. (2008). Occupational therapy practice framework: Domain and process. *American Journal of Occupational Therapy 62,* 625–683.

Borcherding, S. (2005). *Documentation manual for writing SOAP notes in occupational therapy* (2nd ed.). Thorofare, NJ: Slack.

Borcherding, S. & Kappel C. (2002). The OTA's guide is writing SOAP notes. Thorofare, NJ: Slack.

Centers for Medicare and Medicaid Services. (2008). *Pub100-02 Medicare benefit policy: Transmittal 88.* Retrieved May 8, 2008, from http://www.cms.hhs.gov/transmittals/ downloads/R88BP.pdf

Kettenbach, G. (2004). *Writing S.O.A.P. notes* (3rd ed.). Philadelphia: F. A. Davis.

Moyers, P. (1999). The guide to occupational therapy practice. *American Journal of Occupational Therapy, 53,* 247–322.

Moyers, P. A., & Dale, L. M. (2007). *The guide to occupational therapy practice* (2nd ed.). Bethesda, MD: American Occupational Therapy Association.

SECTION IV

School System Documentation

▼ INTRODUCTION ▼

In school systems the requirements for documentation are different than for occupational therapy services provided in clinical settings. There are clear federal guidelines about what to document and when. In this section of the book, we look at the documentation requirements for services provided to children through the school system. Minimal information about the actual delivery of services is covered.

▼ OVERVIEW OF SCHOOL SYSTEM DOCUMENTATION ▼

The Individuals with Disabilities Education Act (IDEA) dictates how educational services are provided to children with disabilities from birth to age 21 (United States Department of Education [USDE], 2006). IDEA also provides guidelines about how to document those services. Under IDEA, there are three types of documents: notice and consent forms, the Individualized Family Service Plan (IFSP), and the Individualized Education Program (IEP). IDEA allows each state to develop guidelines for service delivery to children that further refine the federal law. In most states, services to these children are provided by local school districts. For children birth to age 2, some states provide services to children with special needs through the school district (coordinated by the state Department of Education), but in others, the primary provider of these services could be a home health agency or welfare agency (coordinated by the state Department of Health or Department of Human Services).

Throughout this section of the book, federal laws and regulations will be cited. However, examples of how these laws and regulations are implemented will come from individual states. This is because federal law requires states to offer certain services, document them, and inform families, but allows the states to determine the exact method of implementation and documentation of these services. States used as examples in this section of the book represent those in which information is more readily available on the Internet. It is not meant to imply that the states whose forms or regulations are cited have better systems than those that are not cited. I have tried to present information from different states representing a geographic cross section of this country.

One of the biggest differences between school system documentation and clinical documentation is that school system documentation is intended to be shared with the child's family/guardian. When you document in a school system, you know that the parent or guardian will receive a copy of the document, and will read what you write. In a clinical setting, you know the physician and other team members will read the document, but only if a family asks for access to the documents will they be allowed to read what you wrote.

School systems may bill third-party payers (insurance companies, managed care organizations, or Medicaid), but not every district has elected to do so, yet. Billing third-party payers may, but does not always, impact the type and frequency of documentation completed by occupational therapy personnel.

▼ ROLE DELINEATION IN SCHOOL SYSTEM DOCUMENTATION ▼

In school systems, most of the documentation is written through a team effort. The team may include teachers, special education teachers, school nurses, speech clinicians, school psychologists, and administrators, along with occupational and physical therapists. As a member of the team, the occupational therapist may write or verbally contribute to sections of the notice and consent forms, IFSP, or IEP. Occupational therapy assistants may also contribute to development of the IEP and IFSP. If the occupational therapist is serving as the service coordinator for an infant or toddler, he or she will be responsible for ensuring that all required documentation is completed within established timelines. As described in the *Guidelines for Documentation of Occupational Therapy* (AOTA, 2007), the occupational therapist is responsible for completing the evaluation; an occupational therapy assistant may participate in the process. Specific rules for documentation written by the occupational therapist or occupational therapy assistant in school systems may vary from state to state. You can find these rules by checking with your state education agency (i.e., Department of Education). As always, the AOTA *Standards of Practice for Occupational Therapy* (2005) for role delineation in documentation apply (see Appendix C).

▼ STRUCTURE OF THIS SECTION OF THE BOOK ▼

Under IDEA, the contents of educational documentation, including notice and consent forms, the IFSP, and the IEP, are specified: however, the specific forms may be developed by the state education agency or the school district/local agency. Just as with documents in medical model settings, these documents are legal documents and can be called into court when there are lawsuits. It seems lately that there are more and more lawsuits involving the provision of special education and related services, especially issues around who will be responsible for paying for what services.

Notice and consent forms are designed to guarantee that the rights of the child and his or her family are respected. Some of these forms provide information or notice to the family; others seek parental consent to evaluate, provide, or change services (USDE, 2006). These are discussed in Chapter 15.

Documentation for children birth through age 2 is covered in Chapter 16. Each infant or toddler who qualifies for services under IDEA must have a written plan, called an Individualized Family Service Plan (IFSP), for the services he or she will receive. This chapter discusses the IFSP.

The last chapter of this section, Chapter 17, discusses the Individualized Education Program (IEP). This is generally written for children with special needs ages 3–21. For these children, occupational therapy is a related service rather than a special education service (AOTA, 2007; USDE, 2006).

REFERENCES

American Occupational Therapy Association. (2005). Occupational therapy standards of practice. *American Journal of Occupational Therapy, 52*, 866–869.

American Occupational Therapy Association. (2007). *Guidelines for documentation of occupational therapy.* Retrieved June 16, 2008, from http://www.aota.org/Practitioners/Official/Guidelines/41257.aspx

United States Department of Education. (2006). *Building the legacy of IDEA, 2004.* Retrieved October 1, 2008 from http://idea.ed.gov/explore/home

CHAPTER 15

Notice and Consent Forms

INTRODUCTION

Whenever you work with children, you are working with a vulnerable population. As such, the federal government has developed regulations that protect the rights and interests of the child and his or her family. The forms that are used to protect the rights of recipients, inform families, and obtain consent are called notice and consent forms. Generally, the school system or agency will have these forms available for obtaining parent signatures and providing legally required notices.

Some states mandate that school districts use a prescribed set of forms; others allow each school district to develop its own set of forms. A survey by the Project Forum of the National Association of State Directors of Special Education (NASDSE) in 2002 showed that 17 states (34%) have mandated procedural safeguard forms and 10 states (20%) have forms for obtaining parental permission prior to initial evaluation of a student (Ahearn, 2002).

Box 15.1 shows the language of the federal law (20 U.S.C. 1400 et seq.) relating to the types of notices and consent forms and their contents (USDE, 2006). No matter what type of form parents are asked to read or sign, they must be provided in the families' native language, including Braille or orally (FAPE, 2001; 34 C.F.R. § 300.503[c]; 34 C.F.R. § 303.403[c]).

BOX 15.1   Procedural Safeguards. (20 U.S.C. 1400.615)

SEC. 615. PROCEDURAL SAFEGUARDS

(a) ESTABLISHMENT OF PROCEDURES. Any State educational agency, State agency, or local educational agency that receives assistance under this part shall establish and maintain procedures in accordance with this section to ensure that children with disabilities and their parents are guaranteed procedural safeguards with respect to the provision of a free appropriate public education by such agencies.

(b) TYPES OF PROCEDURES. The procedures required by this section shall include the following:

(1) An opportunity for the parents of a child with a disability to examine all records relating to such child and to participate in meetings with respect to the identification, evaluation, and educational placement of the child, and the provision of a free appropriate public education to such child, and to obtain an independent educational evaluation of the child.

(2) (A) Procedures to protect the rights of the child whenever the parents of the child are not known, the agency cannot, after reasonable efforts, locate the parents, or the child is a ward of the State, including the assignment of an individual to act as a surrogate for the parents, which surrogate shall not be an employee of the State educational agency, the local educational agency, or any other agency that is involved in the education or care of the child. In the case of—

(i) a child who is a ward of the State, such surrogate may alternatively be appointed by the judge overseeing the child's care provided that the surrogate meets the requirements of this paragraph; and

(ii) an unaccompanied homeless youth as defined in section 725(6) of the McKinney-Vento Homeless Assistance Act (42 U.S.C. 11434a(6)), the local educational agency shall appoint a surrogate in accordance with this paragraph.

(Continued)

(B) The State shall make reasonable efforts to ensure the assignment of a surrogate not more than 30 days after there is a determination by the agency that the child needs a surrogate.

(3) Written prior notice to the parents of the child, in accordance with subsection (c)(1), whenever the local educational agency—

(A) proposes to initiate or change; or

(B) refuses to initiate or change, the identification, evaluation, or educational placement of the child, or the provision of a free appropriate public education to the child.

(4) Procedures designed to ensure that the notice required by paragraph (3) is in the native language of the parents, unless it clearly is not feasible to do so.

(5) An opportunity for mediation, in accordance with subsection (e).

(6) An opportunity for any party to present a complaint—

(A) with respect to any matter relating to the identification, evaluation, or educational placement of the child, or the provision of a free appropriate public education to such child; and

(B) which sets forth an alleged violation that occurred not more than 2 years before the date the parent or public agency knew or should have known about the alleged action that forms the basis of the complaint, or, if the State has an explicit time limitation for presenting such a complaint under this part, in such time as the State law allows, except that the exceptions to the timeline described in subsection (f)(3)(D) shall apply to the timeline described in this subparagraph.

(7) (A) Procedures that require either party, or the attorney representing a party, to provide due process complaint notice in accordance with subsection (c)(2) (which shall remain confidential)—

(i) to the other party, in the complaint filed under paragraph (6), and forward a copy of such notice to the State educational agency; and

(ii) that shall include—

(I) the name of the child, the address of the residence of the child (or available contact information in the case of a homeless child), and the name of the school the child is attending;

(II) in the case of a homeless child or youth (within the meaning of section 725(2) of the McKinney-Vento Homeless Assistance Act (42 U.S.C. 11434a(2)), available contact information for the child and the name of the school the child is attending;

(III) a description of the nature of the problem of the child relating to such proposed initiation or change, including facts relating to such problem; and

(IV) a proposed resolution of the problem to the extent known and available to the party at the time.

(B) A requirement that a party may not have a due process hearing until the party, or the attorney representing the party, files a notice that meets the requirements of subparagraph (A)(ii).

(8) Procedures that require the State educational agency to develop a model form to assist parents in filing a complaint and due process complaint notice in accordance with paragraphs (6) and (7), respectively.

(c) NOTIFICATION REQUIREMENTS.

(1) Content of prior written notice. The notice required by subsection (b)(3) shall include—

(A) a description of the action proposed or refused by the agency;

(B) an explanation of why the agency proposes or refuses to take the action and a description of each evaluation procedure, assessment, record, or report the agency used as a basis for the proposed or refused action;

(C) a statement that the parents of a child with a disability have protection under the procedural safeguards of this part and, if this notice is not an initial referral for evaluation, the means by which a copy of a description of the procedural safeguards can be obtained;

(D) sources for parents to contact to obtain assistance in understanding the provisions of this part;

(E) a description of other options considered by the IEP Team and the reason why those options were rejected; and

(F) a description of the factors that are relevant to the agency's proposal or refusal.

(2) Due process complaint notice.

(A) Complaint. The due process complaint notice required under subsection (b)(7)(A) shall be deemed to be sufficient unless the party receiving the notice notifies the hearing officer and the other party in writing that the receiving party believes the notice has not met the requirements of subsection (b)(7)(A).

(B) Response to complaint.

(i) Local educational agency response.

(I) In general. If the local educational agency has not sent a prior written notice to the parent regarding the subject matter contained in the parent's due process complaint notice, such local educational agency shall, within 10 days of receiving the complaint, send to the parent a response that shall include—

(aa) an explanation of why the agency proposed or refused to take the action raised in the complaint;

(bb) a description of other options that the IEP Team considered and the reasons why those options were rejected;

(cc) a description of each evaluation procedure, assessment, record, or report the agency used as the basis for the proposed or refused action; and

(dd) a description of the factors that are relevant to the agency's proposal or refusal.

(II) Sufficiency. A response filed by a local educational agency pursuant to subclause (I) shall not be construed to preclude such local educational agency from asserting that the parent's due process complaint notice was insufficient where appropriate.

(ii) Other party response. Except as provided in clause (i), the non-complaining party shall, within 10 days of receiving the complaint, send to the complaint a response that specifically addresses the issues raised in the complaint.

(C) Timing. The party providing a hearing officer notification under subparagraph (A) shall provide the notification within 15 days of receiving the complaint.

(D) Determination.—Within 5 days of receipt of the notification provided under subparagraph (C), the hearing officer shall make a determination on the face of the notice of whether the notification meets the requirements of subsection (b)(7)(A), and shall immediately notify the parties in writing of such determination.

(E) Amended complaint notice.

(i) In general. A party may amend its due process complaint notice only if—

(I) the other party consents in writing to such amendment and is given the opportunity to resolve the complaint through a meeting held pursuant to subsection (f)(1)(B); or

(II) the hearing officer grants permission, except that the hearing officer may only grant such permission at any time not later than 5 days before a due process hearing occurs.

(ii) Applicable timeline. The applicable timeline for a due process hearing under this part shall recommence at the time the party files an amended notice, including the timeline under subsection (f)(1)(B).

(d) PROCEDURAL SAFEGUARDS NOTICE.

(1) In general.

(A) Copy to parents. A copy of the procedural safeguards available to the parents of a child with a disability shall be given to the parents only 1 time a year, except that a copy also shall be given to the parents—

(i) upon initial referral or parental request for evaluation;

(ii) upon the first occurrence of the filing of a complaint under subsection (b)(6); and

(iii) upon request by a parent.

(B) Internet website. A local educational agency may place a current copy of the procedural safeguards notice on its Internet website if such website exists.

(2) Contents. —The procedural safeguards notice shall include a full explanation of the procedural safeguards, written in the native language of the parents (unless it clearly is not feasible to do so) and written in an easily understandable manner, available under this section and under regulations promulgated by the Secretary relating to—

(A) independent educational evaluation;

(B) prior written notice;

(C) parental consent;

(D) access to educational records;

(E) the opportunity to present and resolve complaints, including—

(Continued)

(i) the time period in which to make a complaint;

(ii) the opportunity for the agency to resolve the complaint; and

(iii) the availability of mediation;

(F) the child's placement during pendency of due process proceedings;

(G) procedures for students who are subject to placement in an interim alternative educational setting;

(H) requirements for unilateral placement by parents of children in private schools at public expense;

(I) due process hearings, including requirements for disclosure of evaluation results and recommendations;

(J) State-level appeals (if applicable in that State);

(K) civil actions, including the time period in which to file such actions; and

(L) attorneys' fees.

▼ SERVICE COORDINATION ▼

Providing educational services to children is a team effort. It includes professionals from several disciplines as well as the parents and, when possible, the child. Because of the many people who could be involved in the team, there needs to be one person who takes responsibility for ensuring that everything that needs to be done gets done in a timely fashion. This person is referred to as the service coordinator (team leader). An occupational therapist can serve as the service coordinator for a child from birth through age 2 if designated as such by the Individualized Family Service Plan (IFSP) team (34 C.F.R. § 303.6). However, because occupational therapy is a related service (rather than a special education service) for children ages 3–21, an occupational therapist is usually not the service coordinator for preschool through school-age children. However, if designated by the Individualized Education Program (IEP) team, the occupational therapist can be the case manager (National Early Childhood Technical Assistance Center [NECTAC], 2008).

The service coordinator prepares the documents for parent notification and consent (NECTAC, 2008). The service coordinator must provide parents with written information about procedural safeguards upon initial referral or evaluation, each notification of IFSP or IEP meetings, every reevaluation, and when the parents request it (34 C.F.R. § 300.504[a]). This information accompanies notice and consent forms presented to families to ensure that families are fully informed about their rights.

Exercise 15.1

Go to the website for the Department of Education for your state. See if you can locate information about the notice and consent forms or procedural safeguards that are used in your state. You are looking for state regulations about special education services. Once you find where the regulations are posted, locate and read the requirements for parental notifications and consents. Some state websites are more difficult to navigate than others, but do not get discouraged. Keep digging until you find what you are looking for.

▼ TYPES OF NOTICE AND CONSENT FORMS ▼

The Individuals with Disabilities Education Act (IDEA) requires that notice be given to parents (or designated surrogates) whenever there is a proposal to initiate or change services, or when the agency refuses to initiate or change services (USDE, 2006; 20 U.S.C. 1400.615[b]). The law requires that notices must be provided in the family's native language (USDE; 34 C.F.R. § 300.503[c]; 34 C.F.R. § 303.403[c]) in writing or by other approved method such as e-mail (USDE). Providing notice means that the agency has notified the parent or guardian; it does not mean that the parent has agreed to anything. Whether you are the service coordinator or not, it is important to know the different types of forms a family might be asked to sign, so that if a family member asks you about a form, you will know how to respond.

Evaluation (and Reevaluation) Notice and Consent

Parental consent is needed before an evaluation or reevaluation can be conducted (USDE, 2006; 34 C.F.R. § 300.505[a][1]; 34 C.F.R. § 300.505[a][1]; 34 C.F.R. § 300.503[b]; 34 C.F.R. § 303.404). The notice has to include what action is being proposed, a rationale for that action, what procedural safeguards are available, and procedures for filing a complaint in that state (34 C.F.R. § 303.403[b]).

The service coordinator completes a form that details what areas are to be evaluated. Areas to be evaluated may vary from state to state in terms of wording, but usually include health, vision and hearing, social/emotional status, general intelligence, academic performance, communication status, and motor abilities (Illinois State Board of Education [ISBE], 2001). For each area to be assessed, the members of the team who will be involved in conducting the evaluation are listed. Finally, a reason for evaluating that area and a plan for doing so are documented. A copy of the form is presented to the child's family, and sometimes to the referral source. An example of a consent form can be found in Appendix G and at http://idea.ed.gov/static/modelForms.

Since the family or guardian will be reading this document, it is imperative that the writer use clear language, avoid abbreviations and jargon, and be especially careful to keep evaluative language out of any written document. The hardest part of the form to word appropriately is the explanation of the reason for assessing a particular area. You do not need to be very specific. You could say that you want to do a motor assessment to "determine student's ability to participate in movement related preschool learning activities." For an older child, you could say that you want to do an assessment of motor function to "determine the student's ability to participate in instructional activities/programs and complete class work requirements" or an assessment of transition skills to "determine vocational skills for possible employment after graduation."

Exercise 15.2

Write a reason for doing the following assessments:

1. Peabody Developmental Motor Scales for a 5-year-old who has difficulty with both gross and fine motor skills, which cause her to stand out as "different" in her kindergarten class.

2. Test of Visual Perceptual Skills on a 6-year-old with attention deficits and mental retardation.

3. Clinical observations of neuromotor skills for a 7-year-old with cerebral palsy.

4. Erhardt Developmental Prehension Assessment for a 2-year-old with Down syndrome.

Meeting Notice

Since parents and guardians are so involved in this process, they need to be notified and invited to participate in all team meetings, especially meetings for developing the IEP or IFSP. Parents/guardians are vital to the success of school-based programs. The service coordinator must be sure that proper forms for notifying parents/guardians of team meetings are completed and delivered to the parents/guardians. At minimum, the notice of a team meeting must include the purpose, time, and place of the meeting, as well as identifying who will be at the meeting in addition to the parents (34 C.F.R. § 300.345[b][1]).

Other Notices

In addition to notifying parents when an evaluation is being conducted or a team meeting is being held, notices are required whenever services are initiated, changed, discontinued, or refused (34 C.F.R. § 300.503; USDE, 2006). For example, if a school district proposes to make significant changes to the IEP or refuses to make changes requested by the family, or proposes to change a student's placement or refuses to change a placement (34 C.F.R. § 300.503; PDE, 2001), notice is required.

Here is a sample list of notice and consent forms used by school districts or state agencies (Minnesota Department of Education [MDOE], 2008; Ahearn, 2002):

- Referral for an initial evaluation
- Procedural safeguards notice
- Parental permission for initial evaluation/reevaluation
- Report of IEP/IFSP meeting
- Manifestation determination form
- Notice of a team meeting
- Consent to release private data
- Documentation of significant changes to Individual Education Program (IEP) plan
- Permission to start the program

Not every state agency or school district will require all of these forms. Complete information on which forms are required where you work can be found on the website for the Department of Education (or whatever agency is the lead agency for early intervention services) of your state.

SUMMARY

In school systems, there are several forms that are used to ensure that a child and his or her family's rights to notice and consent are protected. For children under age 3, an occupational therapist may be the service coordinator, thereby being the person responsible for the completion of notice and consent paperwork. For children over the age of 3, an occupational therapist may contribute to the notice and consent documents, but would not usually be the responsible person (case manager). As with all school system documentation, the writer needs to be sure that they are written so that parents of all educational levels can read them.

REFERENCES

Ahearn, E. M. (2002). *State special education forms*. Retrieved March 28, 2003, from http://www.nasdse.org/FORUM/sped_forms.pdf

Families and Advocates Partnership for Education (FAPE). (2001). *Facts on hand: Informed parent consent for pre-school and school-aged children with disabilities*. Retrieved March 28, 2003, from http://www.fape.org/pubs/FAPE-23%20Informed%20Parent% 20Consent.pdf

Illinois State Board of Education. (2001). *Required special education notice and consent forms*. Retrieved March 28, 2003, from http://www.isbe.state.il.us/speced/PDF/Notice EnglishDataInput3-03.pdf

Minnesota Department of Education. (2008). *Recommended due process forms*. Retrieved October 24, 2008, from http://education.state.mn.us/MDE/Accountability_Programs/ Compliance_and_Assistance/Recommended_Due_Process_Forms/index.html

National Early Childhood Technical Assistance Center. (2008). *Service coordination under IDEA 2004*. Retrieved October 3, 2008, from http://www.nectac.org/topics/scoord/scoord.asp

United States Department of Education. (2006). *Building the legacy: IDEA 2004*. Retrieved October 1, 2008, from http://idea.ed.gov/explore/home

CHAPTER 16

Individualized Family Service Plans

INTRODUCTION

The Individuals with Disabilities Education Act (IDEA), Part C (2004 revision, 20 U.S.C. 1400 et seq.), states that services provided to children with disabilities, birth through age 2, are provided under an Individualized Family Service Plan (IFSP) (Jackson, 2007; Stephens & Tauber, 2005; 20 U.S.C. 1400 Part C Sect. 634). An IFSP is a written document that specifies the unique strengths and needs of a child and his or her family, the steps that will be taken to help the child achieve the outcomes desired by the child's family, and who is responsible for implementing and paying for services needed to meet those outcomes (Stephens & Tauber; 20 U.S.C. 1400 Part C Sect. 636[d]). While the law, IDEA, was revised and reauthorized in 2004, when this textbook was revised in early 2009, the final rules for the provision of services to infants and toddlers, Part C, had not yet been made public. This chapter is based on the proposed rules for Part C under IDEA.

▼ IFSP REQUIREMENTS ▼

Specifically, the IFSP must contain the following eight elements:

1. A statement of the infant or toddler's present level of performance of physical development, cognitive development, communication development, social or emotional development, and adaptive development, based on objective criteria;

2. A statement of the family's resources, priorities, and concerns relating to enhancing the development of the family's infant or toddler with a disability;

3. A statement of the major outcomes (measurable results) expected to be achieved for the infant or toddler and the family, and the criteria, procedures, and timelines used to determine the degree to which progress toward achieving the outcomes is being made and whether modifications or revisions of the outcomes or services are necessary;

4. A statement of specific evidence-based early intervention services necessary to meet the unique needs of the infant or toddler and the family, including the frequency, intensity, and method of delivering services;

5. A statement of the natural environments in which early intervention services shall appropriately be provided, including a justification of the extent, if any, to which the services will not be provided in a natural environment;

6. The projected dates for initiation of services and the anticipated frequency and duration of the services;

7. The identification of the service coordinator from the profession most immediately relevant to the infant's or toddler's or family's needs who will be responsible for the implementation of the plan and coordination with other agencies and persons; and

8. A description of how the toddler with a disability will be transitioned to preschool or other appropriate services (20 U.S.C. 1400.636[d][1–8]).

Under certain circumstances, children who are between the ages of 3 and 5, at the request of their family, can have an IFSP written instead of an Individualized Education Program (IEP), which is the document usually written for children ages 3 through 21 (see Chapter 17) (34 CFR § 300.342[c]).

As noted in Chapter 15, for each IFSP written, there must be a person designated as the service coordinator who is responsible for ensuring the implementation of the IFSP and coordination of care with other service providers (Jackson, 2007; 20 U.S.C. 1400.636[d][7]). If the infant or toddler's needs are best served by intervention from an occupational therapist (e.g., an infant with cerebral palsy or a toddler who had a stroke), then the occupational therapist can serve as the service coordinator. As service coordinator, the occupational therapist would be the person responsible for completing all notice and consent forms as well as the IFSP. The order in which the required information appears on the IFSP document may vary from state to state or agency to agency.

Documentation for services provided under an IFSP minimally consists of the notice and consent forms (see Chapter 15) and the IFSP document. In some states and under some circumstances (such as when a third-party payer is involved) additional documentation may be required. When birth-through-age-2 services are provided in a child's home, it is common for the occupational therapist to also write visit or contact notes that describe what occurred during the intervention session and recommendations for follow-through (i.e., home programs). These notes can be written in either a narrative or a SOAP format.

> **Exercise 16.1**
>
> Get on the Internet and look up the rules governing how services are delivered to infants and toddlers with disabilities in your state. The rules may be posted by your state's Department of Education, Department of Human Services, Department of Health, Department of Public Health, Department of Health and Human Services, Department of Children and Families, Department of Public Instruction, or State Board of Education. Read the section on IFSP services. If you live in a state that mandates or recommends use of a particular form for writing the IFSP, download it to look at as you work your way through the rest of this chapter.

▼ EVALUATION ▼

The evaluation is the first step in preparing the IFSP (after consent to evaluate is obtained). Based on the results of the evaluation, the IFSP is developed and implemented. The occupational therapist and other members of the IFSP team use the evaluation to develop statements of the present level of development in the areas of "physical development (including vision, hearing, and health status), cognitive development, communication development, social or emotional development, and adaptive development" (Clark, Lucas, Jackson, & Nanof, 2008; 34 C.F.R. § 303.344[a]).

If the occupational therapist is the service coordinator for a particular child and family, he or she will be responsible for ensuring the quality of the assessment process (Stephens & Tauber, 2005). This means that the occupational therapist has to ensure that the assessment process meets certain criteria (Clark et al., 2008; Stephens & Tauber):

- The evaluation is conducted by qualified personnel;
- It is based on the criteria established by the state;
- The child's medical and health histories are included;
- The report includes levels of development, unique needs of the child and family, and services recommended to improve the cognitive, physical, communication, social, adaptive and emotional development of the child;
- The evaluation is conducted in the child's natural environment; and
- Evaluation procedures and materials must be administered in the parent's native language (nondiscrimination).

The service coordinator must also gather data about available family resources, family priorities, and the concerns the family has regarding the child's development (Clark et al., 2008; Stephens & Tauber; 30 C.F.R. 303.344[b]).

The evaluation process is conducted by members of a multidisciplinary team (Clark et al., 2008; Stephens & Tauber, 2005). The evaluation must be completed within 45 days after the agency receives the referral for services (Clark et al., Waisman Center, 2008; 30 C.F.R. 303.321[a][2]). If an interim IFSP is developed, the child may begin to receive early intervention services prior to the completion of the evaluation process (Jackson, 2007; 30 C.F.R. 303.345).

▼ PRESENT LEVELS OF DEVELOPMENT ▼

Based on professionally acceptable, objective criteria, the infant or toddler's physical, cognitive, communication, social or emotional, and adaptive (e.g., self-care skills) development are summarized using both descriptive and interpretive statements (34 C.F.R. 303.344[a]). These summaries identify the infant or toddler's present levels of performance and include both strengths and areas in need of improvement. It is important to note that not every child will have needs in every area.

An example of a present level of development in the physical area:

> Barak is rolling to the right and left independently. At this time he requires assistance to move from prone to all fours and prone to sit. Once positioned, he can maintain the sitting position for up to a minute. He uses his whole hand to grasp objects and bring them to midline. He does not weight shift to reach objects; rather, he grasps for only those objects within range of an outstretched arm.

▼ FAMILY INFORMATION, RESOURCES, AND CONCERNS ▼

In addition to what professionals identify as the present levels of development, the family's input is recorded on the IFSP. There is space to identify the resources that the family has, the family's priorities, and concerns the family has related to the child's development (Clark et al., 2008; National Dissemination Center for Children with Disabilities [NICHCY], n.d.; Waisman Center, 2008; 20 U.S.C. 1400.636[d][2]). Families contribute to identifying the child's strengths as well as desired outcomes of early intervention. Because this document is written for families as well as the providers of early intervention services, it can be helpful to use the parent's words to the extent that you can. Family resources can include people, skills, capacities, and assets (such as private health insurance) that can help the family of an infant or toddler with a disability. You can ask the family to share this information with you, but it would be unethical to pressure the family to divulging more than they want to. Whatever concerns, worries, or distresses the family expresses gets recorded on the IFSP. Other members of the team can identify concerns, but unless the family agrees with them, they are not recorded on the IFSP. The family determines the priorities for their infant or toddler. It is not necessary to prioritize every individual concern; only those that are of the greatest concern to the family right now.

Some IFSPs identify each member of the team working with the client, including school system personnel; physician; private physical, occupational, or speech therapists; county social workers; and others involved in the care of that child (Waisman Center, 2008). This page is a wonderful resource for families because it lists names, addresses, and phone numbers of all these key people all on one page.

▼ OUTCOMES ▼

Next, the IFSP documents the expected outcomes for the child and his or her family, based on input from both health or education professionals and the family. These outcomes can be for either the child or the family (Clark et al., 2008; NICHCY, n.d.; Waisman Center, 2008; U.SC. 1400.636[d][5]). The outcomes should be specific and have criteria, procedures, and a timeline for meeting them. While the outcomes are written annually, they are reviewed at 6-month intervals (USDE, 2006). An outcome is a statement of change that relates to the infant or toddler's development, which the family can see. This requires using the family's language rather than professional jargon. For example, use the phrase "brothers and sisters" rather than "siblings" or "sit without support" instead of "improve muscle tone."

The exact format for wording the outcomes will vary from state to state, and perhaps within a state from agency to agency. Usually, there is an annual outcome that identifies what the child will be doing 1 year from the start date of the IFSP, although some states, such as Nebraska, use a 6-month time frame instead (IFSPWeb, n.d.). An annual outcome is sometimes referred to as the annual goal.

One format for writing the annual goal includes both the starting and ending performance. For example, Ebony will appropriately play with a variety of toys, moving from simple manipulation of toys/objects to consistent intentional use of toys/objects as observed by the occupational therapist. Notice that this goal is worded differently than any of the formats talked about in Chapter 11. It does not include a measure of time. The time frame is implied since a new goal is written every year when the IFSP is rewritten. Figure 16.1 shows the elements of an annual goal (outcome) written in this format. The instructional objectives that lead to meeting the annual goal simply state the desired behavior, the contexts under which the behavior will be performed, and the criteria and procedures that will be used to measure attainment (Clark et al., 2008; Southwest/West Central Service Cooperatives [SWCSC], 2006). The goal could be written in ABCD, FEAST, RHUMBA, or SMART format (see Chapter 11).

Annual Goal	State	Examples
Direction of Change	• Increase • Improve • Decrease • Maintain	• Calvin will increase the time he stays engaged in play activities while positioned on his stomach from <1 min to 10 min.
Skill or Behavior	• Measurable skill • Observable behavior • Developmental Milestone	• Marni will improve her tolerance of getting her hair combed from crying immediately when she sees the comb to letting her mother comb her hair for 1 min without crying.
Present level	From _____	
Expected level of achievement	To _____ (measurement)	

Objectives	State	Examples
Context	• Physical environment • Sociocultural environment • Human assistance • Adaptive equipment or assistive technology	• Given an interesting toy while placed prone on his mother's lap, Calvin will play with the toy for 2 min or more on 3 consecutive days as reported in a log kept by his mother.
Skill or Behavior	• Observable behavior • Measurable skill	• When Marni sees her mother pick up Marni's comb, Marni will cry for less than 10 seconds on 50% of trials as recorded in a daily journal kept by her mother.
Criteria for attainment	• Measurement in terms of a number	
Procedure for attainment	• Tool used to measure • Who will measure	

FIGURE 16.1 IFSP Annual Goals and Objectives, Direction of Change Format.

Skill Set	Annual Goal	Objectives
Move around in his environment		
1. Transition between prone on belly and sitting independently 2. Rock while on hands and knees for 30 seconds 3. Crawl forward 10 feet 4. Pull self up to standing independently 5. Walk while holding on to furniture 10 feet in each direction 6. Take 5 steps forward independently	Calvin will improve from performing 0 skills to performing 5 of 6 skills identified.	1. Padrick will perform 2 of the 6 skills identified on 90% of trials as observed and documented by the occupational therapist on an observation checklist. 2. Padrick will perform 4 of the 6 skills identified on 90% of trials as observed and documented by the occupational therapist on an observation checklist.
Play with toys		
1. Hold a toy in one hand for 1 min 2. Hold a toy in each hand for 1 min 3. Remove an object from inside an open container 4 out of 5 times 4. Place an object inside another 4 out of 5 times 5. Push a button to activate a toy 4 out of 5 times 6. Stack 3 objects on 3 out of 5 trials 7. Hand a toy to another person when asked on 90% of trials	Edo will improve play skills by going from performing none of the skills listed to satisfactorily performing 5 of the 7 skills listed.	• When presented with a toy, Edo will successfully complete 3 of 7 skills as observed by the occupational therapist and recorded on a play checklist. • When presented with a toy, Edo will successfully complete 5 of 7 skills as observed by the occupational therapist and recorded on a play checklist.

FIGURE 16.2 IFSP Annual Goals and Objectives, Skill Set Format Examples.

Another format takes a very different approach from the other two. In this format, the team identifies a skill set for each need area that they would like the child to obtain in the next year (SWCSC, 2006). The annual goal then states how much of that skill set the child will obtain during the year. Shorter term objectives identify increasing the number or percentage of the identified skills the child will obtain (SWCSC). Figure 16.2 shows an example of this type of goal setting.

The most important considerations when writing outcomes in an IFSP is that they address both the child's and the family's needs, state why the outcomes are important to the family, and the goals are written so that the family can understand them (Waisman Center, 2008).

Exercise 16.2 Family-Friendly Outcome Statements

For each poorly written outcome statement, translate it into clear, measurable language any parent could understand.

1. Torii will transition from prone to sitting with moderate assistance by the end of the school year.

2. Lynette will don and doff her jacket, including fasteners, in less than 3 minutes by December 1, 2009.

3. Ione will demonstrate improved muscle tone so that she can sit unsupported while engaging in bilateral occupations for 5 minutes or longer by March 1, 2010.

4. Edgar will engage in age-appropriate play activities with a peer on a regular basis within 6 months.

5. Condalisa's parents will access available community support services to take the stress off the family for caring for a child with multiple disabilities.

Exercise 16.3 Writing Outcome Statements

For each child and family, write an outcome statement that is clear, measurable, and written in language any parent could understand. Write an outcome statement for the child and another for the family.

1. Soren's father is in the Army reserve and has just been recalled up for active duty, soon to be deployed for a third time to Iraq. His mother works as a manager at a local fast food restaurant. Soren's grandmother functions as his PCA (personal care attendant). Soren is 2.5 years old; he is nonverbal, and has difficulty attending to any task for more than a few seconds before moving on to something new. The only time he sits still for a few minutes at a time is when grandma puts in a cartoon on TV or DVD. He does not dress himself, but does feed himself finger food. He drinks from a sippy cup. He is a very picky eater and has several food allergies. He walks independently, but cannot jump. Each time his father deploys or comes home, Soren has trouble sleeping, and negative behaviors increase (e.g., throwing things, hitting himself, or biting others).

2. Denay was a normally developing child when her mother's boyfriend got frustrated with her crying while he was babysitting, and he threw her into a wall. She sustained a serious head injury. She is now 18 months old and living with a foster family. The foster family also cares for 4 other children with special needs. She commando crawls to move around a room, but her right leg is dragged behind her while she uses her arms to pull her body forward. When she stands, she puts most of her weight on her left leg and arm, and her right heel does not touch the floor. She has seizures that are not completely controlled by medication. She grasps objects with either hand, but does not cross midline. She is beginning to learn some signs like "more," "please," and "mother."

▼ SERVICES PROVIDED ▼

The specific services provided under the IFSP must, to the extent possible, be based on peer-reviewed research (USDE, 2007). The frequency, intensity, duration, length, and method of intervention provided by each service provider involved in that child's care must be explicitly stated (Clark et al., 2008; NICHCY, n.d.; USDE, 2007; Waisman Center, 2008; 20 U.S.C. 1400.636[d][4]). Frequency refers to how often the child is seen (Waisman Center, 2006). In some states you need to differentiate between direct and indirect minutes. Direct minutes are those in which the service provider spends directly with the child. Indirect minutes are spent on a case but without working directly with the child; it could be time spent in observation and consultation with the child's parents or other caregivers, cooperative planning, or modifying environments (Southwest/West Central Service Cooperatives, 2006). Intensity is stated in terms of the average number of minutes per session the child will receive services; it is stated specifically rather than a range of minutes (Waisman Center, 2006). Duration means how long the service will be offered from the date of the IFSP meeting or the date of initiation of the service (Waisman Center, 2006). The IFSP must include information about the date the plan will take effect and the anticipated length of time the plan will cover (almost always a year) (Waisman Center, 2006). This task usually falls to the service coordinator.

The IFSP also includes a place to document proposed methods of intervention, the location of the services, and any payment arrangements that may affect or be affected by the services provided (Waisman Center, 2006). The methods of intervention would be written just as the methods of intervention are written in clinical settings (see Chapter 12). Methods of intervention are the things you plan to implement when you are working with the child; they are your best guess as to what will work to move the child toward achievement of the established goals and objectives.

▼ ENVIRONMENTAL STATEMENT ▼

Location of service is exactly what it sounds like. You identify where each service will be provided. Often for young children, services are provided in the most natural environment for an infant or toddler, the child's home. Services may also be provided in a clinic, a preschool, on the playground, in an early childhood classroom, or in a day care facility. IDEA does require that services to these young children be provided in natural environments or justification be provided explaining why the natural environment is not the best place to provide a service (USDE, 2007). A natural environment is a setting that would be considered natural or normal for a child that age without disabilities (Waisman Center, 2006).

▼ TRANSITION TO PRESCHOOL SERVICES ▼

Finally, there must be documentation in the IFSP of steps that will be taken to help the child make the transition from home-based or center-based early intervention services to preschool or other appropriate services (Waisman Center, 2006). Transition planning can also address other transitions in the child's life such as moving from hospital to home, biological family to foster care or vice versa, or a move to a new community (IFSPWeb, n.d.). Planning for any transition should begin as soon as a child is identified for transition; there is no need to wait for an IFSP team meeting. The 2004 revision of IDEA allows for changes to the IFSP to be made without a full team meeting, as long as the frequency and intensity of the new or revised services are unchanged from the original IFSP (IFSPWeb). You can view examples of completed IFSP forms by visiting the websites in Table 16.1.

TABLE 16.1   Websites with Sample Completed IFSP Forms

Website	Host
http://www.edis.army.mil/documents/IFSP-Handbook.pdf	US Army
http://www.waisman.wisc.edu/birthto3/EmmasIFSP.pdf	Waisman Center (Wisconsin)
http://www.nectac.org/~pdfs/meetings/nationalDec05/ numerickKate070Dec19-1handout.pdf	National Early Childhood Technical Assistance Center
http://www.isd518.net/district/sped/cimpfiles/01c0ecse.pdf	Independent School District 158, Worthington, MN
http://www.dese.mo.gov/divspeced/FirstSteps/pdfs/ IFSPGuidanceExemplars.pdf	Missouri Department of Elementary & Secondary Education: Special Education
http://www.nectac.org/~pdfs/topics/families/ IFSPRatingScale.pdf	National Early Childhood Technical Assistance Center

Since the natural environment for most infants and toddlers is the home, most IFSP services are provided in the home. Rarely will these services be provided on a daily basis; once or twice a week is usually adequate. However, in providing services only a couple times a week, the occupational therapist may want to see some kind of follow-through on the infant's program by the family or personal care attendant. This is where a visit note comes in.

The occupational therapist can use a visit note to communicate with the child's family. The occupational therapist can document what happened during the intervention session, how the child reacted, and what the family can do to supplement or enhance the occupational therapy program. The note can be written in either narrative or SOAP format.

While the law does not require this documentation, it is recommended because it does create a paper trail should there ever be questions about how a family was instructed. If an occupational therapist does write visit notes, it is a good idea to do it on "magic-carbon" (NCR) paper so that both the family and the occupational therapist can retain a copy.

Preprinted exercise/activity sheets can also be given to families to help them follow through on occupational therapy programs. These may be in addition to or in place of visit notes. Several vendors sell reprintable handouts. Be careful not to copy and distribute pages of books or journal articles that are copyright protected (see Chapter 8).

SUMMARY

The IFSP is written annually to show the child's current level of performance, set goals to move the child's development forward, and determine the frequency and intensity of services. Since an infant or toddler is totally dependent on his or her family, the family plays a big role in the development and implementation of the IFSP. The IFSP must be written in words the family will understand. The goals (outcomes) established in the IFSP can be for the child or the family to achieve. The IFSP contains specific information on what services will be provided, who will provide them, who will pay for them, where they will be provided, and the frequency and duration of those services.

An occupational therapist can be the service coordinator for birth-to-age-2 services. A service coordinator is the person responsible for the development, coordination, and implementation of the plan. Writing the IFSP is a team effort, with the family included as part of the team. While much of the IFSP is similar to an intervention plan in a clinical setting, it differs in that it is written for the family rather than being written for other professionals or third-party payers as the primary audience. While an intervention plan usually represents the services of one provider, an IFSP represents the integrated plan of everyone working with that child.

REFERENCES

Clark, G. F., Lucas, A., Jackson, L., & Nanof, T. (2008, April). *School system annual program: IDEA part C: Early intervention & occupational therapy.* Paper presented at the meeting of the American Occupational Therapy Association Annual Conference, Long Beach, CA.

ISFPWeb (n.d.). *Developing a great IFSP.* Retrieved October 10, 2008, from http://www.ifspweb.org/developing.html

Jackson, L. L. (2007). *Legislative context of occupational therapy practice in schools and early childhood settings.* In L. L. Jackson (Ed.) Occupational therapy services for children and youth under IDEA (3rd ed.; pp. 1–22). Bethesda, MD: American Occupational Therapy Association.

National Dissemination Center for Children with Disabilities. (n.d.). *How to write a services plan.* Retrieved October 10, 2008, from http://www.nichcy.org/babies/ifsp/pages/default.aspx

Southwest/West Central Service Cooperatives. (2006, January). *Related services: Decision-making and service provision.* Paper presented at the DAPE and Related Services Network Meeting. Marshall, MN.

Stephens, L. C., & Tauber, S. K. (2005). Early intervention. In J. Case-Smith, (Ed.), *Occupational therapy for children* (5th ed., pp. 771–793). St. Louis, MO: Mosby.

United States Department of Education. (2006). *Building the legacy: IDEA 2004.* Retrieved October 1, 2008, from http://idea.ed.gov/explore/home

United States Department of Education. (2007). *Federal register May 9, 2007(34 CFR Part 303).* Retrieved October 10, 2008, from http://edocket.access.gpo.gov/2007/pdf/07-2140.pdf

Waisman Center (2006). *Guidelines completing Wisconsin's Individualized Family Service Plan.* Retrieved October 10, 2008, from http://www.waisman.wisc.edu/birthto3/Guidelines.pdf

Waisman Center (2008). *Welcome to unit 3: The IFSP document.* Retrieved October 10, 2008, from http://www.waisman.wisc.edu/birthto3/WPDP/Unit_Three.html

CHAPTER 17

Individualized Education Program

INTRODUCTION

The Individualized Education Program (IEP) is the guiding document for special education and related services for children with special needs. It is written for children with special needs ages 3–21 and administered by the school district. The Individuals with Disabilities Education Act (IDEA) (20 U.S.C. 1400 et seq.) allows children between the ages of 3 and 5 to have an Individualized Family Service Plan (IFSP) written instead of an IEP as long as the IFSP contains the same information as would be contained in an IEP (United States Department of Education, 2006; 34 C.F.R. §303.342[c]). Because the IEP is individualized, it takes a great deal of planning and interdisciplinary coordination to produce and implement the document. Specific information on the content of the IEP is found in Part B of IDEA (Polichino et al., 2007).

The IEP has some similarities to the IFSP: Both are written by a team of professionals and include input from the parents of the child involved; both are written annually and both start with an evaluation of the child. Both require parent notification, consent (see Chapter 15), and involvement throughout the process. There are also some differences. While the IFSP is family-centered, the IEP is student-centered. The IFSP looks at the overall development of the child; the IEP looks at levels of educational development, the ways in which a student's disability affects the child's ability to participate in learning (20 U.S.C. 1400.614[b][2][A]; 20 U.S.C. 1400.614[d][1][A][i][I]; 34 C.F.R. §300.347[a][1]).

Occupational therapy is considered a related service under Part B of IDEA (Jackson, 2007; National Dissemination Center for Children with Disabilities [NICHCY], n.d.; 20 U.S.C. 1400.602[22]). This means that usually the occupational therapist would not be the service coordinator, but rather would be a contributor to the IEP process. In this instance, the child must first qualify for special education before receiving occupational therapy. An IEP is not a guarantee that the maximum amount of service will be provided; it identifies the necessary services to allow the student to participate in learning. In other words, it provides need-to-have services, not want-to-have services.

Every IEP must include certain information. While IDEA does not mandate the use of one particular form or format, it does mandate the content required in each IEP. Box 17.1 shows the minimum content required by IDEA (34 C.F.R. §300.347). The order in which the information appears in the IEP document is irrelevant. Essentially, the minimum content can be summarized as follows:

- Present level of academic achievement and functional performance
- Annual goals
- Special education and related services
- Participation with nondisabled children
- Participation in state- and district-wide tests
- Starting date and location of services
- Transition services
- Measurement of progress

§300.320 DEFINITION OF INDIVIDUALIZED EDUCATION PROGRAM

(a) *General.* As used in this part, the term individualized education program or IEP means a written statement for each child with a disability that is developed, reviewed, and revised in a meeting in accordance with §§300.320 through 300.324, and that must include—

   (1) A statement of the child's present levels of academic achievement and functional performance, including—

   (i) How the child's disability affects the child's involvement and progress in the general education curriculum (i.e., the same curriculum as for nondisabled children); or

   (ii) For preschool children, as appropriate, how the disability affects the child's participation in appropriate activities;

   (2) (i) A statement of measurable annual goals, including academic and functional goals designed to—

   (A) Meet the child's needs that result from the child's disability to enable the child to be involved in and make progress in the general education curriculum; and

   (B) Meet each of the child's other educational needs that result from the child's disability;

   (ii) For children with disabilities who take alternate assessments aligned to alternate achievement standards, a description of benchmarks or short-term objectives;

   (3) A description of—

   (i) How the child's progress toward meeting the annual goals described in paragraph (2) of this section will be measured; and

   (ii) When periodic reports on the progress the child is making toward meeting the annual goals (such as through the use of quarterly or other periodic reports, concurrent with the issuance of report cards) will be provided;

   (4) A statement of the special education and related services and supplementary aids and services, based on peer-reviewed research to the extent practicable, to be provided to the child, or on behalf of the child, and a statement of the program modifications or supports for school personnel that will be provided to enable the child—

   (i) To advance appropriately toward attaining the annual goals;

   (ii) To be involved in and make progress in the general education curriculum in accordance with paragraph (a)(1) of this section, and to participate in extracurricular and other nonacademic activities; and

   (iii) To be educated and participate with other children with disabilities and nondisabled children in the activities described in this section;

   (5) An explanation of the extent, if any, to which the child will not participate with nondisabled children in the regular class and in the activities described in paragraph (a)(4) of this section;

   (6) (i) A statement of any individual appropriate accommodations that are necessary to measure the academic achievement and functional performance of the child on State and districtwide assessments consistent with §612(a)(16) of the Act; and

   (ii) If the IEP Team determines that the child must take an alternate assessment instead of a particular regular State or districtwide assessment of student achievement, a statement of why—

   (A) The child cannot participate in the regular assessment; and

   (B) The particular alternate assessment selected is appropriate for the child; and

   (7) The projected date for the beginning of the services and modifications described in paragraph (a)(4) of this section, and the anticipated frequency, location, and duration of those services and modifications.

(b) *Transition services.* Beginning not later than the first IEP to be in effect when the child turns 16, or younger if determined appropriate by the IEP Team, and updated annually, thereafter, the IEP must include—

   (1) Appropriate measurable postsecondary goals based upon age appropriate transition assessments related to training, education, employment, and, where appropriate, independent living skills; and

   (2) The transition services (including courses of study) needed to assist the child in reaching those goals.

(Continued)

(c) *Transfer of rights at age of majority*. Beginning not later than one year before the child reaches the age of majority under State law, the IEP must include a statement that the child has been informed of the child's rights under Part B of the Act, if any, that will transfer to the child on reaching the age of majority under §300.520.

(d) *Construction*. Nothing in this section shall be construed to require—

(1) That additional information be included in a child's IEP beyond what is explicitly required in section 614 of the Act; or

(2) The IEP Team to include information under one component of a child's IEP that is already contained under another component of the child's IEP.

While IDEA does not require the use of a particular format, the USDE does offer a model form for states or school districts to use (see Appendix G and http://idea.ed.gov/static/modelForms). Many states have developed their own model forms as well.

Exercise 17.1

Get on the Internet and look up the rules governing how services are delivered to children with disabilities in your state. The rules may be posted by your state's Department of Education, Department of Children and Families, Department of Public Instruction, or State Board of Education. Read the section on IEP services. If you live in a state that mandates or recommends use of a particular form for writing the IEP, download it to look at as you work your way through the rest of this chapter.

▼ EVALUATION PROCESS ▼

The IEP process begins with an evaluation. For a student receiving services under an IEP, a reevaluation is done at least every 3 years (NICHCY, .n.d.; USDE, 2006; 20 U.S.C. 1400.614[a][2][A]). The initial evaluation is done to determine the child's disability and educational needs (NICHCY; USDE; 20 U.S.C. 1400.614[a][1][B][i–ii]). Subsequent evaluations identify the child's current level of performance and determine whether the child continues to have a disability, whether the child continues to need special education services, and whether changes or additions to the special education and related services the child receives are needed to enable participation in the general curriculum (NICHCY; USDE; 20 U.S.C. 1400.614[c][1][B][i–iv]). The evaluation must be completed within 60 days of the parents' giving their consent for the evaluation (USDE). At minimum, the evaluation must contain information about the child's

- health,
- vision and hearing,
- social and emotional status,
- general intelligence,
- academic performance,
- communicative status, and
- motor abilities (NICHCY, n.d., *Scope of the Evaluation*)

IDEA contains legal requirements for conducting an evaluation of a child (20 U.S.C. 1400.614[b][2][A–C]):

A. Use a variety of assessment tools and strategies to gather relevant functional, developmental, and academic information, including information provided by the parent, that may assist in determining—

i. whether the child is a child with a disability; and

ii. the content of the child's individualized education program, including information related to enabling the child to be involved in and progress in the general education curriculum, or, for preschool children, to participate in appropriate activities;

B. Not use any single measure or assessment as the sole criterion for determining whether a child is a child with a disability or determining an appropriate educational program for the child; and

C. Use technically sound instruments that may assess the relative contribution of cognitive and behavioral factors, in addition to physical or developmental factors.

In addition, IDEA requires tests and evaluation materials to be nondiscriminatory, or not contain racial or cultural bias, and be administered in the child's native language whenever feasible (Polichino *et al.,* 2007; 20 U.S.C. 1400.614[b][3][A]). Standardized tests have to be valid for the purposes they are being used for, be administered by someone who is knowledgeable and trained in the use of the test, and be administered according to the instructions provided by the test producer (Polichino *et al.,* 2007; 20 U.S.C. 1400.614[b][2][B]). Besides standardized tests, other evaluation methods include information provided by the parents, observation, work samples, interviews, and a review of the student's cumulative educational record (NICHCY, n.d.).

If the results of the evaluation show that the child qualifies for special education services, the school then has 30 calendar days in which to meet with the parents to discuss evaluation findings and write the IEP (USDE, 2006; 34 C.F.R. §300.343[b][2]). Often, the sharing of results of the evaluation and writing the IEP occur at the same meeting. If the evaluation results show that the child does not qualify for special education services, but the parents feel the child should have qualified, the parents have the right to ask for an independent education evaluation or appeal the decision using due process as established in IDEA (USDE).

▼ PRESENT LEVEL OF EDUCATIONAL PERFORMANCE ▼

The results of the evaluation may be incorporated into the IEP, in the section on present level of academic achievement and functional performance. IDEA is quite specific about the kind of information that must be included in the IEP. In the present level of academic achievement and functional performance section, federal law requires the IEP to consider three components (USDE, 2006; NICHCY, n.d.; 614 [d][1][A][i][I][aa–cc]):

I. A statement of the child's present levels of academic achievement and functional performance, including—
   (aa) how the child's disability affects the child's involvement and progress in the general education curriculum;
   (bb) for preschool children, as appropriate, how the disability affects the child's participation in appropriate activities; and
   (cc) for children with disabilities who take alternate assessments aligned to alternate achievement standards, a description of benchmarks or short-term objectives.

Present levels of academic achievement and functional performance reflect what the student is able to do now, regardless of what that child was able to do or not do in the past. In this sense, it is very different from a summary of the client's progress or pertinent history in a clinical setting.

Current evaluation results are shared with the IEP team (including parents/guardians). The specific areas that an occupational therapist looks at include activities of daily living (e.g., toileting, eating lunch, putting a coat on and taking it off), instrumental activities of daily living (e.g., safety, using computers and communication devices), education (e.g., ability to access and use learning materials), work (e.g., vocational exploration, work habits), play (e.g., ability to access and use the playground, participation in games), leisure (e.g., ability to participate in extracurricular activities), and social participation (ability to interact with peers, express a need) (Jackson, 2007). The evaluation results need to show any identified deficits that interfere with the education process. If no connection to the educational needs of the child can be drawn, then occupational therapy services may not be necessary in the school setting. This does not mean that occupational therapy services would not in some way benefit the child; it simply means that those services would not be part of the IEP services provided by the school. An example would be that a child has deficits in tying her shoe. Tying one's shoes is not essential for participating in school. The child could wear slip-ons or shoes with Velcro closures. Occupational therapy to work on shoe tying would not be educationally relevant, so it would not be part of the IEP. However, the child could receive occupational therapy services to work on shoe tying from another provider (other than the school district). If the occupational therapist can make a connection between the child's inability to motor plan the act of tying her shoes to the inability to motor plan in other situations that are necessary for learning (such as handwriting), then occupational therapy services might be justifiable. It is the responsibility of the occupational therapist to show how the deficits identified in the evaluation process have the potential to interfere with the learning process and that occupational therapy services are necessary to help the child overcome those deficits.

Anyone who has spent any time in a school or preschool classroom will tell you that a student's behavior can interfere not only with that child's learning but the learning of other students in the room as well. In the present level of performance section, a clear and specific description of observed behaviors and how they may interfere with learning must be documented (Polichino *et al.*, 2007). For example, you observe that a child is repeatedly getting up and down off his chair, moving around his chair, and jumping up and down whenever he is asked to stand in line. This is distracting to other children in the room, and the teacher questions whether the boy is paying attention when he moves around like that. The present level of educational performance would reflect exactly what the behavior looks like.

As discussed in Chapter 16, the present level of performance can include both a description of the performance and the occupational therapist's interpretation of that performance. The Massachusetts Department of Education (2001) uses the following examples to show proper wording of a present level of educational performance:

> *Less than helpful:* Joe is not committed to his school program.
>
> *More helpful:* Joe submits fewer than half of his required homework assignments. He starts most assignments but lacks the organizational skills to complete them by the required due dates (p. 18).
>
> *Less than helpful:* Jill has a short attention span.
>
> *More helpful:* Jill typically interrupts the work of others five times per hour. She interrupts when she requires teacher assistance (p. 18).

Exercise 17.2

Write a more helpful present level of educational performance for each less helpful statement below.

1. Less helpful: Omar has difficulty cutting with a scissors.
   More helpful:

2. Less helpful: Lucinda does not respect the personal space of other students.
   More helpful:

3. Less helpful: Bethany is very messy and careless with supplies.
   More helpful:

4. Less helpful: Rodney's handwriting is illegible.
   More helpful:

On the IEP, the team writes annual goals for the child. For children with disabilities who will require alternate assessments (of statewide testing in accordance with the No Child Left Behind Act), short-term objectives or benchmarks are required in addition to the annual goals (Jackson, 2007). These short-term objectives or benchmarks help the IEP team, including the parents, to measure the child's progress throughout the year. Benchmarks describe expected progress at a given point in the year. Unlike the IFSP (Chapter 16), the goals and objectives/benchmarks are written to describe only what the student will do; they cannot be written to address family needs (Jackson). The annual goals must relate to the child's needs that result from the child's disability (USDE, 2006). They must enable the child to participate in and make progress in the general education curriculum (USDE; 614 [d] [1] [A] [i][I]).

Goals are not written for each discipline involved in the child's education; rather, they are written to address student's needs and may reflect a multidisciplinary approach to the problem addressed by the goal (Jackson, 2007).

How the goals are worded will vary by state and, to some degree, the school district you work for. You may be the member of the team to draft the wording of the goals, or your services may be provided under a goal written by other members of the team. Either way, the occupational therapist has input into the goal-writing process (Jackson).

The main components of an IEP annual goal, like the IFSP annual goal, are the behavior or skill to be performed, the direction of the change, and the level of performance expected at the end of the year. The present level of performance may be explicit or implied. For example, if the performance level is explicit, an annual goal might read: Jalena will decrease self-stimulating behavior from 10 episodes per day to two episodes per day. If the performance level is implied, the goal could be: Jalena will decrease self-stimulating behavior to two episodes per day. The advantage of making it explicit is that if the goal page gets separated from the rest of the IEP document, you will know where you started from and be better able to identify progress. The advantage of making it implicit is that it takes fewer words to write it.

Once the annual goals have been established, if the child will have alternative testing, the objectives or benchmarks can be developed. While there is no federal legal requirement regarding the number of objectives/benchmarks per goal, two to four for each annual goal seems to be a good range. One objective seems insufficient to allow stepwise progression toward an annual goal, but more than four seems like too many steps to accomplish in 1 year.

Here is an example:

Goal: Anna will consistently maintain her balance while walking on uneven surfaces from walking in a high-guard position and losing her balance five times in 50 feet, to walking in medium-guard without losing her balance at all in 50 feet.

Objective 1: Anna will consistently walk from the playground, up over a curb, to the grassy area around the playground while holding on to an assistant with one hand as observed by teacher or occupational therapist.

Objective 2: Anna will walk from the playground, up over a curb, to the grassy area around the playground without assistance but with arms in high-guard position as observed by the teacher or occupational therapist.

Objective 3: Anna will consistently walk up and down the hill next to the school with arms in high-guard but without assistance as observed by the teacher or occupational therapist.

You may have noticed that the objectives in the above examples contained the phrase "as observed by the teacher or occupational therapist." Not every state or school district requires that the objectives include procedures for evaluation, but some do.

Some states use a checkoff system for identifying how the goal will be measured (Virginia Department of Education [VDOE], 2008). Possible ways that progress could be measured include

- Classroom participation
- Checklist
- Classwork
- Homework
- Observation
- Special Projects
- Test and Quizzes
- Written Reports
- Criterion-referenced test: _____
- Norm-referenced test: _____
- Other:_____ (VDOE, p. 8)

In general, objectives need to include the conditions under which the behavior or activity occurs, what behavior is to be performed, and the criteria (measurement) for the performance (Case-Smith & Rogers, 2005). The conditions can include the environment(s), specialized instruction or cuing, specialized materials or equipment, and any assistance needed. The behavior to be performed needs to be observable; it can be qualitative or quantitative. The criteria have to show how the student will demonstrate successful completion of the goal, which means there has to be a measurement, and, in some states, who will evaluate the student's performance and document it (Case-Smith & Rogers). Figure 17.1 shows a sample goal page from an IEP.

Exercise 17.3

For each goal, list two objectives that would help a student with disabilities meet the goal.

Goal 1: Keyshawn will improve his penmanship so that he can write his name legibly on unlined paper, as observed by his regular classroom teacher.

Objective 1a:

Objective 1b:

Goal 2: Miriam will improve her attention to task from going off task eight times during a 15-minute task to going off task once during a half-hour of task participation, as observed by her special education teacher.

Objective 2a:

Objective 2b:

Goal 3: Paul will improve scissors use from hand-over-hand assistance to independently cutting along a curved line, as observed by the occupational therapist.

Objective 3a:

Objective 3b:

Individualized Education Program for: <u>Tran Vang</u>
IEP Dates: from <u>Sept. 29, 2009</u> to <u>Sept. 29, 2010</u>   DOB: <u>July 17, 2004</u>

Current Level of Performance/Measurable Annual Goals/Benchmarks

Goal # <u>3</u>
Educational need area: _____ Academic/cognitive _____ Behavior _____ Communication
<u>X</u> Motor _____ Self-help _____ Social _____ Vocational

Current Level of Performance:
Tran uses a rolling walker to move around inside the school building, and a wheelchair for longer distances out of doors. He has very high muscle tone in all four limbs. When he gets excited, he throws his head back, arches his back, and straightens his arms and legs. He uses a whole hand grasp with large-diameter writing utensils. His writing is illegible; the letters are misshapen; letters do not rest on the bottom line; letter size varies.

Measurable Annual Goal:
Tran will write his name (first and last) legibly on a line 80% of the time, as observed by his classroom teacher.

Benchmark/Objectives:
1) Tran will write his first name legibly on a line 50% of the time, as observed by the occupational therapist.
2) Tran will write his first name legibly on a line 80% of the time, as observed by the occupational therapist.
3) Tran will write his last name legibly on a line 50% of the time, as observed by the occupational therapist.

Methods of intervention:
Tran will practice writing his name on a large scale, such as on the white board, in sand in a sandbox, and other types of materials.
Tran will be instructed in techniques for forming letters.
Tran's sitting posture will be modified to decrease muscle tone in his trunk and arms.
Tran will try different types of writing utensils and papers (with and without raised lines) to see which feels best to him and which yields the best results.

Location of intervention:
In his regular education classroom and in the occupational therapy room.

Assistive technology needs:
Various writing utensils
Assorted writing papers
Keyboard with key guard for beginning computer use

FIGURE 17.1   Sample IEP Goal Page.

▼ SPECIAL EDUCATION AND RELATED SERVICES ▼

The IEP must specifically state the type and amount of special education, related services, and supplementary aids and services a child will receive, "based on peer-reviewed evidence to the extent practicable" (USDE, 2006; [34 CFR 300.320(a)]; [20 U.S.C. 1414.614(d)(1) (A)(i)(IV)]). This is a new requirement in the 2004 reauthorization. If an IEP says that a special education or related service is needed, there should be evidence in the scholarly literature that shows that the service is effective for a child with disabilities.

School districts will vary in how they want the frequency stated; most will want the number of minutes per week. Often, the minutes per week or per session will be further specified as either direct or indirect or as individual, group, or consultative.

When appropriate for the unique needs of a child, the IEP includes a statement of whether or not the child will need an extended school year or other calendar modification (USDE, 2006; 34 C.F.R. §300.106). Because of special health needs or other reasons, some students may need shorter school days or a shorter school year. Most school districts will have guidelines that explain under what conditions (how to justify it) this service is offered. Federal regulations require that school districts do not limit this option to any particular category of disability or the type, amount, or duration of those services (USDE; 34 C.F.R. §300.106).

Sometimes the recording of the details of this section occurs on the same page as the goals; in other cases it may appear on a page that lists services and supports. Since each school district has forms or a format for what information goes where in the IEP, simply follow the form. Follow the school district's lead in terms of how specific or general to be in describing the intervention plans.

▼ PARTICIPATION WITH CHILDREN WITHOUT DISABILITIES ▼

IDEA requires that the IEP contain specific information on the extent to which a child with a disability will participate with children without disabilities in a regular classroom, the general curriculum, and extracurricular/nonacademic activities (NICHCY, n.d.; USDE, 2006). The IEP must explain why, if participation in the above-mentioned activities is limited in any way, full participation is not possible. Under IDEA, the preference is that the student spend as much time as possible with peers without disabilities, which means that IEP team members must have good reasons for providing services outside of the regular classroom. The IEP team must determine whether the child could participate in a regular classroom or extracurricular activities with the use of supplementary services and aids. Removing a child from a regular classroom cannot be done only because of needed modifications in the curriculum. The child's transportation needs can be addressed in this section or on a separate page (NICHCY; USDE). While the occupational therapist is not usually the person on the team responsible for documenting this, her knowledge and experience in adaptation of tasks and environments make her a great contributor to this process.

▼ PARTICIPATION IN STATE-AND DISTRICT-WIDE TESTS ▼

The IEP needs to explain why the unique needs of that child would make participation in state- or district-wide tests inappropriate (NICHCY, n.d.; USDE, 2006). If the child cannot participate in the state- or district-wide testing, the IEP states the way in which the child will be assessed. Additional rules for which children can be exempt from state- or district-wide tests can be found in the "No Child Left Behind" legislation, President George W. Bush's education reform law.

▼ DATES AND PLACES ▼

The date the IEP takes effect and the location of the services provided are identified in writing. The IEP needs to specify whether the child will receive special education and related services in the regular classroom, special education or other separate room, or a separate setting, such as a hospital, special school, or home (NICHCY, n.d.; USDE, 2006). Decisions about the location of services require discussion of the "least restrictive environment"

(LRE) (Jackson, 2007; NICHCY; USDE). The least restrictive environment refers to the place where a child with a disability has the greatest exposure to children without disabilities yet where the child with a disability can get his or her needs met. For many children, this means they spend some portion of their day in a regular classroom, some in a separate location. The occupational therapist must make a recommendation to the IEP team as to whether occupational therapy intervention will happen in a regular classroom, in a separate room, or both.

▼ TRANSITION ▼

Transition planning and services typically begin when a child is age 16 (NICHCY, n.d.; USDE, 2006). These services are designed to help the child move from school to life after school, such as preparing for a job and independent living (Orentlicher, 2007; NICHCY, n.d.; USDE). These services are based on the student's wants, needs, and preferred lifestyle. Again, the expertise of an occupational therapist can be of great help in planning for such a move. While the occupational therapist may not write this part of the IEP, he or she will have good ideas to contribute to the planning process.

▼ MEASURING PROGRESS ▼

If you set goals, it stands to reason that you would want to do some evaluation of the child's progress toward meeting those goals throughout the year. The IEP team must have a method of reviewing progress and communicating that progress to the child's parents and/or guardians (NICHCY, n.d.; USDE, 2006). If the child is not making the progress that was expected, the IEP must be revised to address that lack of progress (USDE; 20 U.S.C. 1400.614[d][4][A]). Both the occupational therapist and occupational therapy assistant participate in this process. Table 17.1 has links to some websites that have sample completed IEPs.

TABLE 17.1   Websites with Sample IEPs

Website	Host
http://www.vesid.nysed.gov/specialed/publications/policy/iep/sampform.htm	New York State Education Department
https://www.k12.wa.us/SpecialEd/module.aspx?printable=true	Office of the Superintendent of Public Instruction, State of Washington
http://www.familyvillage.wisc.edu/education/iepsamples.html	Family Village School, Wisconsin
http://www.projectspot.org/resources.htm	Supporting Project Outcomes and Teachers (Kansas)
http://www.untangleautism.org/0300hfa1.htm	Untangle Autism
http://sitemaker.umich.edu/special.education/files/sample_elem_iep.pdf	University of Michigan

SUMMARY

The Individual Education Program (IEP) is the guiding document for services provided by school system personnel, including occupational therapy. Careful wording of goals and objectives or benchmarks is essential. Goals and objectives/benchmarks often follow a specific formula for wording. Goals are the outcomes the child is expected to meet a year from when they are written. Objectives are steps to help the child meet the goals. Occupational therapy practitioners contribute to many parts of the IEP, but are usually not responsible for writing the entire document.

All of this demonstrates just how explicit school system documentation is. Nothing can be assumed. Be clear and direct because not everyone reading the IEP will have the same level of education and understanding of the material as you do.

Because of the amount of specificity in goal setting, specifying minutes per week for every service provider involved with the child in the school, identifying the least restrictive environment, and listing curricular, environmental, and programmatic modifications, the IEP can become a lengthy document. Once you participate in writing one, you will be glad to only do one per year per child. You will also be grateful for a chance to revise your goals and objectives at midyear.

REFERENCES

Case-Smith, J., & Rogers, J. (2005). School-based occupational therapy. In J. Case-Smith (Ed.), *Occupational therapy for children* (5th ed., pp. 795–824). St. Louis, MO: Mosby.

Jackson, L. L. (2007). Legislative context of occupational therapy practice in schools and early childhood settings. In L. L. Jackson (Ed.) *Occupational therapy services for children and youth under IDEA* (3rd ed.; pp. 1–22). Bethesda, MD: American Occupational Therapy Association.

Massachusetts Department of Education. (2001). *IEP process guide.* Retrieved March 28, 2003, from www.doe.mass.edu/sped/iep/proguide.pdf

National Center Dissemination for Children with Disabilities (n.d.). *Handouts: Theme D: Individualized Education Programs.* Retrieved Oct 10, 2008, from http://www.nichcy. org/Laws/IDEA/Documents/Training_Curriculum/D-handouts.pdf

Polichino, J.E., Clark, G.F., Swinth, Y & Muhlenhaupt, M. (2007). Legislative context of occupational therapy practice in schools and early childhood settings. In L. L. Jackson (Ed.) *Occupational therapy services for children and youth under IDEA* (3rd ed.; pp. 23–58). Bethesda, MD: American Occupational Therapy Association.

Orentlicher (2007). Legislative context of occupational therapy practice in schools and early childhood settings. In L. L. Jackson (Ed.) *Occupational therapy services for children and youth under IDEA* (3rd ed.; pp. 187–212). Bethesda, MD: American Occupational Therapy Association.

United States Department of Education. (2006). *Building the legacy of IDEA 2004.* Retrieved October 10, 2008, from http://idea.ed.gov/explore/home

Virginia Department of Education. (2008). *Virginia Department of Education's Sample IEP Form.* Retrieved on October 10, 2008, from http://www.doe.virginia.gov/VDOE/sped/ iep_form_doc

Administrative Documentation

▼ INTRODUCTION ▼

In addition to clinical or school-based documentation, there is documentation related to administrative tasks such as getting paid for services, documenting workplace injuries, writing policies and procedures, and similar tasks. Some of these documents may be written by anyone in the department; they are not necessarily the sole domain of supervisory personnel.

Administrative documentation varies greatly from facility to facility and setting to setting. The chapters in the section deal with several different types of administrative documentation, but these are by no means the only administrative documentation that gets done. Specifically, documents like productivity reports and staffing reports are so individualized by each facility/setting it would be impossible to do justice to them here; therefore, they are not included in this book. As you read the chapters in this section, realize that the information is intentionally general. You can expect modifications in form and content by the facility/setting.

▼ STRUCTURE OF THIS SECTION OF THE BOOK ▼

Chapter 18 deals with incident reports. Incident reports are written whenever there is an injury, no matter how slight, to a client, visitor, or a staff member. Incident reports are used by the facility to help learn from accidents or errors in an effort to prevent them from happening again.

Chapter 19 discusses ways to word appeal letters. Appeal letters are used when an occupational therapist or client thinks that a third-party payer (like Medicare or an HMO) has denied reimbursement unjustly. These letters explain why occupational therapy services are needed for a particular client.

Chapter 20 presents various ways to take minutes at a meeting. It has been said that if it was not documented, it did not happen. One way to demonstrate that a supervisor provided instruction to staff or that a policy was reviewed is to document it in meeting minutes. The minutes need to be retained in such a fashion that they can be easily retrieved and that everyone in the department has access to them.

Chapter 21 deals with grant writing. Grants are funds made available to an organization for a specific purpose, such as developing a new program or to fund services for clients who do not have the financial resources to pay for services (like scholarships for occupational therapy intervention). Usually, grants are awarded to facilities, departments, or nonprofit organizations. Grant money does not need to be repaid, but there are usually conditions for the award of the money. There is always a process for applying for grant money. This chapter discusses a common process for requesting grant money, but there may be details that are unique to particular funding sources that are not covered here.

Chapter 22 presents a format for writing policies and procedures. Policy and procedure manuals are used to guide employees in their on-the-job performance. They explain what must be done and how it must be done. Following policies and procedures is essential for the orderly conduct of the workplace. When an occupational therapy practitioner fails to follow policies and procedures, he or she weakens his or her defense if a client should decide to sue.

Finally, Chapter 23 discusses job descriptions. Occupational therapy practitioners may not only write job descriptions for occupational therapy positions, but they might be called upon to assist with writing job descriptions for other disciplines or industries. Because of their expertise and skill in breaking down occupations into specific tasks and identifying environmental factors influencing job performance, occupational therapy practitioners are excellent at writing job descriptions.

CHAPTER 18

Incident Reports

INTRODUCTION

Imagine this scene:

> An occupational therapist is working on toilet transfers with a teenager who recently had a hemispherectomy (to reduce seizures). The client is much taller than the clinician, and when he starts to lose his balance, the occupational therapist tries in vain to lower him gently to the floor. Instead, he falls and hits his head on the sink, causing a gash on his forehead before landing in a heap on the floor with the occupational therapist still holding on to his transfer belt. The occupational therapy assistant immediately summons help.

After attending to the immediate medical needs of the client and the occupational therapy assistant (if he or she is hurt during this event), it will be necessary to document this incident. The person who is most directly involved in the incident is the person who documents it. Generally, the facility will have a form, usually called an incident report, which will have to be completed in addition to documenting the incident in the medical (or school) record. In this case, the occupational therapy assistant would document it. Usually, after the occupational therapy practitioner completes this form, a supervisor will review the form and may complete a section of the form designed for supervisor input. The form is then routed to the person designated by the facility as the risk management coordinator (or someone with a similar title). It will be used to help the facility investigate possible corrective actions to prevent such incidents, sometimes called "adverse events" (Scott, 2006).

If this event had happened in a clinic or medical facility, a copy of the incident report would not be placed in the clinical record or mentioned in any other clinical document; this is confidential information (*Charting,* 2006). Just what should be documented in the clinical record will be discussed later in this chapter. Examples of other types of incidents that should be reported include burns (e.g., from modalities involving heat or cooking), injuries from the use of restraints, bumps on the head (e.g., bumping into a cabinet), or sores that develop from an ill-fitting orthotic or prosthetic device (*Charting*).

If this event had happened in a school setting, an incident report would also be required. An incident report is completed if any student, faculty, visitor, or staff member is injured on school property. If the incident took place on school property, the principal usually needs to be notified as soon as possible, in addition to the designated risk manager for the school district. Schools may also require incident reports to be completed for incidents of fighting, bullying, cheating, or weapons violations. In these cases, the incident reports may become part of the educational record (Hollis/Brookline High School, 2003).

▼ LEGAL CONSIDERATIONS ▼

The facility's liability or property insurance provider often requires the incident report. Whenever a client, visitor, or employee is injured, there is the possibility of a lawsuit. The incident report is the primary source of documentation of what happened (Scott, 2006). However, if the case does go to court, the incident report itself is usually immune (exempt) from discovery by the person who files the lawsuit (plaintiff) and his or her attorney. To be exempt, the incident reports usually have to be clearly labeled as a "'confidential quality assurance/improvement report' or a 'document prepared at the direction of the facility attorney in anticipation of or in preparation for litigation.'" (Scott, 2006, p. 140). If they are not labeled in that way, they can be considered business records (Southwick, 1988). If the plaintiff's attorney thinks that the incident report is essential for proving the case, and would be admissible as evidence in court, business records can be obtained before they are presented in court.

An incident report is completed whenever a client, visitor, or staff member is injured, no matter how big or how small the incident. There may be slightly different forms for when the injured party is a client/visitor or a staff member, but both forms will want similar information. I have always been told that an incident report should be completed for any injury, even a paper cut. One risk manager told me that what looks like a simple paper cut could get infected, and could turn into a big problem, so always fill out the form.

In reality, many staff members fail to complete the report for such a small thing as a paper cut. In cold, dry climates, paper cuts can be a daily occurrence. If a staff member filled out an incident report for each cut, he or she would be doing it several times a week. It seems like a waste of paper and a waste of time. You cannot prevent paper cuts. However, you need to follow the policies and procedures of the facility. If the person in charge of risk management at your facility says it is not necessary to complete an incident report for a paper cut, then that is fine. If the risk manager says that incident reports are necessary regardless of the size of the injury, then you have to do it.

▼ RECORDING INFORMATION ON AN INCIDENT REPORT FORM AND CLIENT RECORD ▼

Any lawyer I've ever talked to has told me that if I am ever questioned about an event that has occurred, simply answer the questions and do not volunteer additional information. I think it would be wise to view the incident report in the same way. Answer the questions directly, but do not volunteer additional information. The more information you provide, the more likely you are to add embellishments, exaggerations, and extraneous information that could be turned against you by a skilled attorney. As concisely as possible, simply provide the necessary facts on the incident report itself. If you are concerned that the incident could wind up in court, there is nothing that prohibits you from recording a more thorough description of what transpired, including your impressions (as opposed to facts), for your own records, as long as you protect the confidentiality of those involved in the incident.

That said, you still have to provide enough information to adequately describe what happened. You must be objective. Remember the "Descriptive, Interpretive, and Evaluative" discussion from the chapter on evaluation reports? Keep it descriptive, but avoid interpretive or evaluative statements. Examples of interpretive or evaluative statements would include speculating on the cause (Scott, 2006), or taking or assigning blame. You can talk to the safety coordinator later about your impressions, but impressions do not belong on the form (*Charting*, 2006). Only record what you experienced, not what others tell you that they saw, unless you put the other statements in quote marks and identify the statement as hearsay. If the incident involves a client or student, and the client or student says something about his or her role in the incident, record it in quote marks and identify the speaker (*Charting*). If there are witnesses, you may be asked to name them (Elkin, Perry, & Potter, 2000). You will also be asked to specify the time, to the nearest minute, that the incident occurred.

Only record what you actually see, what you witnessed, do not assume anything. For example, if you walk into a room and see a client on the floor, simply describe what you saw, not what you think might have happened, no matter how obvious it seems. Describe the position the person was in when you discovered him or her and the time you found the person. Do not say that you walked into the room and it looked like the person had fallen. You do not know that the person fell; that will be determined when the incident is investigated.

If the incident involves a client, then in the clinical record, documentation would reflect the nature of the injury and any aid provided to the client (Scott, 2006). There should be congruence between what is written in the clinical record and in the incident report

(*Charting*, 2006). Document what the client or client's family says about the incident. Do not offer suggestions for how to prevent this type of event from happening again (*Charting*).

Let's look at another case:

Korpo is an occupational therapy assistant who was born in Somalia and immigrated to this country 10 years ago. She has been assigned to work with a man who recently suffered a head injury, dislocated right shoulder, and two cracked ribs as a result of a motorcycle accident. He is in an agitated state, but needs to relearn grooming, hygiene, and dressing skills. He is a large man with many tattoos and body piercings.

When Korpo enters the room, he immediately begins name-calling and refusing to cooperate. His exact words are "Get out of here, you bitch! I don't do nothin' for n-g---s!" As she brings him a warm, wet washcloth, he hurls it at her, and then shoves the overbed table into her stomach, knocking her down hard. His face gets red, his eyes are open wide, his teeth are bared, and the veins in his neck are standing out. He picks up the phone on the bedside table and throws it at her, hitting her in the head. She crawls out of the room, a small cut on her forehead.

What would be documented in the medical record, and what would be recorded in the incident report? Here is one possibility.

In the medical record, a narrative note might read:

2/4/09, 10:00 AM. Patient refused to participate in self-care training at bedside. He swore and a washcloth and threw the telephone at the occupational therapy assistant. He knocked her down with the bedside table. OTA will attempt to work with him again bedside tomorrow as per the plan of care. Korpo Bohla, OTA/L

A SOAP note might look like this:

S: "Get out of here, you b---h! I don't do nothin' for n-g---s!
O: Client refused occupational therapy self-care training at bedside. He swore and threw the telephone at the occupational therapy assistant. He knocked her down with the bedside table.
A: Client is agitated and uncooperative.
P: Continue to attempt bedside intervention 2/5/09.

Korpo Bohla, OTA/L

In the narrative portion of the incident report, you would see:

When I entered the room, he immediately began name-calling and refusing to cooperate. His exact words were "Get out of here, you b---h! I don't do nothin' for n-g---s!" When I brought him a warm, wet washcloth, he hurled it at me, and then shoved the overbed table into my stomach, knocking me down hard. His face got red, his eyes were open wide, his teeth were bared, and the veins in his neck were standing out. He picked up the phone on the bedside table and threw it at me, which hit me in the head. I crawled out of the room. There was a small cut on my forehead. The cut was cleaned, antibiotic cream was applied, and the wound was closed with steri-strips.

There are some obvious differences between what gets written in the clinical record and what is written in the incident report. The progress note (narrative or SOAP format) is very concise, only the bare minimum of information is written (Distasio, 2000; Scott, 2006; *Charting*, 2006). While the progress notes do not convey the entire picture, you do get some sense of the anger expressed by the client. In a client recovering from a brain injury, this is a predictable phase that many clients go through. It is essential that the agitation and anger be documented. Notice that neither progress note mentions the incident report form.

If the incident results in a client needing medical intervention, that intervention must be documented in the client's clinical record (Elkin et al., 2000). If you are working in a setting without a clinical record, such as at a school, then the incident report may be the only document you write on, depending on the facility's (school's) policy. Of course, in either case, you need to talk to your supervisor as soon as possible after the incident, and in a school, you need to notify the principal as well.

The question that remains is, if a trigger for the explosive behavior can be identified, should it be documented? One side of the issue, using this case as an example, is if the trigger is identified, it can be avoided in the future, cutting down on the risk of injury to staff (Distasio, 2000). On the other hand, what if the trigger is identified, but it casts the client in a negative light? For example, what if the trigger in this case is that the client is prejudiced against people of color? To decrease agitation, one could make an argument that only white staff should work with the client. But that would be discriminatory, and might cause staff of all colors to have negative feelings toward the client. This is a really delicate issue. Most facilities have policies on discrimination. Whether or not to document the trigger would not be a decision that occupational therapy staff would make alone.

Clearly, what is written in the incident report is more detailed. The incident report addresses what happened to the staff person whereas a progress note in a client's record would not. As stated earlier in this chapter, do not even make a reference to completing an incident report in the client's record (Scott, 2006; *Charting*, 2006).

An incident report is also likely to include some checklists for the employee to mark. There may be a checklist that asks the writer to check off what precautions were taken, where the incident occurred, what kind of medical attention was required, and what measures could be taken to prevent further incidents. Of course, with any checklist, there is usually a space for "other" with a blank to fill in where the writer could add to the list something that had not been considered before.

Exercise 18.1

1. Using the case from the beginning of this chapter (post-hemispherectomy client during toilet transfer training), write a narrative progress note and a narrative entry for the incident report.

   Narrative progress note:

   Incident report:

2. Using the following case, write a SOAP note and a narrative entry for the incident report.

   You are working in a community-based program for persons with mental health disorders. The program focuses on development of job skills. The client you are working with on completing job applications begins to get frustrated with the number of errors she is making. On the second application, she begins to scribble across the whole page, saying "Dammit" repeatedly. You calm her down and have her try again. This time, about halfway through, she picks up the application and begins to tear it into pieces while yelling, "I quit. I can't do this. I'm never going to get a job." Before you can stop her, she gets a paper cut. Then she starts cursing, "F---ing S---, A--hole moron, S---" and then more of the same. She starts to hit the wall with her fist. You interrupt her tirade to tell her she has a cut, and when she sees it, she stops and stares at it. You take her to the sink, run it under cold water for a bit, gently dry it off, and then put an adhesive bandage on it. You have her sit calmly for a while before engaging her in another task.

   S:

   O:

   A:

P:

Incident report:

3. Write either a SOAP or narrative progress note and a narrative portion of an incident report about the following scene.

You are an occupational therapist working in a preschool program. You are coleading a group of 3-year-olds. It is snack time. There will be sliced apples and peanut butter. While you are putting peanut butter on the plates, the special education teacher is sitting at the table with the children, showing them what the inside of an apple looks like. She is using a 10-inch cook's knife to cut the apple. Her hands are getting sticky from the apple's juice, so she gets up to get a napkin, setting the knife down on the table. You are at the other end of the table. Just as you are about to remind the teacher to take the knife with her, 3-year-old Tyla picks it up by the blade end, cutting the palm side of three fingers. The special education teacher never saw anything; her back was turned, so she tells you that you have to fill out the paperwork. You take the screaming child to the sink, but realize the child will need medical attention. You wrap up the hand in a clean towel while the special education teacher calls the child's mom and you keep pressure on the wound. Clearly the special education teacher was negligent and bears full responsibility for what happened.

Progress note:

Incident report:

SUMMARY

When the unexpected happens, it needs to be documented in two ways. First, a concise note explaining the event is written in the client's record. The narrative or SOAP/DAP note must contain only objective information that does not lay blame on anyone. Then there is the incident report. You need to provide all the relevant facts on an incident report, but do not volunteer any extra information. Do not lay blame or accept blame anywhere on an incident report. The information you provide may be used by the facility for quality or risk management purposes.

REFERENCES

Charting made incredibly easy (3rd ed.). (2006). Philadelphia: Lippencott, Williams & Wilkens.

Distasio, C. A. (2000). Workplace violence: Part II: Documentation and reporting—how to paint the picture. *Maryland-Nurse, 1*(2), 12.

Elkin, M. K., Perry, A. G., & Potter, P. A. (2000). *Nursing interventions and clinical skills* (2nd ed.). St. Louis, MO: Mosby.

Hollis/Brookline High School. (2003). *Safe school policy: Incident report.* Retrieved April 7, 2003, from http://www.Hollis/BrooklineHighSchool.k12.nh.us/equitycouncil/harassme.htm

Scott, R. (2006). *Legal aspects of documenting patient care for rehabilitation professionals* (3rd ed.). Sudbury, MA: Jones and Bartlett.

Southwick, A. F. (1988). *The law of hospital and health care administration* (2nd ed.). Ann Arbor, MI: Foundation of the American College of Healthcare Executives.

CHAPTER 19

Appeal Letters

INTRODUCTION

It is not unusual for an occupational therapist and a third-party payer to disagree about a client's need for services. In some cases, the occupational therapist may not know until after the service is delivered that the payer does not think that occupational therapy services were medically necessary (or whatever that payer's standard is). Third-party payers may deny payment based on medical necessity, or on a technicality such as not properly completing a required form, not sending in the billing in a timely manner, errors in completing the billing forms, or "claim overlap with another provider's claim for the same or similar service" (Shamus & Stern, 2004). Most occupational therapy services must be paid for in order for the provider to stay in business, to continue to serve other clients. If the claim is denied on the basis of a technicality, correcting the error may be all that is required. If the occupational therapy practitioner thinks that a client needs services and that those services reasonably fall within the scope of what the payer customarily pays for, he or she can appeal the decision not to pay for services. In addition to providing additional clinical documentation (if there is any that was not submitted with the initial claim), the occupational therapist writes an appeal letter that explains the rationale for occupational therapy for that particular client, describes the nature of the skilled service needed, and makes an explicit request to overturn the denial (Brennan & Robinson, 2006).

Medial necessity is a concept that has been embraced by government (Medicare and Medicaid) and nongovernmental agencies (private health insurance, managed care, or worker's compensation insurance) as the standard for determining whether or not to pay for a service. Every payer uses a slightly different definition of medical necessity, so it is important to find out what the definition is for the specific payer to whom you want to appeal a denial. Medicare defines medically necessary as follows: "Services are medically necessary if the documentation indicates they meet the requirements for medical necessity including that they are skilled, rehabilitative services, provided by clinicians (or qualified professionals when appropriate) with the approval of a physician/NPP, safe, and effective (i.e., progress indicates that the care is effective in rehabilitation of function)" (Centers for Medicare and Medicaid Services [CMS], 2008, p. 23).

▼ APPEAL LETTERS AS OPPORTUNITIES TO EDUCATE ▼

It is critically important that the appeal letter is clear, to the point, and states what you want done about the original denial. In some cases, the person reading the appeal letter may be the same person who wrote the denial in the first place, so you have to be very careful to appear professional and respectful of the initial decision. In other cases, there may be levels of review, and a nurse, an occupational therapist, or a physician may conduct the second or third review.

It is helpful to look at an appeal as a learning process for the reviewer. If the reviewer is not an occupational therapist, this is an opportunity for you to teach him or her something about it. As unbelievable as it sounds in this day and age, there are still people out there who think occupational therapists only work with hand function or only provide diversional therapy. I have heard of some insurers who only pay for physical therapy on an outpatient basis for clients with hand injuries, not occupational therapy, even if the occupational therapist is a certified hand therapist.

Not so many years ago, when I called an insurance company to check on coverage for an outpatient, I was told the insurer did not cover occupational therapy services for outpatients (only for inpatients) because "who needs underwater basket weaving anyway?" The person actually said that! After a few calming breaths and a couple more phone calls to the insurer and the client's employer (the insurance was through the client's work), the insurer did pay for occupational therapy, explaining that it had inadvertently left occupational therapy out of the policy. Since it was not listed specifically as an excluded service, they had to cover it.

You have a fighting chance of getting coverage for occupational therapy if the insurance policy is silent on occupational therapy coverage. The insurer can be convinced of the need for occupational therapy and save face by saying the omission of occupational therapy was simply an oversight. If the policy specifically says that occupational therapy services are excluded from coverage, then it is hard to get the insurer to pay for occupational therapy services no matter how strong your arguments are.

Case Study

You are working with an elderly man in his home. He has coverage through Medicare. The Medicare contractor determines that occupational therapy services are no longer medically necessary and should have been discontinued. You had continued to work with the man until you heard that the last 2 weeks of occupational therapy were not paid for. He is recovering from a hip replacement on his left side (6 weeks ago), complicated by a below-knee amputation of his left leg (5 years ago), diabetic neuropathy (decreased sensation in all remaining limbs), and cataracts in both eyes. Occupational therapy services have been provided twice a week for 6 weeks to improve self-care skills. Physical therapy has also been involved with this client, working on ambulation and transfers. Physical therapy had discontinued services, saying the client has plateaued; he is not making any more progress. You want to continue to see the client in his own home to work on more kitchen skills, lower-extremity dressing, and problem solving related to day-to-day challenges he faces. He lives with his wife of 60 years who has been his caretaker but has recently begun to show signs of Alzheimer's. Their children live 3 hours away and do not visit often. You have seen the client make good progress in all areas. Since it is inappropriate for you to write about another person in your client's documentation, you have not documented his wife's deteriorating cognitive state. Your client is cognitively intact. However, you know that the client needs to learn to cook because he has expressed concern about his wife leaving the gas stove on when cooking is done, burning food, and misplacing food items. You decide to appeal this decision.

▼ WRITING AN APPEAL LETTER ▼

In the above case, you are privy to information that the payer does not know. The payer has read all your intervention plans, but is unaware of other environmental factors affecting this case. You have done a good job documenting the client's progress in the stated need areas. The payer has assumed that since the client reached a plateau in physical therapy, a plateau in occupational therapy cannot be far behind, and in most cases, 6 weeks of occupational therapy is usually sufficient. In your letter you will outline progress made so far, what additional progress you expect in the next 4 weeks, and justify it by explaining the social environmental factors that affect this case. Your letter will be formal and professional. Figure 19.1 shows an example of what it might look like.

Part B Reviewer
Best Deal Health Plan
1234 Frugal Street
New Money, NJ 07666-7666

April 15, 2009

Dear Reviewer,

I am the occupational therapist working with Mr. J. Doe, case #246810. I am writing to request that the decision to deny further occupational therapy services be reversed on the basis of the following additional information.

Mr. Doe has been making steady gains in lower extremity dressing, meal preparation and cleanup, and problem solving. He has progressed from being totally dependent in lower extremity dressing to needing minimal assist and adaptive equipment. Meal preparation has progressed from needing step-by-step instruction to Mr. Doe initiating meal planning and preparation. He still has difficulty transporting food from the stove to the table or counter and opening some packaging. He provides instruction to his wife in cleaning up after meals. Mr. Doe has expressed concern for allowing his wife to use the stove. She is showing significant episodes of memory loss and confusion about daily chores leading to some dangerous situations in the kitchen. Mr. Doe wants to take over some of her kitchen responsibilities. Teaching Mr. Doe to plan and prepare meals is essential in order for the Does to live in their own home safely.

In addition to the plans of care you have already reviewed, I am enclosing copies of the visit notes for each of the occupational therapy sessions from the last 6 weeks. If I can provide you with any additional information, please let me know.

Sincerely,

Carin Provider, OTR/L
Carin Provider, OTR/L

FIGURE 19.1   Sample Appeals Letter.

▼ MEDICARE APPEALS ▼

Medicare made significant changes to its appeal processes in 2005 (AOTA, 2005; Brennan & Robinson, 2006). The biggest change is that the process is the same for both Part A and Part B Medicare. Timelines for responding to appeals have been shortened (AOTA, 2005; Brennan & Robinson). This means that occupational therapy practitioners need to be timely in their responses to denials if they want to get paid for their services. All appeals must be done in writing (CMS, 2006). Minor errors or omissions that cause an initial denial are handled through a reopening process rather than the appeals process (CMS, 2005)

Medicare sends a determination of coverage called a Medicare Summary Notice (MSN) to the beneficiary (AOTA, 2005). It is important to have a mechanism for the beneficiary to share this information with you, the provider, since you will not receive this notice (AOTA, 2005). A beneficiary can transfer his or her right to appeal to the provider, as long as Form CMS-20031 is completed and signed by the beneficiary and provider (CMS, 2006). Under Medicare rules, a provider or client has 120 days to send a request for a redetermination (form CMS 20027) to the office that sent the MSN (AOTA, 2005; CMS, 2006). The redetermination is an examination of the request by the Medicare contractor (formerly called the fiscal intermediary [Part A] or carrier [Part B]) (CMS, 2006). To request the redetermination, complete form CMS-20027 (CMS, 2006). The Medicare contractor who will make the redetermination has 60 days to do so. The notice of redetermination can be sent to the beneficiary or beneficiary's representative (AOTA, 2005).

The notice of redetermination must include information on the facts in the case, the laws and policies which apply to the case, and the rights to and process for further appeal (AOTA, 2005). If there is missing documentation, it will be identified in the notice of redetermination. The burden of supplying missing documentation is given to the provider, not the beneficiary. All information must be provided at this level of review because after this level, no new information can be presented (AOTA, 2005). If the provider or beneficiary are not satisfied with the outcome of the redetermination review, they can file form CMS 20033 to request a reconsideration (CMS, 2006).

The reconsideration is conducted by Medicare Qualified Independent Contractors (QICs), independent physician or other health care professional reviewers (AOTA, 2005; CMS, 2006). The beneficiary, the beneficiary's representative, or the provider has 180 days to request reconsideration of the redetermination from the office that is specified on the notice of redetermination. This is a paper review only, so the documentation has to speak for itself. The request has to explain why the provider or beneficiary disagrees with the redetermination. The QIC has 60 days to make a determination based on any new evidence, as well as the original claim. If the QIC does not rule within the 60-day limit, the beneficiary or provider may request the claim be automatically reviewed at the next higher level (AOTA, 2005; CMS, 2006).

An administrative law judge (ALJ) conducts the next level of the appeals process (AOTA, 2005; CMS, 2006). A claim can only get to this level if the amount of the claim is over $110. The ALJ must decide the appeal within 90 days of receiving the appeal. The hearing can be conducted in person, by video conference, or by phone; however, a request for an in-person hearing creates an automatic waiver of the 90-day time limit (AOTA, 2005; CMS, 2006).

There are additional levels of appeal, including going to court, and the reader can learn more by visiting the AOTA or CMS websites. Since no new evidence, no new documentation, can be submitted at these levels, they are not addressed here.

Always make a copy of all documents associated with the appeal to keep for your records. In wording your reasons for appealing the decision, be clear and direct. Do not imply anything, say it explicitly. If the MSN says that your services are not medically necessary, say that you feel the services are medically necessary and give a clear and concise reason you feel the services are necessary. The reasons you feel your services are medically necessary include the fact that the services require the skills of an occupational therapist or occupational therapy assistant under the supervision of an occupational therapist (no other professionals or aides could safely and effectively provide the service), that the service is required for the patient's progress, and that the patient's functional goals can be achieved in a reasonable amount of time. Explain how the specific services you are providing have functional outcomes, usually in areas of occupation such as activities of daily living (ADLs) or instrumental activities of daily living (IADLs) and are appropriate to the setting, the client's condition, and the skills of the person providing the services.

Obviously, the Medicare appeals process is complicated and time-consuming. The best option is to document so well that there are no questions of medical necessity or the need for skilled services. Submit your documentation on time and in the right place.

▼ APPEALS TO PRIVATE INSURERS (INCLUDING HMOs) ▼

Insurers have appeals processes written into each of their health plans (and worker's compensation plans, auto insurance plans, etc.). If it is at all possible, a good first step is to contact the insurer and find out exactly why the claim was denied (Appeal Solutions, 2002). Find out what the insurer's definition of medical necessity is and build your arguments for covering the service around that definition. For example, some insurers routinely deny coverage for sensory integration intervention. They say it is experimental (often insurers say experimental procedures are not medically necessary), that there is not conclusive evidence that it is an effective, medically acceptable intervention. I know of one insurer who will deny an entire claim if even one unit of sensory integration intervention shows up on a claim, even if there are other procedures used during the same intervention session.

The occupational therapist could do one of two things here. One is that he or she could find as much evidence in the literature supporting the use of sensory integrative techniques and attach those to the letter of appeal. This could be a lengthy process, and you have no guarantee the reviewer will read any of the supporting literature since it does not relate specifically to this case. But it is better than doing nothing. Another would be to make an argument that the other procedures used during that intervention session are reasonable and necessary for the child's condition, and that the insurer has paid for those services in the past. In this case you might get paid for some of the session, but probably not the whole session. If I were going to fight an insurer who considers sensory integration to be experimental, I would also enlist the support of the parent and referring physician, asking them to write letters explaining the potential benefits of the denied services.

If you find out that the denial is for all services of a type, such as sensory integration, you can enlist the support of your state occupational therapy association (if you are a member). The association can try to work with the insurer's medical director to change corporate policy. The American Occupational Therapy Association also has resources for members to help in challenging insurance companies.

Insurers deny payment for occupational therapy services for many reasons, not just because they consider an intervention experimental. Other reasons for denial include exceeding coverage limits (e.g., number of allowed visits), failure to complete the required forms in a timely manner, and poor documentation that does not demonstrate medical necessity (Glomstad, 2006). Many insurers post their documentation requirements online, so ignorance of the rules is no excuse. For example, Aetna posts its policy on occupational therapy coverage, including the type and frequency of documentation required at its website (http://www .aetna.com/cpb/medical/data/200_299/0250.html). Be aware that not all private insurance or managed care plans cover the same services. One managed care company in Minnesota will cover occupational therapy services for ADLs, but not for IADLs. This company feels that help is easily available for people with deficits in IADLs, such as grocery shopping. There are home delivery services, so a person would not need to be able to go to the store for food.

Just as with Medicare appeals, a well-written letter of appeal and supporting documentation are needed to try to reverse a denial of coverage. Make sure that your documentation supports your claim of medical necessity and that the skills of an occupational therapist or occupational therapy assistant under the supervision of an occupational therapist are required to address the client's needs. The best defense is a good offense, so take the offensive and use principles of good documentation all the time.

Exercise 19.1

Give reasons to overturn a coverage decision for each of the two cases below.

Case 1: Shevan

Shevan is a 6-year-old child with fetal alcohol syndrome seen for occupational therapy at an after-school program. She has trouble concentrating and is quite active. She is tactilely defensive and fearful of movement through space when both feet are not on the ground (i.e., swings, slides, etc.). She does receive special education services at school, but there are reports that she hits other children and frequently gets off her chair to walk around when she should be sitting and listening. At the after-school program, you have observed her improve at sitting for longer stretches of time, up to 5 minutes sometimes. She has been in the program for 2 months. She is beginning to appear more relaxed on a swing, as long as her feet can touch the ground and she can control the distance the swing goes with her feet. Just yesterday she allowed the swing to go back and forth gently twice before stopping it. She was scribbling on a coloring book page when she first came to the program, but now she attempts to stay roughly within the lines.

The insurance company said that the services of an occupational therapist are not medically necessary. They say that the services could be provided by lesser-skilled personnel.

Case 2: Seiki

Seiki is an elderly man who had a brain tumor removed from the right side of his brain 2 weeks ago. He is now at a long-term care facility for rehabilitation and then plans to return home to his farm after 4 to 6 weeks of rehab. He has a grandson who is looking after his cows for him. His grandson lives on a neighboring farm. As a result of the surgery, Seiki has some limitation in the movement and coordination of his left arm and side. He also has left side neglect. He is beginning to accept that he has left neglect, but at the time of the last evaluation report/plan of care the neglect was strong, and he denied he had it. His left arm is flaccid, but in the last 2 days you have noticed some spasticity has set in. Seiki is making steady gains in dressing, feeding, grooming, and hygiene. His wife visits everyday, but she is a worrier, and says they will have to give up the farm if he does not get better. This agitates Seiki. He is sure that he will recover and be able to go back to farming. In fact, he says that where there is a will, there is a way, and he will rig something up to help him do the work. He has always been a bit of an inventor, and has invented several helpful farm implements in his day. You gave your word to Seiki that you would help him come up with some adaptation that would allow him to do some of the work he used to do in the barn. Then the denial notice came.

The Medicare contractor says that Seiki's potential for recovery is poor at best. The contractor says that Seiki should move to a lower RUG level with fewer therapy minutes.

SUMMARY

You have the right to appeal any payer's decision to deny coverage for occupational therapy services. Each payer will have a process for appealing such a decision. Writing a letter of appeal requires tact, clarity, and the powers of persuasion. You have to remain respectful regardless of how angry the decision makes you. You have to clearly state your reasons for wanting a coverage determination to be overturned. You have to construct sound arguments for the necessity of occupational therapy interventions in this specific case. Well-written appeal letters are extremely important to getting a denial overturned. You cannot overturn a denial unless you appeal it.

REFERENCES

American Occupational Therapy Association. (2005). *Know your Medicare appeal rights: The new landscape for appealing Medicare claim denials.* Retrieved June 5, 2007, from http://www.aota.org/members/area5/links/link16.asp?PLACE=/members/area5/links/link 16.asp

Appeal Solutions. (2002). Case study: Responding to insurance denials due to lack of medical necessity. *The Appeal Letter.* Retrieved November 21, 2002, from http://appealsolutions .com/tal/medical-necessity-case-study/htm

Brennan, C & Robinson, M (2006). Documentation: Getting it right to avoid Medicare denials. *OT Practice 11*(14), pp. 10–15.

Centers for Medicare and Medicaid Services. (2005). *MLN Matters Number MM4019.* Retrieved June 2, 2007, from http://www.cms.hhs.gov/mlnmattersarticles/downloads/mm4019.pdf

Centers for Medicare and Medicaid Services. (2006). *The Medicare appeals process: Five levels to protect providers, physicians, and other suppliers.* Retrieved June 6, 2007, from http://cms.hhs.gov/MLNProducts/downloads/MedicareAppealsProcess.pdf

Centers for Medicare and Medicaid Services. (2008). *Pub 100-02 Medicare benefit policy: Transmittal 88.* Retrieved May 9, 2008, from http://www.cms.hhs.gov/transmittals/downloads/R88BP.pdf

Glomstad, S. (2006). Keeping it covered. *Advance for Occupational Therapy Practitioners 22* (11) 16.

Shamus, E. & Stern, D, (2004). *Effective* documentation *for physical therapy professionals.* New York: McGraw-Hill.

CHAPTER 20

Meeting Minutes

INTRODUCTION

As has been said many times before, if it isn't documented, it didn't happen. While taking minutes may make some meetings feel more formal than the actual tone of the meeting, it is necessary to keep a record of what was discussed. When surveyors of any type (JCAHO, CARF, Department of Health, Department of Education, etc.) come to evaluate a facility or department, they usually ask to see copies of meeting minutes. Sometimes they are looking to verify that staff have been instructed in certain policies and procedures; other times they may be looking to see that continuing education has occurred. Meeting minutes also "give all group members the chance to see how issues that were discussed were finally resolved" (Mosvick & Nelson, 1987, p. 169).

▼ OVERVIEW OF MEETING MINUTES ▼

Most facilities, departments, or organizations have an already established system for taking minutes. For the sake of tradition, that system is continued. This is fine most of the time, but occasionally a new note taker will look for a different system. This chapter presents a couple of systems. Which system is used is often a reflection of the management style of that facility, department, or organization.

Meeting minutes can also be used as evidence in legal proceedings. There may be a question of when staff was informed about an administrative decision or policy change. Often, if there is a question about the level of training received by staff, meeting minutes can be used to see how much training (i.e., about a new policy or procedure) was provided and when.

Sometimes, the minutes are documentation of decisions made by a department, facility, or organization. It is not unusual for a topic of discussion that is raised today to have been discussed last year or a couple years ago. By going back over the minutes, time can be saved and the results of the last discussion shared. If there is nothing new to add, the group can move on to the next topic.

▼ COMMONALITIES ▼

All meeting minutes contain certain information, but the format may vary. One very important piece of information on every meeting minute is the date, including the year. Meeting minutes are not much good if you cannot tell when the meeting occurred. Minutes should also reflect who was present at the meeting. If the names of attendees and the date of the meeting are documented, then there is proof that a particular person was informed of whatever the topic was on that date. That person cannot claim ignorance as a means of defending him- or herself.

Topics of discussion are a main component of meeting minutes. Obviously, minutes are more than just a listing of people and dates. They have to contain something of substance. Some minutes try to capture the entire discussion; some summarize the discussion. How much of the discussion is captured in the minutes will vary from place to place.

Finally, the action items are included in the minutes. Action items are the tasks that people must do as a result of the discussion. Examples of action items include the following:

- Ellie will clean the refrigerator and Chris will clean the microwave.
- Jane will meet with the nursing staff to present our program revisions for post-mastectomy patients.
- Arica will represent the department on the interdisciplinary quality improvement team looking at improving customer service.
- Tanya will contact the vendor for splinting materials about presenting an in-service for the department.

▼ TAKING MINUTES ▼

If you are the person taking minutes at a meeting, the recorder, you have some special responsibilities. Because of the amount of concentration that it takes to record the discussion, it is difficult for one person to both lead a discussion and write minutes at the same time. The recorder is responsible for asking for clarification when discussions seem confusing or start going off on tangents (Mosvick & Nelson, 1987). The recorder can ask the group to verify the conclusions or summaries he or she draws at the end of a discussion. At the same time, the recorder needs to be ready to read back portions of the minutes to the group at the request of a group member.

If you are the recorder, be prepared with proper materials and be on time. If the agenda is provided ahead of time, use it to prepare the format or outline for taking minutes (meetingwizard.org). Be careful that your opinions on a particular subject do not color the minutes that you are taking. Use as few adjectives and adverbs as possible; it is fine if the minutes are dull to read (basic-learning.com). Words that signal that your opinions are surfacing include "inspiring," "interesting," "wonderful," "proud," or "antagonistic."

You may take minutes by writing longhand, using a laptop computer, or by tape-recording the meeting and transcribing it later. If you take minutes with paper and pen, be sure to number your pages. If you have a tendency to abbreviate words or use your own cryptic system, be sure to transcribe the minutes into usable form as soon as possible after the meeting. If you wait too long, you may not be able to make sense of your own minutes (meetingwizard.org). If the minutes refer to other documents, be sure to attach these documents to the official set of minutes or state where the documents can be found (effectivemeetings.com).

While you may make copies of minutes to distribute to each person who attended or should have attended the meeting, there is usually one set of minutes that is kept as the official record of the meeting. In some places, it may be a three-ring binder kept in the office. In others, it may be a website or folder on a shared drive on a computer. If a paper copy of the minutes is kept, some organizations require that the official minutes contain the signature of the minute-taker. In some organizations, the minutes do not become official until the Board of Directors or the membership of the committee approves them.

▼ FORMATS ▼

The simplest, but perhaps the wordiest way to take minutes is to keep a narrative record of the meeting. In this format, after the date and list of attendees, the minute-taker writes down as much of what happened at the meeting as possible. It may include who said what. The paragraphs may be numbered when they represent a new topic.

Figure 20.1 shows an example of narrative minutes of a department meeting.

You can see that taking minutes like this could lead to writer's cramp. It is a lot of writing, and not all of it is important to note. Perhaps some things would be better left undocumented (e.g., getting cut out of parking spaces by an aggressive lab employee) in departmental meeting minutes. On the other hand, if someone in the department missed the meeting, he or she could have a pretty good idea of what transpired at the meeting simply from reading the minutes.

Date: 11-25-08
Present: E. Bay, J. Kay, G. Whiz, and A. Ging

1. Announcements
   • Ellie announced that she would be taking Friday off and a sub would be called in.
   • Jane announced that the United Way fund drive would be starting next week.
   • Gina reminded staff that rounds this week are changed to Thursday at 9:00 a.m.

2. New patient transportation policy
   Jane presented the proposed new hospital policy on patient transportation. Rehabilitation therapies are to send the next day's schedule to each nursing unit, medical imaging, the lab, and the transportation pool by 3:00 p.m. each day. Unless otherwise noted on the schedule, nursing will have the patients dressed, in a wheelchair, with hearing aids and glasses on as needed by the scheduled pick-up time. Transportation pool personnel will transport those patients who are ready at their appointed time. If a patient is not ready, the transporter may wait for up to 5 minutes. If the patient is still not ready, then nursing will be responsible for finding a volunteer or aide to do the transporting. Patients must be finished with therapy at the time they are scheduled to go back to their rooms (or to other appointments), the transporter can only wait up to 5 minutes if the patient is not ready. After that, therapy is responsible for finding a volunteer or aide to do the transporting. Jane said the new policy was designed to encourage everyone to try to stick to the schedule. The policy is expected to go into effect in 30 days unless there is overwhelming negative feedback. The transportation improvement team is accepting written comments for the next 2 weeks. Gina asked if compliance to the policy would be tracked. Jane said yes, there would be forms that transporters fill out whenever they complete a transportation. Jane asked for a show of hands of people who were supportive of the proposed new policy. The department gave unanimous support to the policy. The policy is attached to these minutes.

3. Infection control
   Jane conducted the annual review of infection control policies and procedures for the department. We reviewed hand washing, and each member was asked to demonstrate proper technique. We discussed cleaning of supplies and equipment, including which cleaning solution is used for which items we clean and which items need to be sent to central sterile supply to be cleaned. We reviewed policies for working with patients in isolation rooms, when to wear protective gear (gloves, masks, and gowns), and proper technique for donning and doffing them. Finally, universal precautions were reviewed in detail. Each member of the department signed an annual review of infection control training confirmation sheet. Jane will forward these to the human resources department for placement in employee files.

4. Parking
   Jane asked for a volunteer to serve on a task force looking into issues regarding employee parking. Parking complaints have risen dramatically in the last year. Everyone in the department agrees that parking has gotten worse lately. Ellie said she tries to get to work 20 minutes early to find a decent spot. Arica said she has noticed that some employees get really competitive about parking spaces and that she has been cut out of a space on several occasions by an aggressive parker who works in the lab. The task force will look at existing parking options and consider alternatives for parking in the future. Arica volunteered to serve on the task force. The first meeting is next Friday at 2:30 p.m.

5. Budget request
   Ellie asked if there was any room in the budget for buying the newest revision of the Peabody Motor Scales. The test has new norms and a few new test items. Our competitors have all switched to the newer version. We use the test about 2–3 times per month, more often in summer. It would be a good investment. Jane said that she would need more information about the cost of the test and ordering information. There is some money in the budget, but there may not be enough for the test kit. We may have to delay or eliminate other expenses if we want it this year. If we cannot fit it in this year's budget, we should make it a priority for next year's budget.

FIGURE 20.1 Sample Narrative Meeting Minutes.

```
Date: 11-25-08
Present: E. Bay, J. Kay, G. Whiz, and A. Ging

1. Announcements
   a. Ellie announced that she would be taking Friday off and a sub would be called in.
   b. Jane announced that the United Way fund drive would be starting next week.
   c. Gina reminded staff that rounds this week is changed to Thursday at 9:00 a.m.

2. New patient transportation policy
   Jane presented the proposed new hospital policy on patient transportation, which was designed
   to encourage everyone to try to stick to the schedule. The policy is expected to go into effect in
   30 days unless there is overwhelming negative feedback. The transportation improvement team
   is accepting written comments for the next 2 weeks. Jane asked for a show of hands of people
   who were supportive of the proposed new policy. The department gave unanimous support to the
   policy. Policy is attached.

3. Infection control
   Jane conducted the annual review of infection control policies and procedures for the department
   as per hospital policy. We signed annual review of infection control training confirmation
   sheets, which Jane will forward to the human resources department for placement
   in employee files.

4. Parking
   Jane asked for a volunteer to serve on a task force looking at issues around employee parking.
   The task force will look at existing parking options and consider alternatives for parking
   in the future. Arica volunteered to serve on the task force. The first meeting is next Friday
   at 2:30 p.m.

5. Budget request
   Ellie asked if there was any room in the budget for buying the newest revision of the Peabody
   Motor Scales. Jane said that she would need more information about the cost of the test and
   ordering information. If we cannot fit it in this year's budget, we should make it a priority for next
   year's budget.
```

FIGURE 20.2   Example of Summary Format Meeting Minutes.

Another way to take minutes also involves a narrative format, but it uses summaries instead of trying to capture everything that was said. Figure 20.2 is an example of the same meeting, but a different format for the minutes.

You can see that minutes like this take up less space, but they also have less information. The summary format gives minimal information about what was discussed. It is enough to get the essence of what was discussed, but nothing is very substantial.

Minutes can use different numbering systems. Sometimes a typical outline format is used (I., A., 1., a.) but numerical systems are also used (1., 1.1., 1.1.2.). While I have seen minutes that were not numbered at all, a numbering system of some kind does make it easier to refer back to specific items.

Another format is to list agenda items at the top of the page, and then only document action items. This format definitely saves space. It is sort of a "just the facts ma'am" kind of format. If the minutes from the above meeting were done in an action format, they would look something like Figure 20.3. You can see what a sparse format this is. It is best used for very long meetings.

```
Date: 11-25-08
Present: E. Bay, J. Kay, G. Whiz, and A. Ging

1. Agenda
    1.1. Announcements
    1.2. New patient transportation policy
    1.3. Infection control
    1.4. Parking
    1.5. New budget request

2. Announcements
    2. 1. Ellie announced that she would be taking Friday off and a sub would be called in.
    2. 2. Jane announced that the United Way fund drive would be starting next week.
    2. 3. Gina reminded staff that rounds this week is changed to Thursday at 9:00 a.m.

3. Action Items
    3.1. New patient transportation policy
        3.1.1. The department gave unanimous support to the policy.
        3.1.2. See attached policy
    3.2. Infection control
        3.2.1. We reviewed and signed annual review of infection control confirmation sheets,
               which Jane will forward to the human resources department for placement in
               employee files.
    3.3. Parking
        3.3.1. Arica volunteered to serve on the task force.
    3.4. Budget request
        3.4.1. Ellie will provide Jane with ordering information for the new Peabody Motor Scales.
        3.4.2. It will be ordered if it fits within the department's budget.
```

FIGURE 20.3   Sample Action Format Minutes.

Another format is a combination of the last two. It summarizes a topic, and then identifies the action item. For example, the parking discussion might look like this:

4. Parking
Jane asked for a volunteer to serve on a task force looking at issues around employee parking. The task force will look at existing parking options and consider alternatives for parking in the future.
Action: Arica volunteered to serve on the task force.

The last format that will be presented here is using a preprinted form. Figure 20.4 shows an example of this format. This form requires some preparation before the meeting, but simplifies taking minutes during the meeting (meetingwizard.org). Names of the people expected to attend the meeting can be listed on the form and a checkmark placed in front of the ones who attended the meeting (effectivemeetings.com).

There are many other formats. Some facilities have forms that get filled out with columns for discussions and action items. There can be lots of other variations. When taking minutes, the important thing is to listen for the most important information and record it accurately.

OT Department Meeting Minutes

Date/Time: 11-25-08/3:00 p.m.

Members Present _____ E. Bay _____ J. Kay _____ G. Whiz _____ A. Ging

Topic	Discussion	Action	Person Responsible
Announcements	Ellie announced that she would be taking Friday off and a sub would be called in. Jane announced that the United Way fund drive would be starting next week. Gina reminded staff that rounds this week is changed to Thursday at 9:00 a.m.	N/A	N/A
New Policy	The proposed new hospital policy on patient transportation was presented. It was designed to encourage everyone to try to stick to the schedule. The policy is expected to go into effect in 30 days unless there is overwhelming negative feedback. The transportation improvement team is accepting written comments for the next 2 weeks.	The department gave unanimous support to the policy (attached).	Jane
Infection Control	The annual review of infection control policies and procedures for the department as per hospital policy was conducted.	We signed annual review of infection control training confirmation sheets that will be forwarded to HR for placement in employee files.	Jane
Parking	The hospital is looking for a volunteer to serve on a task force looking at issues around employee parking and existing parking options and consider alternatives for parking in the future.	Arica volunteered to serve on the task force.	Arica
New Budget Request	A request was received to buy the newest revision of the Peabody Motor Scales.	Ellie will find information about the cost of the test and ordering options. Jane will see if it fits in this year's budget.	Ellie and Jane

FIGURE 20.4 Sample Meeting Minutes Form.

Exercise 20.1

Summarize the following meeting topics using the combined format (the last one presented):

Riva gave an update on the actions of the committee that is planning the 50th anniversary celebration of the hospital. The celebration committee is looking for success stories for a weeklong series (a 4-minute segment each day) on the 11:00 p.m. local news. They would like to highlight a different department each day, but they cannot cover every department in the 5-day series. Rhonda suggested Mr. Sayed who recovered from Guillian-Barré syndrome 2 years ago. He still sends a holiday card each year. Rolanda suggested Mr. Hernandez who had extensive rehab following a head injury, but eventually went home and back to work part time. Robert suggested Mrs. Hellenberger who lost six toes and three fingers to frostbite. The committee is also planning an open house in the cafeteria, and each department can put together a display table promoting programs in the department. After much discussion, the department agreed to talk with the other departments in the rehabilitation area about sharing a segment on Mr. Hernandez. Rhonda volunteered to work with the occupational therapy fieldwork students on a display table for the open house.

1. 50th Anniversary Committee Report

Action:

The head of the department, Barb, said she had noticed a decrease in productivity lately. There has been a downward trend over the last 6 weeks. The company's financial picture is not looking as good as was hoped. Ours is not the only department that is falling below projections. The president of the company is asking each department to develop a plan for cutting expenses for the rest of the year by 10%. Barb would like input from the staff as to what cuts would be the least painful to make. Bob suggested that we could cut out doughnuts and coffee for the morning department meetings. Belinda suggested that we could use coupons and buy generic brands for the occupational therapy kitchen. Becky suggested being more careful about walking off with each other's pens, and try to conserve paper. Bob suggested that they be more conscientious about remembering to bill for adaptive equipment. Barb said those were good suggestions, but they wouldn't come anywhere near 10% of the budget. She asked each person to meet with her privately to discuss other possibilities.

1. Budget

Action:

SUMMARY

Taking accurate meeting minutes is an essential function of any occupational therapy department. There is a delicate balance between recording too much information and too little. The names of the people present at the meeting, the date of the meeting, and the outcomes of the meeting in terms of actions and decisions need to be recorded. There are several formats for recording these meetings. While each has some advantages and disadvantages, choose one that fits your facility's needs.

REFERENCES

Basic-learning.com. *Bull's eye business writing tips: Getting to your writing target.* Retrieved April 7, 2003, from http://www.basic-learning.com/wbwt/tip134.htm

Effectivemeetings.com. *Meeting basics, how to record useful meeting minutes.* Retrieved April 7, 2003, from http://www.effectivemeetings.com/meeting/basics/minutes.asp

Meetingwizard.org. *Taking minutes—Useful tips.* Retrieved December 30, 2007, from http://www.meetingwizard.org/meetings/taking-minutes.cfm

Mosvick, R. K.,&Nelson, R. B. (1987). *We've got to start meeting like this! A guide to successful business meeting management.* Glenview, IL: Scott Foresman.

CHAPTER 21

Grant Writing

INTRODUCTION

Occupational therapy services are generally paid for by third-party payers such as Medicare and managed care companies. However, these sources of payment are often inadequate to cover the costs of providing occupational therapy services. While many occupational therapy programs may be part of not-for-profit organizations, that does not mean that the program can afford to continue year after year without at least breaking even financially. Without covering at least the cost of providing services, it is hard for an organization to make the investment needed to develop new programs or expand existing ones. Perhaps there are clients who cannot afford needed services or equipment. Grants can be written to help underwrite the costs of new programs or to set up fund accounts to help clients pay for services and/or equipment. Rarely will grants be awarded to cover ongoing expenses of existing programs.

▼ WHAT GRANTS ARE ▼

Grants are awards of specific amounts of money for specific purposes. Grants can be awarded by either governmental agencies or private organizations. Regardless of the source of the grant, grants are only awarded to those who apply for them. Grants may be awarded to school districts, hospitals or other medical facilities, rehabilitation agencies, community-based organizations, and other for-profit or not-for-profit organizations (Prabst-Hunt, 2002). The organization requesting the grant must demonstrate in writing that there is a purpose and a plan for using the funds.

▼ WHERE TO FIND GRANT OPPORTUNITIES ▼

There are several places to look for grant funding opportunities. The Internet has literally millions of sites related to grant writing. Some sites focus more on tips for writing grants, but many others contain specific instructions for applying for particular grants. Table 21.1 lists selected websites and the type of information found on those sites.

If you work at a facility that has a development office, the people working in that office can be of great assistance. Hospitals and nonprofit corporations often have development offices. The staff of these offices can help you locate funding sources, help you write the grant, and in some cases, actually solicit funds for you. These people have lots of experience working with funding agencies. They know the tricks of the trade. It helps to have a friendly working relationship with development staff if you are going to be seeking grant money from any source. Few things make development staff angrier than staff from other departments going out and seeking funds without their knowledge. It is critical that development staff be aware of every time an outside source is asked to make a donation or fund a grant so they can know which funding agency has been asked for what contribution this year. In this sense, they act as gatekeepers for soliciting funds.

TABLE 21.1 Grant-Related Websites

Website Address	Agency or Organization	Type of Content
www.grants.gov	Federal government	Searchable listing of federal grant opportunities
www.foundationcenter.org	Foundation Center	Directory of foundations Offers online and classroom training programs on seeking foundation money Has subscription service Has a foundation finder Free tutorials on grant seeking Online library has a glossary of terms used in grant-writing process
www.fundsnetservices.com	Grant Writing Resources	Fundraising and grant-writing resources Grant applications Proposal writing guides
www.tgci.com	The Grantsmanship Center	Grant information and grantsmanship training Includes grant sources by state search engine
http://grants.nih.gov/grants/oer.htm	National Institutes of Health (federal govt.)	Lots of information on applying for NIH grants
www.middlebury.edu/administration/grants/proposal	Middlebury College	Provides advice on grant preparation Links to sites with information on grant writing
www.npguides.org/	SeaCoast Web Designs	Lots of information on writing grants

▼ GENERAL GRANT WRITING TIPS ▼

The awarding of grants is a competitive process. Granting organizations usually have less money to award than the total amount requested by grant applicants. This means there will be criteria established to help guide the decision making. It is critical that anyone applying for a grant know exactly what criteria will be used to determine who will receive the grant, and then to use that information in writing the grant (Fazio, 2001). Criteria for awarding grants vary significantly so it is critical to match the reason you want funding to the criteria used by the funder to make award decisions. For example, if you want funding to help start a program for teenage children of immigrant families to learn work skills, it would be a waste of your time, and the funder's, to apply for a grant for such a program from a funder whose main purpose is to fund programs for adults with chemical dependency. Although some of the teens you propose to serve might have chemical dependency issues, it would be more likely that a funding agency that supported programs focused on self-sufficiency would take an interest in your proposed program.

The two most important things to remember when applying for a grant are to follow the instructions and to proofread, proofread, and then proofread some more. While these seem like simple and obvious tips, they are absolutely critical to the grant application process. Granting agencies provide instructions to those interested in applying for grants. There is usually a good reason why they instruct applicants to organize the grant application in a certain way, so even if the applicant thinks it would look better if organized differently the instructions, including deadlines, have to be followed. You want the reader of your grant proposal to look favorably at your proposal. A proposal that does not follow the grant agency's instructions may be discarded without being reviewed (J. C. Downing Foundation, 2000; Middlebury College, 2000).

Proofreading will ensure there are no typos, no grammatical or spelling errors, and no sloppy formatting or bad copies (i.e., printer running low on ink). As mentioned several times in this book, people form impressions of you and your program based on your written work. To be seen as competent and able to implement the proposed program, you have to write like a competent and polished professional. Not only does the proposal writer need to proofread the proposal, but it is a good idea to get a couple of other people to proofread it as well. You want the application to look good. Be careful to choose words that the funding agency will understand. The person reading your grant request will probably not be an occupational therapist.

While specific instructions for the organization of the grant application will vary, a cover letter will be the first thing the granting agency representative will read. A cover letter needs to provide enough information to interest the reader and make the reader want to read the rest of the proposal. Be sure your cover letter is addressed to the right person. A phone call to the funding agency can tell you who to address the letter to (name, credentials, and title) and how to correctly spell that person's name (Genesee Intermediate School District [GISD], 2000). Be sure the cover letter is on appropriate letterhead and is signed by the person in the highest authority as possible for your program/employer. Strive to keep the letter to one page (J. C. Downing Foundation, 2000; SeaCoast Web Design, 1999). The layout and visual qualities of this page can set the tone of the reader's disposition toward your proposal.

Begin your grant application with an abstract or executive summary (GISD, 2000). The abstract describes the need your proposal intends to meet, what the project involves, who will benefit from this project, why this project is important, and the total cost of the project in greatly condensed form. This is a lot of information to squeeze into one or two pages, but it can be done if you are clear, direct, and do not elaborate on anything. You have the rest of the proposal to do that.

▼ WRITING A GRANT TO FUND A NEW PROGRAM ▼

According to Middlebury College (2000), in general there are seven key topics that are addressed in the narrative portion of the grant application, as shown in Box 21.1.

In your proposal, you need to describe what it is you hope to accomplish in a few sentences without oversimplifying and avoiding jargon (Middlebury College, 2000). Make it easy for the readers to understand what you want to do. You may want to include subheadings to make it easier to find certain information. Suggested section headings include:

- Program Description
- Goals and Objectives
- Operational Plans
- Financial Plans
- Marketing Plans
- Supplemental Materials

Program Description

It is important to establish why you want to do what you are proposing to do. You need a reason to do what you are proposing, and it has to be better than "Because no one else has done it before." A needs assessment can be used to demonstrate the need for this project.

Show data that supports your claim of need (GISD, 2000). Describe how you became aware of the need. Do not make any claims of need that you cannot support. Be sure that the need you hope to address is not so huge that your proposed program could not make a reasonable dent in it. In other words, as a quality improvement coordinator used to tell me, "You can't boil the ocean one teaspoon at a time."

In addressing how your proposal will meet an existing need, you will need to explain what steps you will take to implement your plan. Explain the mission of the program. By reading the mission and a description of the proposed program, the reader should have a good idea of what you are hoping to accomplish. Include a timeline for which activities will be done by what date leading up to and including providing the services you propose (GISD, 2000; Middlebury College, 2000).

In your grant proposal, you need to explain why you are the one(s) to do it (Middlebury College, 2000). Here is where you clearly state your commitment to the proposal. Do not assume the readers will know much about your agency or organization, so tell them why you are in a position to address the stated need (GISD, 2000). If you have developed other similar projects in the past, explain the success you have had with them. It can be helpful to demonstrate how some aspect of the proposed program could be continued after grant funding ends.

You need to explain what good will come from this proposed program (Middlebury College, 2000). This is where it is helpful to know what the mission and goals of the funding agency are. You can explain what would happen if the proposal is not funded. Most funding agencies need to know that their money is going to support an activity that will benefit some portion of society in some way. It is up to you to clearly demonstrate that your proposed program will do that.

Goals and Objectives

The goals and objectives of the proposed program need to be clearly articulated (Prabst-Hunt, 2002). The goals are overarching, long-range program goals, while objectives are specific and measurable. These will be the yardsticks by which your program's success or failure will be measured. They can be written in ABCD, FEAST, RHUMBA, or SMART format (see Chapter 11). For example, if you are developing a program for musicians with hand injuries, your goal might be to provide musicians with a program to help their recovery that is sensitive to their unique needs for very precise finger movements. The objectives of the program might be:

- 90% of the musicians participating in the program will rate their satisfaction with the program as very helpful or outstanding.
- 85% will report a decrease of pain while playing of at least two points on a 1–10 scale.
- The reinjury rate will be 20% or less 6 months after intervention ends.

This would be an appropriate place to describe any program evaluation activities you plan to conduct, and how the data you collect will be used. Explain how you will use this information to modify the project during the grant period and beyond (GISD, 2000). Make sure the evaluation plan relates to the goals and objectives stated earlier in your proposal. Be specific about who will do what as part of the evaluation process.

Exercise 21.1

Write a measurable goal for the following programs.

1. Your clinic is developing a summer program for school-age children who will not be receiving school-based services during the summer break. It will focus on handwriting, movement, and socialization skills.

2. You want to start a not-for-profit agency to help adults with developmental disabilities develop work skills.

3. The hospital would like you to develop a program for women who have had mastectomies and breast reconstruction surgeries.

Operational Plans

Operational plans include information on space, supplies and equipment, staff, and methods of service delivery. Specify any space, equipment, and supplies that you will need. If you already have any supplies or equipment that will help in the implementation, describe them (Middlebury College, 2000). You can be general and lump similar items into a category. For example, for the musician's rehabilitation program, you could say you need assorted splinting materials and various intervention modalities. This is usually sufficient for small items. For higher-priced items, such as test materials, list them separately. Describe your space needs in terms of square feet required and the purpose for each required space. If you are so inclined, you can describe your vision of how the space will look.

Include information that demonstrates the training and experience (related to the program) of staff that will be involved in the program (GISD, 2000). Full resumes of staff can be included in an appendix, so just summarize here. If you are going to use the grant to fund the salaries for the start of the program, explain how salaries will be paid in future years when the grant money is gone.

Financial Plan

The budget section of the grant needs to include dollar amounts requested as well as a justification for those amounts (GISD, 2000; Middlebury College, 2000). The funding agency may require budget forms to be submitted with the proposal. Every budget item for which you request funding needs to be justified in the narrative portion; there should be no surprises on the budget forms. Your budget is an estimate of costs to deliver the program to consumers. As an estimate, you do not need to record costs down to the last penny; you can round to the nearest dollar, or if you are dealing with large amounts of money, the nearest $100. If some items of the budget for the proposed program will be paid for in some other way (not from the grant), explain the source of that funding. When calculating salaries, remember to include benefits such as health insurance, paid time off, and so on. Do not include any unexplained budget items such as "miscellaneous" or "other" expenses. Never ask for more money than you realistically need.

Marketing Plan

You will have to explain how you will spread the word about your program. If someone is going to fund a program, they want to know that the program will have participants. This means that you have to explain how referral sources will find out about your program and how the public will find out about it.

Supplemental Materials

In addition to whatever forms are required by the funding agency and the narrative proposal, you may want to supplement your proposal with supporting materials. These materials belong in appendices at the back of the proposal package. Some of the kinds of items that might be helpful to include in appendices are included in Box 21.2.

Obviously, it takes careful planning and lots of time to put together a solid grant proposal. The more work you can do before you start writing, the better off you will be in the long run. Understand what the funding agency is looking for in a proposal. If possible, read the proposals of programs the agency has funded in the past. Do not hesitate to ask the funding agency questions throughout the process. Always keep copies of everything you send out. A paper copy is usually preferred to an e-mailed or faxed one; however, a paper copy can take longer than you think to reach the funding agency. Always allow twice as much time as you think you will need for a paper proposal to be delivered to the funding agency.

▼ WRITING OTHER TYPES OF GRANTS ▼

Other types of programs for which you might write a grant include setting up a fund for clients who have no insurance to pay for services, a fund to help families buy needed equipment that third-party payers will not pay for, or to help fund research you are planning to do for your thesis or dissertation. You might write a grant to enable your clinic to purchase a particularly expensive piece of equipment. A grant request for these purposes would be less cumbersome to write than a grant to fund a new program.

BOX 21.2   Suggested Contents for Appendices.

- Documents showing the type of business (for-profit, not-for-profit, charitable, etc.) the proposed program will be operated as. This could be in the form of an IRS determination letter to verify tax-exempt status, certificate of incorporation, and by-laws of the organization.
- Listing of corporate officers and board of directors
- Financial statement for the last completed fiscal year
- Current operating budget
- Résumés or biographies of key personnel
- Letters of support from people outside the organization (only a couple)
- Floor plan for space that will be used for the program
- Equipment and supply lists in detail (summarized in body of proposal)

Source: SeaCoast Web Design, 1999.

As with a new program grant, you would begin by following the funding agency's grant application process. You would want to choose your words carefully so that any reader will understand the purpose of your grant. A cover letter and executive summary would accompany the narrative part of your proposal.

The narrative portion of the grant proposal for funding noncovered services or equipment would be shorter than a new program grant. You will be asking for a lump sum of money, so there will not be a need for any kind of detailed budget. Instead, you would explain why you think the amount of money you are asking for will be sufficient to meet the need. If the grant will enable your clinic to purchase a particular piece of equipment, be sure to include the cost of shipping, handling, and any training required to use it. There may be less of a need to create a marketing plan, unless the new equipment will allow you to provide some kind of service that you currently do not provide. Usually, if there is a fund to help cover the cost of services for the uninsured or underinsured, it is not advertised to the public. You may or may not let referral sources know that you have such a fund. The reason is that if you make too big of a deal about having this fund, you may find yourself overwhelmed with people who need your services.

The narrative of these types of grants should explain the need for creating the fund or buying the piece of equipment. Provide whatever data you can collect that demonstrate a demand for the services or equipment. You may make both arguments of fact (based on data) and emotions (based on feelings, appealing to the heartstrings) in demonstrating the demand. For example, if you are trying to create a fund for uninsured clients, you could argue on the basis of the percentage of people without insurance in your community, the number of clients who were unable to pay for services. You could also argue that without access to your services, these clients will live in pain, may be more likely to reinjure themselves, and may become a burden to their families.

Since organizations donating money for grants want to know what benefit to the community will result from granting their money to your program, you will need to be very explicit in stating the benefits expected. Perhaps the new equipment will enable you to be more precise in your measurements of dysfunction. Perhaps the fund will enable families to purchase custom-made seating devices for children with multiple disabilities. Perhaps the fund will allow a client to be fully rehabilitated before going back to work, decreasing the likelihood of reinjury.

Rather than setting specific objectives and conducting a comprehensive program evaluation, these kinds of grants require less accountability. Setting an overall goal may be sufficient. Instead of a comprehensive program evaluation system, it may be enough to collect data on how the money was spent during the year, a simple accounting of expenditures.

If you are seeking funding for your research, then your grant application might look a little different. Research is usually for a specific period of time, and there is not a need to demonstrate how the program will continue after the funding is discontinued. You will need to explain the purpose of the research, the potential benefits and risks of the research, the cost of the research, where the results will be presented or published, and why you are qualified to do the research. Depending on whether you are applying for a research grant from your college or university, the American Occupational Therapy Foundation (AOTF), or the National Institutes of Health, the amount of information and level of detail required will vary.

Exercise 21.2

1. Visit the AOTF website (www.aotf.org) and locate the grant application for dissertation research.

2. Next, find the research priorities for AOTF.

3. Visit the Minnesota Council of Foundations common grant application form (www.mcf. http://org/mcf/grant/applicat.htm) and locate both the form and the types of information needed for each section of the form.

4. Compare and contrast the two grant applications for both the application process and the types of information each requires.

Exercise 21.3

Which of the following statements are true and which are false, relative to the grant-writing process?

1. _____ In the abstract, take the time to thoroughly explain the purpose of your proposal.
2. _____ Address all the review criteria established by the funding agency in your proposal.
3. _____ It is a good idea to ask lots of questions throughout the process.
4. _____ It is better to present a good-looking proposal than one that is well written.
5. _____ The timeline can be general rather than specific.
6. _____ Goals can be broad and not measurable.
7. _____ Objectives need to meet RHUMBA criteria.
8. _____ You must demonstrate that your project will have an impact on the target population.
9. _____ Program evaluation criteria need to be as detailed as the rest of the proposal.

SUMMARY

When seeking grant money to fund a new program, it is important to present a well-written, thorough, and specific proposal. The proposal needs to contain the information that the funding agency is requesting. While there are some general similarities in the information and format that most funding agencies want, each has some unique requirements, and the proposal needs to be tailored to fit the funding agency. It is vital that someone applying for a grant follow the instructions of the grant funding agency. A cover letter can help create interest on the part of the funding agency in your proposed program. Somewhere in your proposal, you have to be explicit in what you propose to do, why you propose to do it, how you will do it, why you are the one(s) to do it, and how much it will cost to do it. A grant proposal has to be tailored to the funding agency and to the type of grant being requested.

REFERENCES

Fazio, L. S. (2001). *Developing occupation-centered programs for the community: A workbook for students and professionals.* Upper Saddle River, NJ: Prentice Hall.

Genesee Intermediate School District—Grants and Development Department. (2000). *Grants development summary: Do's and don'ts of grant writing.* Retrieved May 5, 2000, from http://web/gisd.k12.mi.us/gisd/Dos_and_Donts_Chart.htm

J.C. Downing Foundation. (2000). *General guidance.* Retrieved May 5, 2000, from http://www.jcdowning.org/resources/generalguide.htm

Middlebury College. (2000). *Grant preparation advice: Questions your grant proposal must address.* Retrieved May 5, 2000, from http://www.middlebury.edu/~grants/advice.htm

Prabst-Hunt, W. (2002). *Occupational therapy administration manual.* Albany, NY: Delmar.

SeaCoast Web Design. (1999). *Grant writing guide: 10-point plan for standard grant funding proposal.* Retrieved May 5, 2000, from http://www.seacoastweb.com/resource/grant1.htm

CHAPTER 22

Policies and Procedures

INTRODUCTION

In any organization there is a need for everyone to understand what is expected of them. People need to know what company policy is, and the acceptable ways to do things. This is where policy and procedure manuals come in. They help employees to know what the company wants employees to do without them having to ask a superior before doing anything. A policy and procedure manual can be used as a training tool and as a resource when any problems or questions arise (Kenny, 2000). Policies and procedures provide written guidance about decision-making from both the employer's and the employees' perspectives (Page, 2002).

Before facilities, agencies, or programs are credentialed (licensed, certified, or accredited), the surveyors who make the recommendation on credential status will always ask to see policy and procedure manuals. The manuals show what the organization has communicated to employees, in writing, regarding expectations in the workplace. Large organizations may have many policy and procedure manuals. Often, they will have one for human resource policies and procedures, and then one for each department. Smaller organizations may have one manual that has sections for various departments.

A member of the occupational therapy staff may serve on a facility-wide committee drafting policies and procedures. Occupational therapy staff usually write their own departmental policies and procedures. There is likely some sort of approval process for the development of new policies and procedures. Organizations in which occupational therapy practitioners are members also are guided by policies and procedures. Medicare, Medicaid, and other payers have policy and procedure manuals that describe what occupational therapy practitioners and the companies that employ them must do in order to submit bills in the right way so the company can get paid.

▼ POLICIES ▼

Policies tell employees what the company's position is on a particular issue. Some policies are required by law or by the credentialing agency. For example, federal law requires that employers have policies on nondiscrimination. A credentialing agency may require a policy on infection control.

In addition to explaining what is expected, policies often state who is responsible for complying with the policy. Individual names are not used, but it might list a job title or state that all employees are responsible for compliance. For example, a policy on infection control would be the responsibility of all employees while a policy on calibration of electronic equipment may be the responsibility of an electrical engineer.

Usually, policies include a statement that explains the purpose of the policy (Page, 2002). The purpose of a policy on safety may be to protect the health of employees. The purposes of a policy on scheduling of clients are to be fair to both clients and staff and to make the most efficient use of resources (staff and space). The purpose is not always explicitly stated. If the policy is the result of a law or a credentialing requirement, the number of the law or standard can be cited in the purpose statement.

Finally, each policy needs an effective date (Page 2002). Any policy revisions also need to be dated. Sometimes, there is a signature page at the front or back of the manual that the department head or head of the organization signs to indicate that all the policies and procedures have been approved by the organization.

▼ PROCEDURES ▼

Procedures explain, in great detail, what steps need to happen to comply with the policy. A procedure for infection control would include instructions on hand washing, use of protective clothing (e.g. masks, gowns, gloves), disposal of infected waste, cleaning up blood or body fluid spills, and so on. A procedure for scheduling would describe how clients are assigned to a particular staff person, where the schedule is recorded, how appointments are made and canceled, and so on. A policy tells what, a procedure tells how. Because of occupational therapy practitioners' background in task analysis, they are good at breaking down the steps of a task, a necessary skill in writing procedures.

▼ WRITING POLICIES AND PROCEDURES ▼

It is essential that policies and procedures be written clearly, explicitly, and thoroughly to avoid any misinterpretations of policy. Readers should be able to find the important information as quickly and easily as possible. As technology and laws change, it is necessary to revise the policy and procedures. Figure 22.1 shows a sample policy and procedure for timeliness of documentation. Figure 22.2 and Figure 22.3 show sample templates for writing policies and procedures.

Timeliness of Documentation
Occupational Therapy Department

Policy: Documentation will be completed in a timely fashion according to the schedule below.

Responsible party: All occupational therapists and occupational therapy assistants.

Purpose: To ensure timely completion of the medical record.

Effective date: January 1, 2004, rev January 2, 2009

Procedure:
1. Orders will be acknowledged in the client's medical record by an occupational therapist within 24 hours of receipt of the order.
2. Evaluation summaries will be completed by an occupational therapist and filed in the medical record within 48 hours of the first client visit.
3. Progress notes are written at time of the visit by either the occupational therapist or the occupational therapy assistant, whoever conducted the visit.
4. Missed visits will be documented on the same day as the missed visit by the occupational therapist or occupational therapy assistant who was scheduled to work with the client.
5. Reevaluations/revised plans of care will be written by the occupational therapist at least every 30 days.
6. Discontinuation summaries will be written by the occupational therapist and filed in the medical record within 48 hours of discontinuation.
7. Occupational therapy documentation may be filed by any member of the occupational therapy department or by the unit coordinator on the nursing station.

FIGURE 22.1   Sample Policy and Procedure.

Title of Policy and Procedure		
Effective date (revisions):		
Policy:		
Responsible party:		
Purpose:		
Procedure:		

FIGURE 22.2 Sample Policy and Procedure Template, Simple.

Title of Policy and Procedure	Number	
	Original date	
	Dates of revisions	
	Approval	
Purpose		
Definitions (*or omit here and put a section for definitions in the back of the manual*)		
Policy		
Positions affected		
Responsibilities		
Procedures		

FIGURE 22.3 Sample Policy and Procedure Template, Formal. *Source: Page, S. (2004).*

Notice that the sample policy and procedure is written in straightforward, simple terms. The policy addresses the rule, while the procedure describes the tasks required to meet the rule (University of California, Santa Cruz [UCSC], 1994). Make sure you avoid words or names that can become quickly outdated. Any words that may not be understood by a reader (especially a new employee) need to be defined right in the policy. Some people suggest that there be a section on definitions written into each policy, including defining abbreviations and acronyms, as well as technical terms (Page, 2004). Others create a section in the policy and procedure manual that provides the definitions of terms, and spells out the abbreviations and acronyms used in the manual.

It is useful to begin writing your policy and procedure by gathering up the documents that already exist within the organization, such as the vision, mission, and strategic plan (Page, 2002). An organizational chart will help in determining who reports to who within the organization. These documents answer questions such as

- What business are we in?
- Who are our customers?
- What do our customers want?
- What position within the marketplace do we want to be in?

Best practices suggest that the policy reflects the vision, mission, and strategic plan of the organization (Page, 2002). These documents, along with discussions among leaders and managers within the organization can assist in identifying guiding principles (values and beliefs) for the development of policies and procedures (Page, 2002).

Once you have all the materials that can provide guidance for the development of policies and procedures, you can develop the overall structure of your policy and procedure manual. This is the point at which you need to decide if you want to separate your policies and your procedures in separate manuals or write one combined manual. The rest of this chapter assumes you want a combined policy and procedure manual. It also assumes that you will have a separate section at the end of the manual for definitions, abbreviations, and acronyms.

Next you develop the table of contents. This requires you to name and organize the policies and procedures you need to write. This is done using a drafting process. Only after all the policies and procedures are written and approved will the final table of contents be written, (Page, 2002). Each policy and procedure may also be assigned a number to make locating the policy and procedure easier. Figure 22.4 shows a sample table of contents for a policy and procedure manual for a private practice occupational therapy clinic. Stephen Page (2002), an expert in writing policies and procedures, suggests that you might want to have three tables of contents so that readers have three ways to find the policy and procedure they are looking for:

- Functional categories (e.g. personnel, clinical, documentation)
- Alphabetical by title
- Numerical by policy/procedure number (e.g. I.A. 2, V.12, III-1.5)

When the draft of at least one format of table of contents is complete, identify a format for writing each policy and procedure. The format needs to make sense for the type, size, and complexity of the organization for which the policies and procedures are written.

Cover page

Approvals

Section I: Supporting Documents
1. Mission Statement
2. Vision Statement
3. Strategic Plan
4. Organizational Chart
5. Guiding Principles

Section II: Personnel Policies
1. Hiring
2. Background checks
3. Salary and benefits
   a. Pay schedule
   b. Direct deposit
   c. Paid time off (PTO)
   d. Health and dental insurance
   e. Life insurance
   f. Disability insurance
   g. Continuing Education
   h. Maternity leave
   i. Jury duty
   j. Leave of absence

FIGURE 22.4   Sample Table of Contents for a Policy and Procedure Manual for a Private Practice Occupational Therapy Clinic. *Sources: Nolo.com (2009); Page, S. (2002).*

4. Drug and alcohol abuse
5. Sexual harassment
6. Overtime
7. Work scheduling
8. Non-discrimination
9. Conflict of interest
10. Confidentiality
11. Discipline
12. Complaints
13. Workplace civility
14. E-mail and internet access
15. Performance appraisal
16. Employee safety
17. Keys
18. Dress code
19. Gifts
20. Termination

Section III: Clinical
1. Infection control
   a. Cleaning schedule
   b. Use of cleaning materials
   c. Laundry
   d. Gloves, gowns, and masks
   e. Blood or body fluid spills
2. Equipment maintenance
3. Documentation
   a. Referrals/orders
   b. Evaluation
   c. Intervention
   d. Discontinuation
4. Communication with physicians, QRCs, and other professionals involved in the client's care
5. Communication with clients
6. Evidence-based practice
7. Charging for services
8. Charging for supplies
9. Program evaluation

Section IV: Administrative
1. Intake
2. Attendance
3. Billing
   a. Services
   b. Supplies
   c. Appeals
   d. Medicare
   e. Medicaid
   f. Managed care
   g. Private insurance
   h. Self-pay
   i. Other payers
4. Services for the uninsured
5. Ordering supplies and equipment
6. Confidentiality of client information
7. Records retention
8. Storage of discontinued charts

FIGURE 22.4 (Continued)

The order of the items may be different from one organization to another, but within an organization the order should be uniform and consistent (Page, 2002). Figure 22.2 and Figure 22.3 show two possible formats for writing policies and procedures.

Policies and procedures usually undergo some kind of approval process. Depending on the size and complexity of the organization, the individual policies and procedures may be approved by the owner of the business, a board of directors, or a committee formed for the purpose of approving policies and procedures. The approval may be documented on a cover page for the manual, or on the first page of each policy and procedure.

Exercise 22.1

Write a procedure for the following policy.

Effective date: January 1, 2004, rev. January 1, 2010

Policy: Occupational therapy personnel will wash their hands between client visits.

Responsible party: All occupational therapists and occupational therapy assistants.

Purpose: To try to prevent the spread of infectious diseases.

Procedure:

Exercise 22.2

Write a policy for the following procedure.

Effective date: January 1, 2004, rev. January 1, 2010

Policy:

Responsible party: All occupational therapists and occupational therapy assistants.

Purpose: To ensure that documentation meets with regulatory standards.

Procedure:

1. Document each individual intervention session.
2. An occupational therapist or occupational therapy assistant may write and file the visit/contact note.
3. The visit/contact note must include a description of the activities or techniques engaged in along with the degree of participation by the client.
4. The visit/contact note must include a description of any adaptive equipment, prosthetic or orthotics device that is provided to the client and whether the client or client's caregiver appeared to understand instructions in the use and care of the devices.

5. All notes must be signed with first initial, full last name, and credentials of the writer.

6. All notes must be dated and the time it was entered into the record noted.

7. All notes must be written in black ink.

SUMMARY

Policies and procedures tell employees what to do and how to do it. They need to be kept up to date. They are written in simple, direct, and clear wording. Any member of an occupational therapy department may be asked to write a policy and procedure. Some policies and procedures are required by law or by credentialing standards. In addition to complying with laws and standards, policy and procedure manuals can be used as training tools and as resources for questions or problems.

REFERENCES

Kenny, C. J. (2000). Policy and procedure manual should portray well-organized system. *ADVANCE for Medical Laboratory Professionals*, (March 13, 2000). Retrieved December 5, 2002, from http://www.deltasci.com/kenny3.htm

Page, S. (2002). *Best practices in policies and procedures*. Westerville, OH: Process Improvement Publishing.

Page, S. (2004). *7 Steps to better written policies and procedures*. Westerville, OH: Process Improvement Publishing. University of California Santa Cruz, (1994). *Guide to writing policy and procedure documents*. Retrieved December 5, 2002, from http://www.ucsc.edu/ppmanual/pdf/guide.pdf

CHAPTER 23

Job Descriptions

INTRODUCTION

"That's not in my job description."

"I didn't expect to be doing this!"

"She can't really expect me to do all that."

"You want me to do what?"

None of the people who are quoted here seems very happy. They all appear to have a problem related to the reality of their job compared to what they thought their job was. Perhaps they didn't read their job description when they were hired. Perhaps they read a description of their job, but it wasn't a current or accurate one. Maybe no job description exists for their position. Whatever is going on here, it's clear that the supervisor needs to work with the employee to develop or revise the job description. A current and well-written job description can help avoid situations that lead to such comments.

Job descriptions (also called position descriptions) are formal documents that identify the qualifications, duties, and responsibilities of specific positions within a department, organization, or company. They are used in the hiring process to match a candidate for the job to the requirements of the job, and to develop interview questions (Mader-Clark, 2007; Liebler & McConnell, 2004). Workforce Central Florida (2007) says, "For the employee, the job description is a road map and a safeguard" (p. 1). Job descriptions are used in the employee review process to compare employee's performance to the expected performance for that position. Other uses for job descriptions include employee orientation, training, and compensation decisions (Mader-Clark; Liebler & McConnell).

Occupational therapists who work in ergonomics, injury prevention and risk management, or functional capacity and worker rehabilitation may be called on to write job descriptions or consult with those writing job descriptions. An essential skill in writing job descriptions is being able to break a task or activity down to its most basic parts. Occupational therapists are excellent at doing this because of our skills in activity (or task) analysis.

▼ LEGAL AND REGULATORY REQUIREMENTS ▼

Job descriptions are legal documents. They can be used in court in lawsuits involving reasonable accommodations (e.g., alleged violations of the Americans with Disabilities Act [ADA]), employment discrimination, termination of employment, and in other employment-related court cases. External accrediting agencies can review a facility's job descriptions as part of the accreditation process. As legal documents, it pays to review existing job descriptions on a regular basis to make sure they are current and consistent with today's practices (Mader-Clark, 2007). Box 23.1 is a list of dos and don'ts for writing job descriptions that comply with legal and regulatory requirements.

The Fair Labor Standards Act (FLSA) requires employers to document which employees are exempt (professionals paid on a salary basis of at least $455 per week) from federal wage and hour regulations and which ones are nonexempt (often paid on an hourly basis)

237

BOX 23.1   Dos and Dont's for Writing Job Descriptions.

Dos	Don'ts
• Do use action verbs in labeling the job duties • Do be specific, precise, and clear in describing the duties • Do clearly identify which job duties are essential to the position • Do include the physical, mental, and environmental requirements of the job • Do specify the scope of supervisory responsibility of the position (if any) • Do chose your words carefully • Do get feedback on the content of the job description and the wording of it before putting it into use • Do interview people who have similar jobs to help identify the essential functions of the job	• Don't make the list so detailed that it contains every possible task that could be part of it (the kitchen sink approach) • Don't make the job so big it looks impossible for one person to do • Don't include anything that could be contrary to a collective bargaining agreement • Don't use abbreviations that might not be understood by job applicants • Don't include subjective requirements or requirements that only describe one person • Don't make the qualifications so tight they unreasonably restrict who can fill the position

Sources: Loy, B. (2007); NEA (2006); Workforce Central Florida (2007).

(United States Department of Labor [USDL], 2008). The best place to document this is in the job description. The more responsibility and independence a position has, the more likely that position is to be exempt.

Federal laws regarding pay equity require that employers prove that jobs requiring similar skill, effort, and responsibility are paid similarly. The skills, effort, and responsibility required for each position within an organization should be clearly spelled out in a job description (Rice University, 2009). Attention also needs to be paid to the qualifications specified for each position description so that laws relating to nondiscrimination (e.g., race, age, gender) are not violated.

Many job descriptions include sections that describe the working conditions so that employees know what to expect in terms of the work environment. Employees need to know if they will be exposed to any temperature extremes, exposure to toxic chemicals, or loud noises. Not only is this morally correct, but it shows compliance with Occupational Safety and Health Administration (OSHA) regulations. Job descriptions that describe working conditions can serve as a starting point for employee safety training and for the development of safety policies and procedures (Rice University, 2009).

In settings where there are union employees who work under a collective bargaining agreement, job descriptions must not conflict with the collective bargaining agreement (Rice University, 2009). A well-written job description can also help employers properly classify positions into different pay and benefit levels as allowed within the contract.

▼ GATHERING INFORMATION FOR JOB DESCRIPTIONS ▼

If the job description is being written for an existing job, the first step in gathering the needed information is to talk with the people who are currently working in that job/position (Braveman, 2005). Find out how these workers typically spend their day. Ask them what they typically do on an hourly, daily, weekly, or monthly basis. Try to estimate the amount of time spent in each activity, or if exact time varies, estimate the percentage of time spent on each activity on a weekly basis (Braveman).

One danger in writing a job description for an existing position is that there is a possibility that the job description will be written with a particular person in mind, designing the job to utilize that person's strengths to the maximum extent possible. It is really important, especially to avoid allegations of unfairness, that the position be clearly separated from the person in the position (Drafke, 1994). A job description that is specific to a person will make it very hard to hire a new person when the current person leaves. Refer to Box 23.1 for a list of dos and don'ts when writing job descriptions.

If the job description is being written for a new position, start by looking at positions that are similar to the new position and the people who will interact with the new position (Braveman, 2005). Determine what the person in the new position will do on an hourly, daily, weekly, or monthly basis. Make a best guess as to the percentage of time one would spend in each major task. Identify the minimum qualifications for hiring a person to fill this position (education, certification, experience, and special skills). To the ethical and legal extent possible, gather job descriptions from other employers, websites, or textbooks that would be similar to the position you are writing about.

The State of Minnesota has a website, *Career Onestop,* that will help you write a job description electronically using a template for hundreds of job titles (USDL, 2007). The site walks you through the process of developing a job description, including the work tasks and activities, contexts, knowledge and skills, and tools and technology. Using a site like this can be a great first step in the process of developing a job description for your work site. While the site offers some options for customization, further refinement of the job description may be necessary. Figure 23.1 shows a sample job description for an occupational therapy assistant and an occupational therapist generated from this website.

Title: Occupational Therapist, Pediatric

Reporting Relationships:
1. Reports to Supervisor of Pediatric Rehabilitation
2. Supervises occupational therapy assistant, occupational therapy students, volunteers

Job Specifications:
1. Qualifications
   a. Required:
      1. 1-year experience as a pediatric occupational therapist
      2. Bachelor's degree in occupational therapy
      3. NBCOT certification
      4. State OT license
   b. Preferred:
      1. 3 years' experience as a pediatric occupational therapist
      2. Master's degree in occupational therapy
      3. Bilingual (Spanish-English)
      4. SIPT or NDT certification
2. Skills
   a. Reading at college level
   b. Writing at professional level
   c. Clinical reasoning
   d. Complex problem solving
   e. Listening comprehension
   f. Public speaking
   g. Time management
   h. Computer (word processing, EMR, spreadsheet, database)
   i. Splinting
   j. Constructing and modifying adaptive equipment
   k. Cooperation, negotiation, persuasion, and social perceptiveness

---

FIGURE 23.1   Sample Jobs Descriptions. *Sources: Braveman (2005); Liebler & McConnell (2004).*

Gathering Information for Job Descriptions   **239**

3. Knowledge
    a. OT theories and frames of reference
    b. Human behavior and performance
    c. Activity analysis
    d. Conditions and diseases
    e. Anatomy and physiology
    f. Teaching and learning theory and techniques
    g. OT intervention strategies appropriate for children

Essential Functions:
1. Evaluates child's level of developmental, physical, behavioral, sensory, and adaptive functions, interprets findings, and generates evaluation/reevaluation reports.
2. Establishes individualized goals to improve child's occupational performance.
3. Develops and implements intervention plans.
4. Develops home programs for children and instructs caregivers on ways to implement the home programs.
5. Documents clinical interventions and the child's response to those interventions.
6. Determines when to terminate services and generates discontinuation plans and summaries.
7. Provides families with orientation to clinic and clinic policies.
8. Schedules appointments.
9. Directs and supervises OTA in accordance with state law and reimbursement criteria.
10. Orders or fabricates splints, adaptive equipment, assistive technology, and instructs in the use and care of these items.
11. Coordinates service delivery with other team members and outside service providers.
12. Contributes to continuous quality improvement program.
13. Maintains a safe and efficient work space.
14. Informs supervisor of equipment and supply needs.
15. Maintains competency in pediatric occupational therapy.
16. Demonstrates compliance with client health and safety standards.
17. Completes all documentation in a timely manner.
18. Participates in at least 80% of department meetings.

Additional Responsibilities:
1. Attends non-mandatory in-service educational events.
2. Participates in occupational therapy month activities.

Title: Occupational Therapy Assistant, Adult Psychiatry

Reporting Relationships:
1. Reports to Occupational Therapy Supervisor.
2. Supervises occupational therapy assistant students, volunteers.

Job Specifications:
1. Qualifications
    a. Required:
        1. 1-year experience as an occupational therapy assistant
        2. 2-year degree in occupational therapy assistant
        3. NBCOT certification
        4. State OT license
    b. Preferred:
        1. 2 years' experience in mental health setting
2. Skills
    a. Grade 12 reading level
    b. Writing at professional level
    c. Complex problem solving
    d. Listening comprehension
    e. Public speaking
    f. Time management

FIGURE 23.1   (Continued)

g. Computer (word processing, EMR, spreadsheet, database)

h. Cooperation, negotiation, persuasion, and social perceptiveness

3. Knowledge

a. Psychiatric OT frames of reference

b. Human behavior and performance

c. Activity analysis

d. Psychiatric conditions and diseases

e. Teaching and learning theory and techniques

f. OT intervention strategies appropriate for adults with mental illness

Essential Functions:

1. Contributes to the evaluation of client's level of developmental, physical, behavioral, sensory, and adaptive functions, interprets findings, and generates evaluation/reevaluation reports.

2. Contributes to the establishment of individualized goals to improve client's occupational performance.

3. Implements intervention plans.

4. Instructs caregivers on ways to implement the home programs.

5. Documents clinical interventions and the client's response to those interventions.

6. Contributes to the determination of when to terminate services and the generation of discontinuation plans and summaries.

7. Provides families with orientation to clinic and clinic policies.

8. Schedules appointments.

9. Directs and supervises OTA students in accordance with state laws, reimbursement criteria, and AOTA fieldwork evaluation criteria.

10. Coordinates service delivery with other team members and outside service providers.

11. Contributes to continuous quality improvement program.

12. Maintains a safe and efficient work space.

13. Informs supervisor of equipment and supply needs.

14. Maintains competency in psychiatric occupational therapy.

15. Demonstrates compliance with client health and safety standards.

16. Completes all documentation in a timely manner.

17. Participates in at least 80% of department meetings.

Additional Responsibilities:

1. Attends non-mandatory in-service educational events.

2. Participates in occupational therapy month activities.

FIGURE 23.1 (Continued)

▼ PARTS OF JOB DESCRIPTIONS ▼

Job Title

The job title is the formal name of the position for which the description is being written. If there is only one occupational therapist at the place of work, then the simple job title of occupational therapist may be sufficient. If there are multiple occupational therapy practitioners, and the work duties required of each is different, then the title may need to be more specific. Examples of job titles include:

- Occupational therapy aide
- Occupational therapy assistant I
- Occupational therapy assistant II
- Staff occupational therapist
- Lead occupational therapist

- Occupational therapy specialist
- Occupational therapy supervisor
- Occupational therapy manager

The title is usually just a few words long. It is possible for several people to have the same job title, but be differentiated by a specialty practice area or unit name after the title. A hospital might have eight staff occupational therapists, but some might work primarily in rehabilitation, while others work primarily in mental health. In this instance, some of the staff occupational therapists might call themselves "staff occupational therapist, rehabilitation," while others call themselves "staff occupational therapist, mental health." Officially, they could all have the job title of staff occupational therapist.

Job Purpose

The job purpose (sometimes called the job function, job objectives, or job summary) provides an overview of the job and explains why this position exists: the purpose of the job (Mader-Clark, 2007). It should only be a sentence or two long, describing the scope of the position, without a lot of detail. It should contain just enough information to provide an overview of the position and to distinguish it from other positions in the organization (Liebler & Mc Connell, 2004; National Education Association [NEA], 2006). The details of the job will be described elsewhere in the job description, so keep this as concise as possible.

Reporting Relationships

In this section, identify which job title/position the person in this position will report to and which job titles/positions will report to this person (Bravemen, 2005). Do not name names, since people change jobs fairly often, and you do not want to rewrite the job description every time a supervisor or supervisee leaves. Most often, the reporting relationships can be found on the organizational chart for the organization, business, or agency (Liebler & McConnell, 2004).

Job Specifications

This is where you provide detail about the qualifications required for this position, the working conditions, level of responsibility and autonomy, and types of equipment the person in the position will need to be proficient in using (NEA, 2006). In some organizations, the working conditions may be identified on a checklist attached to the job description. Figure 23.2 contains a list of possible working conditions that an occupational therapy practitioner may have to work under.

There are two types of qualifications that are used to determine whether an applicant is a good fit for a particular job. Required qualifications reflect the minimum education, skills, and experience necessary for anyone to possess in order to do the job. Preferred qualifications are those that the employer would like an employee to possess above and beyond those that are required. For example, a job as a lead occupational therapist may require 2 years of clinical experience, but 5 years of experience would be preferred. An entry-level occupational therapist position might require a bachelor's degree in the field, but a master's degree may be preferred.

When writing a job description, it is very important to carefully evaluate the education, skills, and experience necessary to do the job. As each qualification is identified, it is helpful to ask, "Is this really necessary, or is this something it would be nice to have?" Do not set the required qualifications so high that it will limit the number of applicants, particularly if it would eliminate all people of a certain age, gender, or race, but not so low that everyone meets all the qualifications (Western Kentucky University, n.d.). The qualifications need to

1. General Physical Requirements

- ❑ Sedentary work: Mostly (90–100%) sitting; occasional walking or standing; occasional lifting, pushing, pulling, or carrying up to 10 lbs.
- ❑ Light work: Mostly (75–89%) sitting; occasional walking or standing; occasional lifting, pushing, pulling, or carrying up to 20 lbs.
- ❑ Medium work: Some sitting (50–74%); some walking or standing; occasional lifting, pushing, pulling, or carrying up to 50 lbs; frequent lifting, pushing, pulling, or carrying up to 20 lbs.
- ❑ Heavy work: Mostly standing or walking (75–89%); occasional sitting; occasional lifting, pushing, pulling, or carrying up to 100 lbs.; frequent lifting, pushing, pulling, or carrying up to 50 lbs.
- ❑ Very heavy work: Mostly standing or walking (75–89%); occasional sitting; occasional lifting, pushing, pulling, or carrying in excess of 100 lbs.; frequent lifting, pushing, pulling, or carrying in excess of 50 lbs.

2. Physical Activities

- ❑ Bending
- ❑ Climbing
  - ❑ Stairs
  - ❑ Ladders
  - ❑ Ramps
- ❑ Crouching
- ❑ Crawling
- ❑ Fingering
- ❑ Grasping
- ❑ Kneeling
- ❑ Leaning
- ❑ Lifting
- ❑ Maintaining balance
- ❑ Placing
- ❑ Pulling
- ❑ Pushing
- ❑ Reaching
- ❑ Standing
- ❑ Stooping
- ❑ Talking
- ❑ Touching
- ❑ Turning or twisting
- ❑ Walking

3. Mental/Intellectual Activities

- ❑ Attention to detail
- ❑ Categorization
- ❑ Complex mathematics
- ❑ Cooperating following directions
- ❑ Generalization
- ❑ Listening
- ❑ Memory
  - ❑ Short-term
  - ❑ Long-term
- ❑ Prioritizing
- ❑ Problem solving
- ❑ Reading at _____ grade level

FIGURE 23.2 Sample Working Conditions Checklist. *Sources: Wake Forest University (2001); AOTA (2008).*

- ❏ Sequencing
- ❏ Simple mathematics

4. Environmental conditions
- ❏ Atmospheric conditions
  - ❏ Dust
  - ❏ Fumes
  - ❏ Gases
  - ❏ Odors
  - ❏ Poor ventilation
  - ❏ Steam or mist
- ❏ Exposure to infectious diseases
- ❏ Exposure to sharp instruments (e.g., needles, scissors, knives)
- ❏ Exposure to toxic chemicals/agents
- ❏ Extreme cold indoors (below 32 for 1 hr. or more)
- ❏ Extreme heat indoors (above 100 for 1 hr. or more)
- ❏ Exposure to weather extremes outdoors (e.g., wind, humidity)
- ❏ Frequent temperature changes
- ❏ Loud noise
- ❏ Proximity to electrical current
- ❏ Proximity to moving mechanical parts
- ❏ Proximity to moving vehicles
- ❏ Vibration
- ❏ Working in high places (e.g., on scaffolding)
- ❏ Work with volatile people (e.g., people with head injuries, mental illness, or prisoners)
- ❏ Work in small, enclosed places

FIGURE 23.2   (Continued)

be commensurate with the level of responsibility the job carries. Types of qualifications can include (Liebler & McConnell, 2004):

- Minimum education level
- Licensure, certification, or registration required
- Amount and type of experience
- Physical skills required
- Communication skills required

Be as specific as possible in listing qualifications. Avoid vague terms such as good skills, appropriate degree, and several years. Describe the kind of work experience and mention the number of years—for example, three years of experience working with children and families, one year of hospital experience. When listing the types of skills required or preferred, be sure they are job related. While it might be nice to have only optimists working in your department, optimism is not usually a job-related skill. Be wary of listing skills that are open to interpretation, such as being a team player or a quick learner (Spechler, 1996; NEA, 2006).

Essential Functions

The ADA defines essential functions as those functions that an employee is required to do, or are fundamental to the job (the nature of the job would change if it was removed, or the whole reason the job exists is to do that function) (Spechler, 1996; Equal Employment Opportunity Commission [EEOC], 2005; Workforce Central Florida, 2007). If it is something that a person spends very little time doing or it is done rarely (once a year), then it is not essential. The ADA requires that the essential functions be identified (although the ADA does not specifically require written job descriptions); this information is used in determining if discrimination has occurred. If a candidate is otherwise qualified, and can perform the essential functions of the job with or without accommodations, that person is protected under the law (EEOC). This does not mean the employer has to hire that person, but only that the person's disability or perceived disability cannot be used as a reason not to hire the person. An employer can hire the most qualified applicant for a job (EEOC).

The EEOC (2005) does provide some guidance for determining the essential functions of the job. In addition to the criteria already discussed, the EEOC also considers the level of specialization required, the number of other employees among whom a particular task could be divided or reallocated, the work experience of current and previous employees in the same position, and the terms of the collective bargaining agreement if that position is covered under a union contract (EEOC; Loy, 2007).

In some places, the essential functions, along with marginal functions or additional responsibilities, are listed as job duties (Braveman, 2005; Workforce Central Florida, 2007). Job duties sometimes include specific tasks that may or may not be essential. Depending on the nature of the job being described, this could be a very long list. Some suggestions are to list the job duties in order of importance (NEA, 2006), by separating the routine duties from the periodic duties (Braveman), or by separating the essential functions from the marginal functions or additional responsibilities (Workforce Central Florida; Loy, 2007). Describe the job duties using action verbs (Workforce Central Florida).

Some people recommend using a "catchall" or "elastic" sentence in order to avoid having employees claim a particular task is not in their job description (Workforce Central Florida, 2007). This seems to run counter to all the advice to be specific and clear. This is an example of a "catchall" sentence: Performs other duties as assigned by supervisor. While on the one hand this might cover just about anything a supervisor could throw at a supervisee, it might be vague enough that it could be challenged in court.

SUMMARY

Job descriptions are an essential part of any employment situation. They outline what an employee is expected to do. They help guide hiring, performance review, compensation, and disciplinary actions of employers and provide employees with a clear set of performance expectations. A well-written job description should include the job or position title, purpose of the position, reporting relationships, job specifications (qualifications, working conditions, equipment used, and responsibility and autonomy), and essential functions or job duties.

REFERENCES

American Occupational Therapy Association. (2008a). Occupational therapy practice framework: Domain and process. *American Journal of Occupational Therapy, 62,* 625–683.

Braveman, B. (2005). *Managing and leading in occupational therapy: An evidence-based approach.* Philadelphia: F. A. Davis.

Drafke, M. W. (1994). *Working in health care: What you need to know to succeed.* Philadelphia: F. A. Davis.

Equal Employment Opportunity Commission (2005). *The ADA: Your responsibilities as an employer.* Retrieved July 24, 2007, from http://www.eeoc.gov/facts/ada17.html

Liebler, J. G. & McConnell, C. R. (2004). *Management principles for health professionals* (4th ed.). Sudbury, MA: Jones and Bartlett.

Loy, B. (2007). *Job descriptions.* Retrieved July 24, 2007, from http://www.jan.wvu.edu/media/JobDescriptions.html

Mader-Clark, M. (2007). *Writing and using job descriptions.* Retrieved June 6, 2007, from http://www.nolo.com/article.cfm/ObjectID/7D40564D-E366-49E5-8F7C42399A6D071F/

National Education Association (2006). *Job descriptions.* Retrieved July 23, 2007, from http://www.nea.org/esphome/nearesources/jobdodon.html

Rice University (2009). *How to hire handbook: Guidelines for writing job descriptions.* Retrieved July 23, 2007, from http://people.rice.edu/jobs.cfm?doc_id=7333

Spechler, J. W. (1996). *Reasonable accommodation: Profitable compliance with the Americans with Disabilities Act.* Delray Beach, FL: St. Lucie.

US Department of Labor (2007). *Career Onestop.* Retrieved July 12, 2007, from http://www.careerinfonet.org/acinet/JobWriter/default.aspx

US Department of Labor (2008). *Fact Sheet #17A: Exemption for executive, administrative, professional, computer & outside sales employees under the fair labor standards act (FLSA).* Retrieved January 27, 2009, from http://www.dol.gov/esa/whd/regs/compliance/fairpay/fs17a_overview.pdf

Western Kentucky University (n.d.). *How to hire handbook: Guidelines for writing job descriptions.* Retrieved July 23, 2007, from http://www.wku.edu/CareerServ/welcome/students/handouts/hiring.pdf

Workforce Central Florida (2007). The importance of a properly written job description [electronic version]. *Workforce Watch, 1*(47), 1–2.

Answers to Selected Exercises

▼ EXERCISE 2.1 ▼

1. Jennifer attended three sessions this week. She needed encouragement to participate in the group discussion. She rarely made eye contact with the therapist or other group members. She mumbled incoherently and occasionally picked at something unseen in the air around her. When given a sorting task to do, she refused to participate. Her attention span was less than 2 minutes. She smiled while listening to classical music and the mumbling and picking at the air stopped. When asked specific questions at different times on different days, she was not oriented to person, place, or time.

▼ EXERCISE 2.2 ▼

2. Andrea has been referred to OT for work on self-care skills, following a TBI and fractured Ⓛ clavicle, humerus, and pelvis. Visited Andrea in her room to introduce her to OT and explain the schedule of visits. She has no memory of the accident or first week in the hospital. In the 5 minutes I spent with her, she asked my name six times. She knows she is married, but cannot remember the names of her four children. She appears to tire easily, yawning often. She is agreeable to therapy, but states she has no idea what she'd like to accomplish in OT, and does not know what would be realistic for short-term goals. For a long-term goal, she would like to go home and live life like she did before her accident.

▼ EXERCISE 3.1 ▼

1.	A	Combing one's hair
4.	P	Making one's needs known
5.	C	Hand strength
8.	C	Understanding nonverbal communication
9.	P	Posture
12.	A	Balancing a checkbook
15.	P	Taking turns during a card game
19.	C	Finding items in a hidden picture puzzle

▼ EXERCISE 4.1 ▼

2. Bottom-up
6. Top-down
8. Top-down

10. Bottom-up
13. Top-down
15. Bottom-up

▼ EXERCISE 4.2 ▼

1. No. This would be appropriate for the biomechanical frame of reference. To be consistent with Bobath, the goal would address patterns of movement.
4. Yes.
6. No. With this frame of reference, goals would describe client expression of self-worth or use of stress management techniques.

▼ EXERCISE 5.1 ▼

Case 1

C: What is there is clear and free from jargon; spelling and grammar seem OK.

A: Probably is accurate, but it seems incomplete; interpretations not clearly separate from findings.

R: It is unclear how anything in this note is relevant to her goals; it jumps around a lot.

E: Documented refusal on an activity (slide).

Case 3

C: This note is not very clear. Probably meant hand therapy not hard therapy. How much progress is steady progress? What can he do now that he could not do at the time of his last note?

A: There are no good measurements in the note, but there may be in the flow sheet. It is OK to do this.

R: Note is relevant to client's condition.

E: No exceptions noted; there may not have been any to document.

▼ EXERCISE II.1 ▼

Problem	Solution
Illegibility	Use word processor or electronic medical record
Cannot tell which patient the note is about	
Notes written out of sequence	
Pencil or colored ink	
Erasures or white out	Stop doing this immediately and correct errors with a line through error.
Blank spaces	
Incomplete signatures	

Problem	Solution
Notes written by students are not cosigned by supervisor	Go back in and cosign them, but with today's date
Poor grammar/spelling	
Poor word choices	
Unknown abbreviations	Use only approved abbreviations from now on; use fewer abbreviations; put line through and replace with full word
Missing documents	
Computer screen with client information displayed left unattended	Develop habit of closing documents every time you leave the computer. As a backup, have the screen saver set to come on after a minute of idle time, but do not depend on this option; it is not sufficient protection of privacy since the slightest mouse movement removes the screen saver
Chart left unattended	

▼ EXERCISE 6.1 ▼

1. If the wording of the release is limited to the discontinuation summary, this is a breach. In addition, providing such subjective information would leave the hospital occupational therapist open to allegations of defamation of character or slander.
2. This is OK; the case manager is contracted to the insurer.
3. This is a breach of confidentiality.

▼ EXERCISE 7.1 ▼

2. Carelessness
3. Fraud
5. Fraud and carelessness

▼ EXERCISE 8.2 ▼

1. In client-centered therapy, the client actively participates in the evaluation and intervention processes (Schwartzberg, 2002).
4. Freud is credited with developing classical psychoanalysis in the early 1900s (Hagedorn, 1997).
6. Occupational therapy helps people do the things that are important to them when circumstances create barriers to getting them done (Niestadt & Crepeau, 1998).

▼ EXERCISE 9.1 ▼

2.
May 31, 2008	Date of referral	Dr. Don Touchme	Name of physician
Kyle Beback	Name of client	unknown	Frequency
unknown	Duration	unknown	Intensity

<u>Work on ADLs.</u>   Reason for referral

Is this an adequate referral?   Yes   (No)

Why or why not?

There is not enough information. Judging by the age of the client, Medicare may be the payer. In that case, more detailed information is needed. It would be OK to do the evaluation and then call the physician with a recommendation for clearer orders. Having the physician sign the plan of care provides written evidence that the physician certifies that the plan is appropriate. I would not provide any intervention beyond the evaluation without written or oral orders from the physician.

▼ EXERCISE 9.2 ▼

2. OK.
3. This would be questionable. Before doing the screenings, decide if you have the knowledge and expertise to work with this population and know who would provide the services should they be needed.

▼ EXERCISE 10.1 ▼

1. Descriptive
2. Interpretative
4. Descriptive, although more professional wording could be used.
5. Interpretive
8. Descriptive
10. Interpretive

▼ EXERCISE 10.2 ▼

2. R
3. I
6. I

▼ EXERCISE 10.3 ▼

1. *Interpretation:* Client is at risk for choking with thin liquids. Client needs to slow down his eating, swallow after chewing each bite, and learn to use utensils.

▼ EXERCISE 11.1 ▼

3. A: Bobby
   B: Retrieve tools
   C: Independently
   D: 3 out of 5 sessions

▼ EXERCISE 11.2 ▼

2. F: Write
   E: Consistently
   A: Write

S: Each letter correctly formed

T: June 15, 2009

▼ EXERCISE 11.3 ▼

1. R: Relates to using mouse with nondominant hand, result of the stroke

   H: By 1/2/10

   U: I would know what to do if I stepped in to work with this client

   M: Cut and paste 8 individual letters in 5 minutes or less

   B: Cutting and pasting is observable

   A: You do not have enough information to answer this, but I assure you it is achievable.

▼ EXERCISE 11.4 ▼

2. S: This would make a difference in her life

   M: Spilling two or fewer times per meal while using a fork or spoon

   A: I think it is achievable in the time frame given

   R: Relates to arthritis and vision difficulty

   T: By April 22, 2010

▼ EXERCISE 11.5 ▼

1. **ABCD:** Client will independently don and doff splint within 2 days of receiving splint.
2. **FEAST:** The client will participate in a craft of her choosing for 10 minutes without moving around the room or shouting at other clients within 3 days.
3. **RHUMBA:** The client will maneuver her wheelchair from the front door of the school to her classroom without bumping into walls or people by 11-2-09.
4. **SMART:** By one month from now, the client will independently obtain a coffee mug on the bottom shelf of the above counter cabinet.

▼ EXERCISE 12.2 ▼

2. *Three suggested activities:* Practice feeding himself breadsticks or other large finger food, sort clothes for the laundry, and Velcro checkers.

   Rationale: The more he uses it, the more comfortable he will be. May need to do both one-handed and two-handed activities.
3. *Three suggested activities:* Practice using a dressing stick, practice using long-handled shoehorn, and practice using a sock-aid.

   Rationale: Trying different adaptive equipment will allow client to see which is the most practical and useful.

▼ EXERCISE 13.1 ▼

2. _X_ Client said she is hearing voices telling her to cut her hair.
5. _X_ "I am fat and ugly."
6. ___ Client is resistant to all suggestions.
9. ___ Saji's shirt was misbuttoned, untucked, and stained.

▼ EXERCISE 13.2 ▼

1. _X_ The client's eyes were red and watery.
2. ___ Bob seemed to be frustrated.
3. _X_ He pushed away from the table and left the room.

▼ EXERCISE 13.3 ▼

1. I think the list (the middle way) is the easiest to read and compare the two sides of the body. The narrative is by far the most difficult way to read and understand the information.
2. Present your idea to a colleague.

▼ EXERCISE 13.4 ▼

1. _X_ She has to be told to come out of her room.
3. ___ Client completed 75% of the task without assistance.
4. _X_ Usha does not interact with peers.
9. _X_ Willow is making good progress.

▼ EXERCISE 13.5 ▼

1. A: Client has limited active range of motion in both hands. There is significant ulnar drift and swan neck deformity present in both index fingers. These limitations interfere with his ability to keyboard.
2a. A: Deshaun demonstrates sensitivity to tactile stimuli, but responds well to deep pressure and traction.

▼ EXERCISE 13.6 ▼

3. ___ She should be more careful in the kitchen.
4. _P_ Increase repetitions as tolerated.
7. _P_ Client will work on chewing food at least 10 times before swallowing.

▼ EXERCISE 13.7 ▼

Case 3: Client with left side neglect

P: Videotape client swinging a golf club and eating. Discuss evidence of left-side neglect. Teach compensatory techniques. Continue 2x/wk home visits as per plan of care.

▼ EXERCISE 13.8 ▼

1. O
5. S
7. O
8. P
9. A

▼ EXERCISE 13.9 ▼

Case 1

> S is OK.
> O included some A terms by generalizing and analyzing performance.
> A is supported by O.
> P seems appropriate.

▼ EXERCISE 13.11 ▼

Case 2

Client received OT for 45 min. in a home visit today. She used a plastic bag hanging from her forearm near her elbow to collect supplies for a dinner salad and cottage cheese. She prepared the salad while seated on a tall stool at the counter. Client reported less fatigue than carrying one item at a time. Instructed client in use of bath bench. Client demonstrated proper use of the seat. She tried a sock-aid and was successful in donning socks half the time. She said she was not sure she liked it but was willing to work with it for a couple of days. She was shown card holders, but did not like using either one. Plan to continue to work on meal prep, dressing, and leisure occupations 2x/wk at her home.

▼ EXERCISE 14.1 ▼

Case 1

Client received occupational therapy services as an outpatient 3x/wk for 3 wks and 2x/wk for 3 wks, for a total of 15 visits. Initially, she had severely limited shoulder flexion and abduction on her right side. She currently has nearly full range of motion in both directions. She was initially dependent in grooming and hygiene; now she is independent. When she started receiving occupational therapy intervention, she needed moderate assistance in feeding and dressing; now she is independent in these occupations. She is also now completing meal preparation on her own. She reports pain on movement of her right arm has decreased from a rating of 9 (on a 1–10 scale, 10 being excruciating) to a rating of 4.

▼ EXERCISE 15.2 ▼

2. To determine if the way he is interpreting what he sees is different than other children his age.
3. To determine the ways in which her muscle tone and movement limitations interfere with her ability to play with peers and participate in school activities.

▼ EXERCISE 16.2 ▼

1. Torii will move from lying on her stomach to sitting, getting help for half the process, by the end of the school year.
5. Condalisa's parents will contact 2 agencies that provide support to families of children with disabilities to obtain information about their services by January 2, 2010.

▼ EXERCISE 16.3 ▼

2. Denay needs to be able to stand, reach, and grasp toys in order to interact with and learn from her environment.

▼ EXERCISE 17.2 ▼

1. More helpful: Omar is able to make snips with a scissors, but not make successive cuts along a line. He moves the paper with the hand not using the scissors, rather than move the scissors to a new place to cut.

2. More helpful: Lucinda bumps into other children when they are standing in a line. She often will reach out and touch other children's hair or clothing, rubbing the hair or fabric between her thumb and index finger.

▼ EXERCISE 17.3 ▼

3. Objective 3a: Paul will cut single snips on short lines across a page without assistance by November 1, 2010.

   Objective 3b: Paul will cut an 8 1/2×11 piece of paper in half independently by March 1, 2011.

▼ EXERCISE 18.1 ▼

1. **Narrative progress note:**

   While practicing toilet transfers in the occupational therapy clinic bathroom the client fell, hitting his head on the sink. He returned to the unit under nursing care. Rest of session canceled today. Will resume intervention tomorrow.

   Incident Report:

   While attempting to teach the client a pivot transfer in the occupational therapy bathroom, the client fell, hitting his head on the sink. The client was wearing a transfer belt at the time, and I was holding on to it at the time of the incident. The client received a 1/2-inch cut on his forehead. Emergency call button activated, help came within 2 minutes. No loss of consciousness. I was not injured.

▼ EXERCISE 19.1 ▼

Case 1

1. The child is making good progress right now, so this is the best time for skilled intervention.

2. While she is making progress, she has not yet met her goals.

3. Providing graded sensory experiences requires the skilled judgment of an experienced occupational therapist.

▼ EXERCISE 20.1 ▼

2. **Budget**

   The department needs to trim 10% of our expenses from the budget. We can trim some by being more conscientious about remembering to bill for adaptive equipment, conserving paper and food, and not walking off with each other's pens.

   Action:

   Each person needs to meet with Barb to discuss other ways to cut the budget.

▼ EXERCISE 21.1 ▼

3. Monthly client satisfaction surveys will show that 85% of women will say they were satisfied or very satisfied with the occupational therapy services they received.

▼ EXERCISE 21.3 ▼

2. _T_ Address all the review criteria established by the funding agency in your proposal.
3. _F_ It is a good idea to ask lots of questions throughout the process. It is a good idea to ask questions as needed, but to not ask so many that you begin to be a bother to the agency.
6. _T_ Goals can be broad and not measurable.
7. _T_ Objectives need to meet RHUMBA criteria.

▼ EXERCISE 22.1 ▼

Procedure

1. Turn on warm water.
2. Wet hands thoroughly.
3. Use two squirts of soap from the dispenser, pushing the dispensing bar with the back of one's hand.
4. Massage hands with soap so that entire surface of both hands, front and back, and under nails are covered with soap suds. Keep massaging for 15 seconds.
5. Rinse hands under warm running water for 15 seconds, completely removing soap. Leave the water running.
6. Dry hands on paper towels. Use paper towels to turn off faucets.
7. Discard paper towels in waste basket.

▼ EXERCISE 22.2 ▼

Policy

Each client visit will be documented appropriately in the client's record.

▼ EXERCISE B.1 ▼

Corrected words are in **bold**.

calendar	**a lot**	definitely	sense	professor
accepted	**benefited**	necessary	against	develop

▼ EXERCISE B.2 ▼

Corrected versions are in **bold**.

Occupational Therapy 101	**a foundations of occupational therapy course**
Professor Susan Jones	**Susan Jones, our professor**

▼ EXERCISE B.3 ▼

Correct answers are in **bold.**

I am	I were	**I was**	I are	I is
He is	She are	She were	**She was**	She am
They were	**They are**	They is	They was	They am

▼ EXERCISE B.4 ▼

1. The client prepared a meal of toast and tea. **Yes**

2. The <u>balls was</u> placed into the container one at a time. **No**

▼ EXERCISE B.5 ▼

Errors are underlined and comments are in italics.

2. Bobby crawled <u>6</u> feet without assistance. He used a reciprocal <u>pattern</u> of arm and leg movement. He laughed when he finished and reached the toy. Bobby seems motivated. Then he tried to carry the toy back with him while he crawled but it kept falling, frustrating him. *You need a subject for the fourth sentence; Bobby, the client, or he could be used.*

Grammar and Spelling Review

▼ INTRODUCTION ▼

All of us have read something that made us laugh because we misinterpreted the writer's intention. For example, a student of mine once wrote in a progress note, "Patient was born at 36-week gestation with no significant pregnancy." While this is humorous to the reader, it is not funny when you are the one who wrote the laughable note in a client's official record. Then it's embarrassing. Beyond that, if it happens often enough the other professionals on the team may begin to think that you are not the brightest bulb on the tree. They may start to doubt your professional skills and knowledge. However, the impressions they form do not stop there. They may also view you as a typical representative of your profession or the academic program you attended. If they begin to doubt your professional skills and knowledge, they may project that and doubt the integrity of your profession or your alma mater. That is a heavy burden to bear.

Realistically, very few people are always accurate spellers or constantly grammatically correct. Occasional mistakes are normal. However, repeated mistakes need attention. Most colleges and universities have writing centers where students can go to get help with writing skills. There are also things you can do on your own to improve the quality of your writing.

I strongly recommend purchasing and keeping (do not sell this book at the end of the semester!) some kind of guide to writing. By this I mean a book like *The Everyday Writer* (Lunsford, 2009) or *A Pocket Style Manual* (Hacker, 2008). Most occupational therapy journals use the American Psychological Association (APA) writing style, so the *APA Publication Manual* (2001) is also a good resource. Find a book that explains and has examples of such things as punctuation and capitalization. A dictionary is also helpful to check your spelling.

In the next few pages, I will show you common errors in spelling and grammar and how they affect the way others perceive you. I will also show you a few simple rules to remember to help your writing look more professional.

Here are some examples of documentation gone bad, taken from http://www. medleague.com/Articles/humor/charting_bloopers.htm (*Charting bloopers,* n.d.):

"On the second day the knee was better and on the third day it had completely disappeared."

"Patient was released to outpatient department without dressing."

"I have suggested that he loosen his pants before standing, and then, when he stands with the help of his wife, they should fall to the floor."

"No mobility limitations noted except for difficulty with transfers, standing, turning and ambulating."

"Patient was alert and unresponsive."

"The patient lives at home with his mother, father, and pet turtle, who is presently enrolled in day care three times a week."

"I saw your patient today, who is still under our car for physical therapy."

"She is numb from the toes down."

"Skin intact, red, and broken."

"The patient is tearful and crying constantly. She also appears to be depressed."

The anonymous writers did not intend these to be funny. These are supposedly taken directly from medical records. A lawyer would have a field day in court with the writer of these statements, "And yet you claim to be competent at your job..."

▼ COMMON ERRORS ▼

Spelling and Proofreading

When one is writing quickly, it is very easy to drop a letter or blur two letters. As in the example of the patient "under our car" in the list of sentences just given, leaving the end "e" off of a word is a frequent occurrence. However, there is a big difference between car and care, mad and made, or scar and scare. Spell-checkers on your computer will not catch these errors because all are real words. Only careful proofreading will catch this kind of error. Spell-checkers do not catch misused words.

As found in *The Everyday Writer* (Lunsford, 2009), the rules you learned in grade school, such as "I before e, except after c, and when it sounds like an 'a' as in neighbor and weigh" still hold true today. Prefixes usually do not change the original spelling of a word. For example, by adding the prefix "un" to the word "necessary," it becomes "unnecessary." However, adding a suffix may change the last letter of the word to which it is added. When you want to make a noun ending in "y" into a plural, change the "y" to an "i" and add "es" (rather than simply adding an "s," unless the "y" is preceded by a vowel). For example, "key" becomes "keys" but "therapy" becomes "therapies." The silent "e" is dropped when adding a suffix that starts with a vowel, such as "ing," "able," or "istic." For example, "believe" becomes "believable." If the root word ends in a vowel–consonant combination, double the consonant before adding the suffix, but only if it is a single-syllable word or a word in which the last syllable is accented (Lunsford, 2009). If the accent is on another syllable, or the word ends in vowel–vowel–consonant or vowel–consonant–consonant, do not double the last consonant. For example, "stop" becomes "stopped," but "start" becomes "started."

Exercise B.1

Identify the words that are spelled correctly.

calander	alot	definitely	sense	professor
accepted	benifitted	necessary	against	develop
independent	maybe	truely	thoroughly	occasion
immediately	untill	categorically	tomatoe	committee
noticeible	cheif	beleive	roommates	apparantly

Homonyms are words that sound the same, but are spelled differently and have different meanings. The words in Box B.1 are examples of some commonly confused homonyms.

I keep a small pocket dictionary next to my computer. If I am at all unsure whether a word is spelled with an "ea" or "ee," or if it ends with "able" or "ible," I look it up. When I am writing in a chart and I am unsure of a spelling, I will write the word a couple of different ways on a scratch piece of paper. Sometimes seeing it written two ways helps to find the right way. I do not depend on a spell-checker to catch my errors.

There is a poem that was written by Jerrold H. Zar and has been widely adapted and circulated on the Internet, sometimes under the name "Ode to a Spelling Checker" or "Ann Owed Two the Spelling Checker" (http://tenderbytes.net/rhymeworld/feeder/teacher/pullet. htm on 5/8/02). Every word of this poem passes the computerized spelling checker programs but most of the words are used incorrectly.

▼ CAPITALIZATION ▼

The first word of a sentence, names of people, cities, states, and countries are all capitalized. Names of companies, organizations, specific historical events, specific languages, and academic institutions are also capitalized (Lunsford, 2009). Names of seasons or professions are not capitalized (Lunsford, 2009). A common error that I've found in student writing is capitalizing the words "occupational therapy" in the middle of a sentence.

Exercise B.2

Which phrases are correctly capitalized?

Lake Superior	The Lincoln Memorial
A Monument to Creativity	A Prayer Book
The Bible	The Library of Congress
The School Library	a Foundations of Occupational Therapy
Occupational Therapy 101	Course
Professor Susan Jones	Susan Jones, our Professor
My Mother	Aunt Sylvia
Up at the Lake	Aunt Sylvia

▼ PUNCTUATION ▼

There are so many punctuation marks to choose from (,. /;: -!?). How do you know which one to use when? In clinical documentation, most sentences will end with a period. There are few instances where you would use an exclamation point or question mark, unless you are quoting a client.

It is easy to get confused about when to use commas, semicolons, and colons. Colons are used for three purposes: to add an explanation, to introduce a series or list, or to separate elements (Lunsford, 2009). According to APA style (APA, 2001), there should be one space after a colon, and it is usually not necessary to capitalize the first word after the colon. A semicolon is used to link clauses of a sentence that are either closely related or joined by transitional phrases (Lunsford, 2009). Semicolons can also be used to separate words in a series that contain other punctuation, as in the example below:

The patient is independent in feeding; dressing, grooming, and hygiene; meal preparation, serving, and cleanup; and medication management.

Commas have multiple uses; however, in every case commas cause the reader to take a momentary break, a pause, in the sentence (Lunsford, 2009). Proper placement of a comma can change the whole meaning of a sentence. Here is an example (author unknown):

Woman, without her man, is nothing.
Woman, without her, man is nothing.

The words are the same, but the simple placement of a comma can change the entire meaning of a sentence.

▼ SUBJECT–VERB AGREEMENT ▼

Essentially, a subject is the primary noun in your sentence. It tells the reader who or what the sentence is about. The verb is the action part of the sentence. In a properly written sentence, the subject and verb will agree with each other in terms of the number of subjects and which person (voice) is being used (Lunsford, 2009). To help me remember, I recite little phrases like "A person does what people do" or "I go where she goes." Here are some examples.

I am writing this sentence. (first-person singular)
The committee is drafting a proposal. (third-person singular)
The committee members are drafting a statement. (third-person plural)
We are writing an interdisciplinary evaluation report. (first-person plural)
You are writing an intervention plan for Ms. Rivera. (second-person singular)

Exercise B.3

In the examples below, identify which verbs agree with which subjects.

I am	I were	I was	I are	I is
We was	We are	We is	We am	We were
You are	You am	You is	You were	You was
He is	She are	She were	She was	She am
They were	They are	They is	They was	They am

Exercise B.4

Identify which sentences have subject–verb agreement.

1. The client prepared a meal of toast and tea.
2. The balls was placed into the container one at a time.
3. The client is seated at the table with her feet on a footrest.
4. After several tries, the group make a successful circle.
5. The client's family have some concerns.

▼ VERB–TENSE AGREEMENT ▼

Within one sentence, as well as within one paragraph, the verb tenses should be the same (Lunsford, 2009). In other words, if the sentence or paragraph starts in the past tense it should stay there. You should not jump from present to past and back again. See if you can spot the verb–tense shifting in the following paragraph.

> The client got out of bed unassisted and sits in her wheelchair. She pushes herself up to the sink and begins to adjust the temperature of the water. The water was too hot, so she turned down the hot water and turns up the cold water. Then she moistens the washcloth and adds soap. Next, she washed her face.

Changing tenses confuse the reader and are distracting when you are trying to make sense out of a note.

▼ PRONOUN–ANTECEDENT AGREEMENT ▼

Another common error is mixing singular and plural pronouns and antecedents in the same sentence (Lunsford, 2009). Pronouns are words that are used to replace other words (antecedents) in a sentence so that the sentence does not become repetitive (Lunsford, 2009). For example, in the sentence "The client sat down when he became tired," the pronoun "he" replaces the antecedent "the client." A pronoun should always agree with the antecedent in gender and in number (Lunsford, 2009). Here is an example of pronoun–antecedent mismatch: *A student* needs to be aware that *they* often have more homework than they anticipated. This is the corrected version: Students need to be aware that they often have more homework than they anticipate. An alternative version would be as follows: A student needs to be aware that he or she will often have more homework than anticipated.

When writing in the singular, choosing the right pronoun can become a challenge. The pronouns he, she, and one can be used. Some people object to the phrase "he or she" or "s/he" as cumbersome. Using "he" is viewed as gender insensitive, while "one" seems contrived or prim. As a writer, it is your prerogative to choose which word you use. Sensitivity does matter, so think things through thoroughly before you put pen to paper.

▼ PLACEMENT OF MODIFIERS ▼

Modifiers are used to clarify a sentence, adding important details or descriptions (Lunsford, 2009). However, when a modifier is used, where it is placed in the sentence can affect the meaning of the sentence. Here is another anonymous example of medical records humor (www.wwnurse.com): "Patient has chest pain if she lies on her left side for over a year." It sounds like she has been lying on her left side for a year. However, by moving the modifier, we can change the meaning of the sentence. *For over a year, the patient has chest pain if she lies on her left side.* It is still not a great sentence, but at least the meaning is clearer.

▼ INCOMPLETE SENTENCES ▼

As mentioned earlier in the chapter, a sentence must have a subject and a verb (Lunsford, 2009). If either one is missing, the sentence is incomplete. Find the incomplete sentence in the following paragraph:

> The client has been out of work for two months. She has difficulty maintaining a firm grasp on writing or eating utensils with her right hand. She can only use a keyboard for a few minutes at a time. Also comb her hair. Recovered mobility in her hand to dress herself with the use of adaptive equipment.

The incomplete sentence fits in the paragraph; it is just missing something. What about combing her hair? Can she do it or not? If she can comb her hair, how well does she do?

▼ WORD CHOICE ▼

I heard an ad on the radio (presumably the speaker was reading from a script) where the store being advertised was trying to get shoppers to spend money in this particular store because of a great January sale. The speaker said something to the effect of "This year, resolute to save money, shop smart at our New Year's Sale." I think the person meant *resolve* to save money, make a resolution to save money. The word resolute is a real word, but it just does not belong in the sentence in the way it was used.

There are many rules for speaking (and writing) English properly. They can be difficult to sort through. According to Lunsford (2001), the 20 most common errors in writing, listed in order of frequency, are:

1. Missing comma after an introductory element (e.g., In fact, the client...)
2. Vague pronoun reference (pronouns should refer to a specific antecedent in the same or previous sentence; if there is more than one possible antecedent, this can be confusing)
3. Missing comma in a compound sentence (i.e., when parts of a sentence could stand as a sentence on their own, but are joined by words such as "and," "but," or "or")
4. Wrong word (using improper homonyms or words with the wrong shade of meaning)
5. Missing comma(s) with a nonrestrictive element (an element not essential to the basic meaning of the sentence)
6. Wrong or missing verb ending (i.e., "ed" or "ing")
7. Wrong or missing preposition (i.e., "at" or "to")
8. Comma splice ("A comma splice occurs when only a comma separates clauses that could each stand alone as a sentence" [p. 16].)
9. Missing or misplaced possessive apostrophe (i.e., "client's" or "clients'")
10. Unnecessary shift in tense (i.e., from past tense to future tense in the same sentence)
11. Unnecessary shift in pronoun (i.e., from using "one" to using "you" or "I")
12. Sentence fragment (a part of a sentence is written as if it was a whole sentence)
13. Wrong tense or verb form (need to clarify whether the action is, was, or will be completed)
14. Lack of subject–verb agreement (subjects and verbs should agree in number and person; not every word that ends in "s" is a plural, so do not trust word-processing grammar-check programs)
15. Missing comma in a series (use commas to separate three or more items in a list)
16. Lack of agreement between pronoun and antecedent (i.e., "the client" and "they")
17. Unnecessary comma(s) with a restrictive element (a part of a sentence that is essential to its meaning)
18. Fused sentence (a run-on sentence with little or no punctuation)
19. Misplaced or dangling modifier (modifiers need to be as close as possible to the word they describe; a dangling modifier is one that does not seem to be attached to anything in the sentence)
20. Its/it's confusion (use an apostrophe only when you mean "it is" or "it has")

Not every reader of your documentation will be bothered by, or even recognize, each of these common errors (Lunsford, 2009). However, some readers might. If any item on this list seems unclear, that is probably a sign that a review of grammar rules would help your writing.

Exercise B.5

Find the errors in the notes below:

1. The client attended three occupational therapy sessions this week. She worked on sequencing the steps to making simple meals such as canned soup cooked on the stove; a frozen dinner cooked in a microwave; and a peanut butter and banana sandwich. The client need multipel verbal cues too complete the tasks in the proper, safe, sequence. She follows one step directions only so far. Next week, will try two step directions.

2. Bobby crawled six feet without assistance. He used a recipricol patter of arm and leg movement. He laughed when he finished and reached the toy. Seems motivated. Then he tried to carry the toy back with him while he crawled but it kept falling, frustrating him.

3. R.L. stated that he slept well last night, but is still tired this morning. He completed ten repetititions of shoulder stretches. Then rests for five minutes before repeating the exercise. He worked on his woodworking project with frequent rest periods. He says the pain is less than before. Continue to work on endurance, strength, and leisure skills.

SUMMARY

There are some general rules for grammar and spelling that are necessary for an occupational therapy practitioner to use in order to be perceived as a professional. Failure to write well can lead people to think the writer is incompetent. Proofreading one's writing is important. While proofreading, check for spelling, capitalization, punctuation, and word use. Watch out for incomplete sentences. Be careful with punctuation, subject–verb agreement, verb–tense agreement, and modifiers. There are many resources to help a person become a better writer, including dictionaries and grammar guides. Easy access to these resources is always helpful.

REFERENCES

American Psychological Association. (2001). *Publication manual of the American Psychological Association* (5th ed.). Washington, DC: Author.

Charting bloopers (n.d.). Retrieved February 18, 2009, from http://www.medleague.com/Articles/humor/charting_symptoms.htm

Hacker, D. (2008) *A pocket style manual (5th ed).* Boston: Bedford/St. Martin's.

Lunsford, A. (2001). *The everyday writer* (2nd ed.). New York: Bedford/St. Martin's.

Lunsford, A. (2009). *The everyday writer* (4th ed.). New York: Bedford/St. Martin's.

APPENDIX C

AOTA Standards of Practice for Occupational Therapy

▼ PREFACE ▼

This document defines minimum standards for the practice of occupational therapy. The *Standards of Practice for Occupational Therapy* are requirements for occupational therapists and occupational therapy assistants for the delivery of occupational therapy services. *The Reference Manual of Official Documents* contains documents that clarify and support occupational therapy practice (American Occupational Therapy Association [AOTA, 2004]). These documents are reviewed and updated on an ongoing basis for their applicability.

▼ EDUCATION, EXAMINATION, AND LICENSURE REQUIREMENTS ▼

All occupational therapists and occupational therapy assistants must practice under federal and state law.

To practice as an occupational therapist, the individual trained in the United States

- has graduated from an occupational therapy program accredited by the Accreditation Council for Occupational Therapy Education (ACOTE®) or predecessor organizations;
- has successfully completed a period of supervised fieldwork experience required by the recognized educational institution where the applicant met the academic requirements of an educational program for occupational therapists that is accredited by ACOTE® or predecessor organizations;
- has passed a nationally recognized entry-level examination for occupational therapists; and
- fulfills state requirements for licensure, certification, or registration.

To practice as an occupational therapy assistant, the individual trained in the United States

- has graduated from an associate- or certificate-level occupational therapy assistant program accredited by ACOTE® or predecessor organizations;
- has successfully completed a period of supervised fieldwork experience required by the recognized educational institution where the applicant met the academic requirements of an educational program for occupational therapy assistants that is accredited by ACOTE® or predecessor organizations;
- has passed a nationally recognized entry-level examination for occupational therapy assistants; and
- fulfills state requirements for licensure, certification, or registration.

▼ DEFINITIONS ▼

Assessment. Specific tools or instruments that are used during the evaluation process.

Client. A person, group, program, organization, or community for whom the occupational therapy practitioner is providing services.

Evaluation. The process of obtaining and interpreting data necessary for intervention. This includes planning for and documenting the evaluation process and results.

Screening. Obtaining and reviewing data relevant to a potential client to determine the need for further evaluation and intervention.

▼ STANDARD I: PROFESSIONAL STANDING AND RESPONSIBILITY ▼

1. An occupational therapy practitioner (occupational therapist or occupational therapy assistant) delivers occupational therapy services that reflect the philosophical base of occupational therapy and are consistent with the established principles and concepts of theory and practice.

2. An occupational therapy practitioner is knowledgeable about and delivers occupational therapy services in accordance with AOTA standards, policies, and guidelines, and state and federal requirements relevant to practice and service delivery.

3. An occupational therapy practitioner maintains current licensure, registration, or certification as required by law or regulation.

4. An occupational therapy practitioner abides by the AOTA *Occupational Therapy Code of Ethics* (AOTA, 2000).

5. An occupational therapy practitioner abides by the AOTA *Standards for Continuing Competence* (AOTA, 1999) by establishing, maintaining, and updating professional performance, knowledge, and skills.

6. An occupational therapist is responsible for all aspects of occupational therapy service delivery and is accountable for the safety and effectiveness of the occupational therapy service delivery process.

7. An occupational therapy assistant is responsible for providing safe and effective occupational therapy services under the supervision of and in partnership with the occupational therapist and in accordance with laws or regulations and AOTA documents.

8. An occupational therapy practitioner maintains current knowledge of legislative, political, social, cultural, and reimbursement issues that affect clients and the practice of occupational therapy.

9. An occupational therapy practitioner is knowledgeable about evidence-based research and applies it ethically and appropriately to the occupational therapy process.

▼ STANDARD II: SCREENING, EVALUATION, AND RE-EVALUATION ▼

1. An occupational therapist accepts and responds to referrals in compliance with state laws or other regulatory requirements.

2. An occupational therapist, in collaboration with the client, evaluates the client's ability to participate in daily life activities by considering the client's capacities, the activities, and the environments in which these activities occur.

3. An occupational therapist initiates and directs the screening, evaluation, and re-evaluation process and analyzes and interprets the data in accordance with law, regulatory requirements, and AOTA documents.

4. An occupational therapy assistant contributes to the screening, evaluation, and re-evaluation process by implementing delegated assessments and by providing verbal and written reports of observations and client capacities to the occupational therapist in accordance with law, regulatory requirements, and AOTA documents.

5. An occupational therapy practitioner follows defined protocols when standardized assessments are used.

6. An occupational therapist completes and documents occupational therapy evaluation results. An occupational therapy assistant contributes to the documentation of evaluation results. An occupational therapy practitioner abides by the time frames, formats, and standards established by practice settings, government agencies, external accreditation programs, payers, and AOTA documents.

7. An occupational therapy practitioner communicates screening, evaluation, and re-evaluation results within the boundaries of client confidentiality to the appropriate person, group, or organization.

8. An occupational therapist recommends additional consultations or refers clients to appropriate resources when the needs of the client can best be served by the expertise of other professionals or services.

9. An occupational therapy practitioner educates current and potential referral sources about the scope of occupational therapy services and the process of initiating occupational therapy services.

▼ STANDARD III: INTERVENTION ▼

1. An occupational therapist has overall responsibility for the development, documentation, and implementation of the occupational therapy intervention based on the evaluation, client goals, current best evidence, and clinical reasoning.

2. An occupational therapist ensures that the intervention plan is documented within the time frames, formats, and standards established by the practice settings, agencies, external accreditation programs, and payers.

3. An occupational therapy assistant selects, implements, and makes modifications to therapeutic activities and interventions that are consistent with the occupational therapy assistant's demonstrated competency and delegated responsibilities, the intervention plan, and requirements of the practice setting.

4. An occupational therapy practitioner reviews the intervention plan with the client and appropriate others regarding the rationale, safety issues, and relative benefits and risks of the planned interventions.

5. An occupational therapist modifies the intervention plan throughout the intervention process and documents changes in the client's needs, goals, and performance.

6. An occupational therapy assistant contributes to the modification of the intervention plan by exchanging information with and providing documentation to the occupational therapist about the client's responses to and communications throughout the intervention.

7. An occupational therapy practitioner documents the occupational therapy services provided within the time frames, formats, and standards established by the practice settings, agencies, external accreditation programs, payers, and AOTA documents.

▼ STANDARD IV: OUTCOME ▼

1. An occupational therapist is responsible for selecting, measuring, documenting, and interpreting expected or achieved outcomes that are related to the client's ability to engage in occupations.

2. An occupational therapist is responsible for documenting changes in the client's performance and capacities and for discontinuing services when the client has achieved identified goals, reached maximum benefit, or does not desire to continue services.

3. An occupational therapist prepares and implements a discontinuation plan or transition plan based on the client's needs, goals, performance, and appropriate follow-up resources.

4. An occupational therapy assistant contributes to the discontinuation or transition plan by providing information and documentation to the supervising occupational therapist related to the client's needs, goals, performance, and appropriate follow-up resources.

5. An occupational therapy practitioner facilitates the transition process in collaboration with the client, family members, significant others, team, and community resources and individuals, when appropriate.

6. An occupational therapist is responsible for evaluating the safety and effectiveness of the occupational therapy processes and interventions within the practice setting.

7. An occupational therapy assistant contributes to evaluating the safety and effectiveness of the occupational therapy processes and interventions within the practice setting.

REFERENCES

American Occupational Therapy Association. (1999). Standards for continuing competence. *American Journal of Occupational Therapy, 53*, 599–600.

American Occupational Therapy Association. (2000). Occupational therapy code of ethics (2000). *American Journal of Occupational Therapy, 54*, 614–616.

American Occupational Therapy Association. (2004). *The reference manual of the official documents of the American Occupational Therapy Association* (10th ed.). Bethesda, MD: Author.

AUTHORS

The Commission on Practice:

Sara Jane Brayman, PhD, OTR/L, FAOTA, Chairperson

Susanne Smith Roley, MS, OTR/L, FAOTA, Chairperson-Elect

Gloria Frolek Clark, MS, OTR/L, FAOTA

Janet V. DeLany, DEd, MSA, OTR/L, FAOTA

Eileen R. Garza, PhD, OTR, ATP

Mary V. Radomski, MA, OTR/L, FAOTA

Ruth Ramsey, MS, OTR/L

Carol Siebert, MS, OTR/L

Kristi Voelkerding, BS, COTA/L

Lenna Aird, COTA/L, ASD Liaison

Patricia D. LaVesser, PhD, OTR/L, SIS Liaison

Deborah Lieberman, MHSA, OTR/L, FAOTA, AOTA Headquarters Liaison

for

The Commission on Practice

Sara Jane Brayman, PhD, OTR/L, FAOTA, Chairperson

Adopted by the Representative Assembly 2005C218

NOTE: This document replaces the 1998 *Standards of Practice for Occupational Therapy.* These standards are intended as recommended guidelines to assist occupational therapy practitioners in the provision of occupational therapy services. These standards serve as a minimum standard for occupational therapy practice and are applicable to all individual populations and the programs in which these individuals are served.

APPENDIX D

AOTA Guidelines for Documentation of Occupational Therapy 2007

Documentation is necessary whenever professional services are provided to a client. Occupational therapists and occupational therapy assistants[1] determine the appropriate type of documentation and document the services provided within their scope of practice. This document, based on the *Occupational Therapy Practice Framework: Domain and Process* (American Occupational Therapy Association [AOTA], 2002, 2007) describes the components and the purpose of professional documentation used in occupational therapy. AOTA's *Standards of Practice for Occupational Therapy* (2005) state, an occupational therapy practitioner[2] documents the occupational therapy services and "abides by the time frames, format, and standards established by the practice settings, government agencies, external accreditation programs, payers, and AOTA documents" (p. 664). In this document, *client* may refer to an individual, organization, or population.

The purpose of documentation is to

- Articulate the rationale for provision of occupational therapy services and the relationship of this service to the client's outcomes
- Reflect the occupational therapy practitioners' clinical reasoning and professional judgment
- Communicate information about the client from the occupational therapy perspective, and
- Create a chronological record of client status, occupational therapy services provided to the client, and client outcomes.

▼ TYPES OF DOCUMENTATION ▼

Box 1 outlines common types of reports. Depending on the service delivery and setting, reports may be named differently or combined and reorganized to meet the specific needs of the setting. Occupational therapy documentation should always record the professional's activity in the areas of evaluation, intervention, and outcomes (AOTA, 2002, 2007).

BOX D.1	Common Types of Occupational Therapy Reports	
Process Areas	**Type of Report**	
I. Evaluation	A. Evaluation or Screening Report	
	B. Reevaluation Report	
II. Intervention	1. Intervention Plan	
	2. Occupational Therapy Service Contacts	
	3. Progress Report	
	4. Transition Plan	
III. Outcomes	1. Discharge/Discontinuation Report	

I. Evaluation
   A. Evaluation or Screening Report
      1. Documents the referral source and data gathered through the evaluation process, including
         a. Description of the client's occupational profile
         b. Analysis of occupational performance and identification of factors that hinder and support performance in areas of occupation
         c. Delineation of specific areas of occupation and occupational performance that will be targeted for intervention and outcomes expected
      2. An abbreviated evaluation process (e.g., screening) documents only limited areas of occupation and occupational performance applicable to the client and to the situation.
      3. Suggested content with examples includes
         a. Client information—name/agency, date of birth, gender, health status, applicable medical/educational/developmental diagnoses, precautions, and contraindications
         b. Referral information—date and source of referral, services requested, reason for referral, funding source, and anticipated length of service
         c. Occupational profile—client's reason for seeking occupational therapy services, current areas of occupation that are successful and problematic, contexts and environments that support and hinder occupations, medical/educational/work history, occupational history (e.g., patterns of living, interest, values), client's priorities, and targeted outcomes
         d. Assessments used and results—types of assessments used and results (e.g., interviews, record reviews, observations, standardized or nonstandardized assessments), and confidence in test results
         e. Analysis of occupational performance—description of and judgment about performance skills, performance patterns, contexts and environments, features of the activities, and client factors that facilitate and inhibit performance
         f. Summary and analysis—interpretation and summary of data as it is related to occupational profile and referring concern
         g. Recommendation—judgment regarding appropriateness of occupational therapy services or other services.
            Note: Intervention goals addressing anticipated outcomes, objectives, and frequency of therapy are listed on the Intervention Plan (see below).
   B. Reevaluation Report
      1. Documents the results of the reevaluation process. Frequency of reevaluation depends on the needs of the setting and the progress of the client.
      2. Suggested content with examples includes
         a. Client information—name/agency, date of birth, gender, applicable medical/educational/developmental diagnoses, precautions, and contraindications
         b. Occupational profile—updates on current areas of occupation that are successful and problematic, contexts and environments that support or hinder occupations, summary of any new medical/educational/work information, and updates or changes to client's priorities and targeted outcomes
         c. Reevaluation results—focus of reevaluation, specific types of assessments used, and client's performance and subjective responses
         d. Summary and analysis—interpretation and summary of data as related to referring concern and comparison of results with previous evaluation results
         e. Recommendations—changes to occupational therapy services, revision or continuation of goals and objectives, frequency of occupational therapy services, and recommendation for referral to other professionals or agencies where applicable

II. Intervention
    A. Intervention Plan
        1. Documents the goals, intervention approaches, and types of interventions to be used to achieve the client's identified targeted outcomes based on results of evaluation or reevaluation processes. Includes recommendations or referrals to other professionals and agencies.
        2. Suggested content with examples include
            a. Client information—name/agency, date of birth, gender, precautions, and contraindications
            b. Intervention goals—measurable goals and short-term objectives directly related to the client's ability and need to engage in desired occupations
            c. Intervention approaches and types of interventions to be used—intervention approaches that include create/promote, establish/restore, maintain, modify, and prevent; types of interventions that include consultation process, education process, advocacy, therapeutic use of occupations or activities, and therapeutic use of self
            d. Service delivery mechanisms—service provider, service location, and frequency and duration of services
            e. Plan for discharge—discontinuation criteria, location of discharge, and follow-up care
            f. Outcome measures—outcomes that include improved occupational performance, adaptation, role competence, improved health and wellness, prevention of further difficulties, improved quality of life, self-advocacy, and occupational justice
            g. Professionals responsible and date of plan—names and positions of persons overseeing plan, date plan was developed, and date when plan was modified or reviewed
    B. Occupational Therapy Service Contacts
        1. Documents contacts between the client and the occupational therapy practitioner. Records the types of interventions used and client's response. Includes telephone contacts, interventions, and meetings with others.
        2. Suggested content with examples include
            a. Client information—name/agency, date of birth, gender, diagnosis, precautions, and contraindications
            b. Therapy log—date, type of contact, names/positions of persons involved, summary or significant information communicated during contacts, client attendance and participation in intervention, reason service is missed, types of interventions used, client's response, environmental or task modification, assistive or adaptive devices used or fabricated, statement of any training education or consultation provided, and the persons present
    C. Progress Report
        1. Summarizes intervention process and documents client's progress toward goals achievement. Includes new data collected; modifications of treatment plan; and statement of need for continuation, discontinuation, or referral.
        2. Suggested content with examples include
            a. Client information—name/agency, date of birth, gender, diagnosis, precautions, and contraindications
            b. Summary of services provided—brief statement of frequency of services and length of time services have been provided; techniques and strategies used; environmental or task modifications provided; adaptive equipment or orthotics provided; medical, educational, or other pertinent client updates; client's response to occupational therapy services; and programs or training provided to the client or caregivers
            c. Current client performance—client's progress toward the goals and client's performance in areas of occupations

        d. Plan or recommendations—recommendations and rationale as well as client's input to changes or continuation of plan

    D. Transition Plan

        1. Documents the formal transition plan and is written when client is transitioning from one service setting to another within a service delivery system.

        2. Suggested content with examples include

            a. Client information—name/agency, date of birth, gender, diagnosis, precautions, and contraindications

            b. Client's current status—client's current performance in occupations

            c. Transition plan—name of current service setting and name of setting to which client will transition, reason for transition, time frame in which transition will occur, and outline of activities to be carried out during the transition plan

            d. Recommendations—recommendations and rationale for occupational therapy services, modifications or accommodations needed, and assistive technology and environmental modifications needed

III. Outcomes

    A. Discharge Report—Summary of Occupational Therapy Services and Outcomes

        1. Summarize the changes in client's ability to engage in occupations between the initial evaluation and discontinuation of services and make recommendations as applicable

        2. Suggested content with examples includes

            a. Client information—name/agency, date of birth, gender, diagnosis, precautions, and contraindications

            b. Summary of intervention process—date of initial and final service; frequency, number of sessions, summary of interventions used; summary of progress toward goals; and occupational therapy outcomes—initial client status and ending status regarding engagement in occupations, client's assessment of efficacy of occupational therapy services

            c. Recommendations—recommendations pertaining to the client's future needs; specific follow-up plans, if applicable; and referrals to other professionals and agencies, if applicable

Each occupational therapy client has a client record maintained as a permanent file. The record is maintained in a professional and legal fashion (i.e., organized, legible, concise, clear, accurate, complete, current, grammatically correct, and objective).

BOX D.2   Fundamental Elements of Documentation

Elements Present in All Documentation

1.   Client's full name and case number (if applicable) on each page of documentation.

2.   Date and type of occupational therapy contact.

3.   Identification of type of documentation, agency, and department name.

4.   Occupational therapy practitioners' signature with a minimum of first name or initial, last name, and professional designation.

5.   When applicable on notes or reports, signature of the recorder directly at the end of the note without space left between the body of the note and the signature.

6.   Countersignature by an occupational therapist on documentation written by students and occupational therapy assistants when required by law or the facility.

7.   Acceptable terminology defined within the boundaries of setting.

8.   Abbreviations usage as acceptable within the boundaries of setting.

9.   When no facility requirements are listed, errors corrected by drawing a single line through an error and by initialing the correction (liquid correction fluid and erasures are not acceptable).

10. Adherence to professional standards of technology, when used to document occupational therapy services.

11. Disposal of records within law or agency requirements.

12. Compliance with confidentiality standards.

13. Compliance with agency or legal requirements of storage of records.

REFERENCES

American Occupational Therapy Association. (2002). Occupational therapy practice framework: Domain and process. *American Journal of Occupational Therapy, 56,* 609–639.

American Occupational Therapy Association. (2004). Guidelines for supervision, roles, and responsibilities during the delivery of occupational therapy services. *American Journal of Occupational Therapy, 58,* 663–667.

American Occupational Therapy Association. (2005). Standards of practice for occupational therapy. *American Journal of Occupational Therapy, 59,* 663–665.

American Occupational Therapy Association. (2006). *Policy 1.41. Categories of occupational therapy personnel. In policy manual* (2005 ed.) Bethesda, MD: Author.

American Occupational Therapy Association. (2007). *Occupational therapy practice framework: Domain and process* (2nd ed.) [Manuscript in preparation]. Bethesda, MD: Author.

AUTHORS

Gloria Frolek Clark, MS, OTR/L, FAOTA
Mary Jane Youngstrom, MS, OTR/L, FAOTA

for

The Commission on Practice
Sara Jane Brayman, PhD, OTR/L, FAOTA, *Chairperson*
Adopted by the Representative Assembly 2003M16
Edited by the Commission on Practice 2007

NOTE: From American Occupational Therapy Association, 2007, *Guidelines for documentation of occupational therapy.* Retrieved June, 16, 2008, from www.aota.org/Practitioners/Official/Guidelines/41257.aspx/.

APPENDIX E

AOTA Code of Ethics

▼ **PREAMBLE** ▼

The American Occupational Therapy Association (AOTA) *Occupational Therapy Code of Ethics* (2005) is a public statement of principles used to promote and maintain high standards of conduct within the profession and is supported by the *Core Values and Attitudes of Occupational Therapy Practice* (AOTA, 1993). Members of AOTA are committed to promoting inclusion, diversity, independence, and safety for all recipients in various stages of life, health, and illness and to empower all beneficiaries of occupational therapy. This commitment extends beyond service recipients to include professional colleagues, students, educators, businesses, and the community.

Fundamental to the mission of the occupational therapy profession is the therapeutic use of everyday life activities (occupations) with individuals or groups for the purpose of participation in roles and situations in home, school, workplace, community, and other settings. "Occupational therapy addresses the physical, cognitive, psychosocial, sensory and other aspects of performance in a variety of contexts to support engagement in everyday life activities that affect health, well being and quality of life" (*Definition of Occupational Therapy Practice for the AOTA Model Practice Act,* 2004). Occupational therapy personnel have an ethical responsibility first and foremost to recipients of service as well as to society.

The historical foundation of this Code is based on ethical reasoning surrounding practice and professional issues, as well as empathic reflection regarding these interactions with others. This reflection resulted in the establishment of principles that guide ethical action. Ethical action goes beyond rote following of rules or application of principles; rather it is a manifestation of moral character and mindful reflection. It is a commitment to beneficence for the sake of others, to virtuous practice of artistry and science, to genuinely good behaviors, and to noble acts of courage. It is an empathic way of being among others, which is made every day by all occupational therapy personnel.

The AOTA *Occupational Therapy Code of Ethics* (2005) is an aspirational guide to professional conduct when ethical issues surface. Ethical decision making is a process that includes awareness regarding how the outcome will impact occupational therapy clients in all spheres. Applications of Code principles are considered situation-specific and where a conflict exists, occupational therapy personnel will pursue responsible efforts for resolution. The specific purpose of the AOTA *Occupational Therapy Code of Ethics* (2005) is to:

1. Identify and describe the principles supported by the occupational therapy profession
2. Educate the general public and members regarding established principles to which occupational therapy personnel are accountable
3. Socialize occupational therapy personnel new to the practice to expected standards of conduct
4. Assist occupational therapy personnel in recognition and resolution of ethical dilemmas

The AOTA *Occupational Therapy Code of Ethics* (2005) defines the set principles that apply to occupational therapy personnel at all levels:

Principle 1. Occupational therapy personnel shall demonstrate a concern for the safety and well-being of the recipients of their services. (BENEFICENCE)

Occupational therapy personnel shall:

A. Provide services in a fair and equitable manner. They shall recognize and appreciate the cultural components of economics, geography, race, ethnicity, religious and political factors, marital status, age, sexual orientation, gender identity, and disability of all recipients of their services.

B. Strive to ensure that fees are fair and reasonable and commensurate with services performed. When occupational therapy practitioners set fees, they shall set fees considering institutional, local, state, and federal requirements, and with due regard for the service recipient's ability to pay.

C. Make every effort to advocate for recipients to obtain needed services through available means.

D. Recognize the responsibility to promote public health and the safety and well-being of individuals, groups, and/or communities.

Principle 2. Occupational therapy personnel shall take measures to ensure a recipient's safety and avoid imposing or inflicting harm. (NONMALEFICENCE)

Occupational therapy personnel shall:

A. Maintain therapeutic relationships that shall not exploit the recipient of services sexually, physically, emotionally, psychologically, financially, socially, or in any other manner.

B. Avoid relationships or activities that conflict or interfere with therapeutic professional judgment and objectivity.

C. Refrain from any undue influences that may compromise provision of service.

D. Exercise professional judgment and critically analyze directives that could result in potential harm before implementation.

E. Identify and address personal problems that may adversely impact professional judgment and duties.

F. Bring concerns regarding impairment of professional skills of a colleague to the attention of the appropriate authority when or/if attempts to address concerns are unsuccessful.

Principle 3. Occupational therapy personnel shall respect recipients to assure their rights. (AUTONOMY, CONFIDENTIALITY)

Occupational therapy personnel shall:

A. Collaborate with recipients, and if they desire, families, significant others, and/or caregivers in setting goals and priorities throughout the intervention process, including full disclosure of the nature, risk, and potential outcomes of any interventions.

B. Obtain informed consent from participants involved in research activities and ensure that they understand potential risks and outcomes.

C. Respect the individual's right to refuse professional services or involvement in research or educational activities.

D. Protect all privileged confidential forms of written, verbal, and electronic communication gained from educational, practice, research, and investigational activities unless otherwise mandated by local, state, or federal regulations.

Principle 4. Occupational therapy personnel shall achieve and continually maintain high standards of competence. (DUTY)

Occupational therapy personnel shall:

A. Hold the appropriate national, state, or any other requisite credentials for the services they provide.

B. Conform to AOTA standards of practice, and official documents.

C. Take responsibility for maintaining and documenting competence in practice, education, and research by participating in professional development and educational activities.

D. Be competent in all topic areas in which they provide instruction to consumers, peers, and/or students.

E. Critically examine available evidence so they may perform their duties on the basis of current information.

F. Protect service recipients by ensuring that duties assumed by or assigned to other occupational therapy personnel match credentials, qualifications, experience, and scope of practice.

G. Provide appropriate supervision to individuals for whom they have supervisory responsibility in accordance with Association official documents, local, state, and federal or national laws and regulations, and institutional policies and procedures.

H. Refer to or consult with other service providers whenever such a referral or consultation would be helpful to the care of the recipient of service. The referral or consultation process shall be done in collaboration with the recipient of service.

Principle 5. Occupational therapy personnel shall comply with laws and Association policies guiding the profession of occupational therapy. (PROCEDURAL JUSTICE)

Occupational therapy personnel shall:

A. Familiarize themselves with and seek to understand and abide by institutional rules, applicable Association policies; local, state, and federal/national/international laws.

B. Be familiar with revisions in those laws and Association policies that apply to the profession of occupational therapy and shall inform employers, employees, and colleagues of those changes.

C. Encourage those they supervise in occupational therapy related activities to adhere to the Code.

D. Take reasonable steps to ensure employers are aware of occupational therapy's ethical obligations, as set forth in this Code, and of the implications of those obligations for occupational therapy practice, education, and research.

E. Record and report in an accurate and timely manner all information related to professional activities.

Principle 6. Occupational therapy personnel shall provide accurate information when representing the profession. (VERACITY)

Occupational therapy personnel shall:

A. Represent their credentials, qualifications, education, experience, training, and competence accurately. This is of particular importance for those to whom occupational therapy personnel provide their services or with whom occupational therapy personnel have a professional relationship.

B. Disclose any professional, personal, financial, business, or volunteer affiliations that may pose a conflict of interest to those with whom they may establish a professional, contractual, or other working relationship.

C. Refrain from using or participating in the use of any form of communication that contains false, fraudulent, deceptive, or unfair statements or claims.

D. Identify and fully disclose to all appropriate persons errors that compromise recipients' safety.

E. Accept responsibility for their professional actions that reduce the public's trust in occupational therapy services and those that perform those services.

Principle 7. Occupational therapy personnel shall treat colleagues and other professionals with respect, fairness, discretion, and integrity. (FIDELITY)

Occupational therapy personnel shall:

A. Preserve, respect, and safeguard confidential information about colleagues and staff, unless otherwise mandated by national, state, or local laws.

B. Accurately represent the qualifications, views, contributions, and findings of colleagues.

C. Take adequate measures to discourage, prevent, expose, and correct any breaches of the Code and report any breaches of the Code to the appropriate authority.

D. Avoid conflicts of interest and conflicts of commitment in employment and volunteer roles.

E. Use conflict resolution and/or alternative dispute resolution resources to resolve organizational and interpersonal conflicts.

F. Familiarize themselves with established policies and procedures for handling concerns about this Code, including familiarity with national, state, local, district, and territorial procedures for handling ethics complaints. These include policies and procedures created by AOTA, licensing and regulatory bodies, employers, agencies, certification boards, and other organizations having jurisdiction over occupational therapy practice.

Note. This *AOTA Occupational Therapy Code of Ethics* is one of three documents that constitute the *Ethics Standards.* The other two are the *Core Values and Attitudes of Occupational Therapy Practice* (1993) and the *Guidelines to the Occupational Therapy Code of Ethics* (2000).

GLOSSARY

Autonomy—The right of an individual to self-determination. The ability to independently act on one's decisions for their own well-being (Beauchamp & Childress, 2001)

Beneficence—Doing good for others or brining about good for them. The duty to confer benefits to others

Confidentiality—Not disclosing data or information that should be kept private to prevent harm and to abide by policies, regulations, and laws

Dilemma—A situation in which one moral conviction or right action conflicts with another. It exists because there is no one, clear-cut, right answer

Duty—Actions required of professionals by society or actions that are self-imposed

Ethics—A systematic study of morality (i.e., rules of conduct that are grounded in philosophical principles and theory)

Fidelity—Faithfully fulfilling vows and promises, agreements, and discharging fiduciary responsibilities (Beauchamp & Childress, 2001)

Justice—Three types of justice are

Compensatory—Making reparation for wrongs that have been done

Distributive justice—The act of distributing goods and burdens among members of society

Procedural justice—Assuring that processes are organized in a fair manner and policies or laws are followed

Morality—Personal beliefs regarding values, rules, and principles of what is right or wrong. Morality may be culture-based or culture-driven

Nonmaleficence—Not harming or causing harm to be done to oneself or others the duty to ensure that no harm is done

Veracity—A duty to tell the truth; avoid deception

REFERENCES

American Occupational Therapy Association. (1993). Core values and attitudes of occupational therapy practice. *American Journal of Occupational Therapy, 47,* 1085–1086.

American Occupational Therapy Association. (1998). Guidelines to the occupational therapy code of ethics. *American Journal of Occupational Therapy, 52,* 881–884.

American Occupational Therapy Association. (2004). Association policies. *American Journal of Occupational Therapy, 58,* 694–695.

Beauchamp, T. L., & Childress, J. F. (2001). *Principles of biomedical ethics* (5th ed.). New York: Oxford University Press.

Definition of Occupational Therapy Practice for the AOTA Model Practice Act (2004). Retrieved April 9, 2005, from http://www.aota.org/members/area4/docs/defotpractice.pdf

AUTHORS

The Commission on Standards and Ethics (SEC):

S. Maggie Reitz, PhD, OTR/L, FAOTA, Chairperson

Melba Arnold, MS, OTR/L

Linda Gabriel Franck, PhD, OTR/L

Darryl J. Austin, MS, OT/L

Diane Hill, COTA/L, AP, ROH

Lorie J. McQuade, MEd, CRC

Daryl K. Knox, MD

Deborah Yarett Slater, MS, OT/L, FAOTA, Staff Liaison

With contributions to the Preamble by Suzanne Peloquin, PhD, OTR, FAOTA

Adopted by the Representative Assembly 2005C202

NOTE: This document replaces the 2000 document, *Occupational Therapy Code of Ethics (2000) (American Journal of Occupational Therapy, 54,* 614–616).

Prepared 4/7/2000, revised draft—January 2005, second revision 4/2005 by SEC.

Medicare Standards

▼ **EXCERPTS FROM COMPREHENSIVE OUTPATIENT REHABILITATION FACILITY MANUAL AND THE MEDICARE PROGRAM INTEGRITY MANUAL** ▼

Excerpts from

CMS Manual System	Department of Health & Human Services (DHHS)
Pub 100-02 Medicare Benefit Policy	Centers for Medicare & Medicaid Services (CMS)
Transmittal 88	Date: May 7, 2008
Change Request 5921	

SUBJECT: Therapy Personnel Qualifications and Policies Effective January 1, 2008

▼ **I. SUMMARY OF CHANGES** ▼

This CR provides guidance on the new regulations discussed in the Federal Register on November 27, 2007, concerning outpatient therapy services including personnel qualifications and the timing of recertification of plans of care. It addresses issues that arose during the comment period.

> New/Revised Material
> Effective Date: January 1, 2008
> Implementation Date: June 9, 2008

> *Disclaimer for manual changes only: The revision date and transmittal number apply only to red italicized material. Any other material was previously published and remains unchanged. However, if this revision contains a table of contents, you will receive the new/revised information only, and not the entire table of contents.*

SUBJECT: Therapy Personnel Qualifications and Policies Effective January 1, 2008

> Effective Date: January 1, 2008
> Implementation Date: June 9, 2008

▼ I. GENERAL INFORMATION ▼

This CR provides guidance on the new regulations published in the Federal Register on November 27, 2007, concerning therapy services including personnel qualifications and the timing of recertification of plans of care for Part B services. It addresses issues that arose during the comment period.

The re-certification for outpatient part B therapy services was required every 30 days until it was changed by the Physician Fee Schedule Final Rule of November 27, 2007.

The re-certification of plans of care for outpatient Part B therapy services is required every 90 days.

▼ 220. COVERAGE OF OUTPATIENT REHABILITATION THERAPY SERVICES (PHYSICAL THERAPY, OCCUPATIONAL THERAPY, AND SPEECH-LANGUAGE PATHOLOGY SERVICES) UNDER MEDICAL INSURANCE ▼

(Rev. 88, Issued: 05-07-08, Effective: 01-01-08,
Implementation: 06-09-08)

A comprehensive knowledge of the policies that apply to therapy services cannot be obtained through manuals alone. The most definitive policies are Local Coverage Determinations found at the Medicare Coverage Database www.cms.hhs.gov/mcd. A list of Medicare contractors is found at the CMS Web site. Specific questions about all Medicare policies should be addressed to the contractors through the contact information supplied on their Web sites. General Medicare questions may be addressed to the Medicare regional offices http://www.cms.hhs.gov/RegionalOffices/.

A. Definitions

The following defines terms used in this section and §230:

ACTIVE PARTICIPATION of the clinician in treatment means that the clinician personally furnishes in its entirety at least 1 billable service on at least *1* day of treatment.

ASSESSMENT is separate from evaluation, and is included in services or procedures, (it is not separately payable). The term assessment as used in Medicare manuals related to therapy services is distinguished from language in Current Procedural Terminology (CPT) codes that specify assessment, e.g., 97755, Assistive Technology Assessment, which may be payable. Assessments shall be provided only by clinicians, because assessment requires professional skill to gather data by observation and patient inquiry and may include limited objective testing and measurement to make clinical judgments regarding the patient's condition(s). Assessment determines, e.g., changes in the patient's status since the last visit/treatment day and whether the planned procedure or service should be modified. Based on these assessment data, the professional may make judgments about progress toward goals and/or determine that a more complete evaluation or re-evaluation (see definitions below) is indicated. Routine weekly assessments of expected progression in accordance with the plan are not payable as re-evaluations.

CERTIFICATION is the physician's/nonphysician practitioner's (NPP) approval of the plan of care. Certification requires a dated signature on the plan of care or some other document that indicates approval of the plan of care.

The **CLINICIAN** is a term used in this manual and in Pub 100-04, Chapter 5, section 10 or section 20, to refer to only a physician, nonphysician practitioner or a therapist (but not to an assistant, aide or any other personnel) providing a service within their scope of practice and consistent with state and local law. Clinicians make clinical judgments and are responsible for all services they are permitted to supervise. Services that require the skills of a therapist, may be appropriately furnished by clinicians, that is, by or under the supervision of qualified physicians/NPPs when their scope of practice, state and local laws allow it and their personal professional training is judged by Medicare contractors as sufficient to provide to the beneficiary skills equivalent to a therapist for that service.

COMPLEXITIES are complicating factors that may influence treatment, e.g., they may influence the type, frequency, intensity and/or duration of treatment. Complexities may be represented by diagnoses (ICD-9 codes), by patient factors such as age, severity, acuity, multiple conditions, and motivation, or by the patient's social circumstances such as the support of a significant other or the availability of transportation to therapy.

A **DATE** may be in any form (written, stamped or electronic). The date may be added to the record in any manner and at any time, as long as the dates are accurate. If they are different, refer to both the date a service was performed and the date the entry to the record was made. For example, if a physician certifies a plan and fails to date it, staff may add "Received Date" in writing or with a stamp. The received date is valid for certification/re-certification purposes. Also, if the physician faxes the referral, certification, or re-certification and forgets to date it, the date that prints out on the fax is valid. If services provided on one date are documented on another date, both dates should be documented.

The **EPISODE** of Outpatient Therapy – For the purposes of therapy policy, an outpatient therapy episode is defined as the period of time, in calendar days, from the first day the patient is under the care of the clinician (e.g., for evaluation or treatment) for the current condition(s) being treated by one therapy discipline (PT, or OT, or SLP) until the last date of service for that discipline *in that setting*.

During the episode, the beneficiary may be treated for more than one condition; including conditions with an onset after the episode has begun. For example, a beneficiary receiving PT for a hip fracture who, after the initial treatment session, develops low back pain would also be treated under a PT plan of care for rehabilitation of low back pain. That plan may be modified from the initial plan, or it may be a separate plan specific to the low back pain, but treatment for both conditions concurrently would be considered the same episode of PT treatment. If that same patient developed a swallowing problem during intubation for the hip surgery, the first day of treatment by the SLP would be a new episode of SLP care.

EVALUATION is a separately payable comprehensive service provided by a clinician, as defined above, that requires professional skills to make clinical judgments about conditions for which services are indicated based on objective measurements and subjective evaluations of patient performance and functional abilities. Evaluation is warranted e.g., for a new diagnosis or when a condition is treated in a new setting. These evaluative judgments are essential to development of the plan of care, including goals and the selection of interventions.

RE-EVALUATION provides additional objective information not included in other documentation. Re-evaluation is separately payable and is periodically indicated during an episode of care when the professional assessment of a clinician indicates a significant improvement, or decline, or change in the patient's condition or functional status that was not anticipated in the plan of care. Although some state regulations and state practice acts require re-evaluation at specific times, for Medicare payment, reevaluations must also meet Medicare coverage guidelines. The decision to provide a reevaluation shall be made by a clinician.

INTERVAL of certified treatment (certification interval) consists of 90 calendar days or less, based on an individual's needs. A physician/NPP may certify a plan of care for an interval length that is less than 90 days. There may be more than one certification interval in an episode of care. The certification interval is not the same as a Progress Report period.

NONPHYSICIAN PRACTITIONERS (NPP) means physician assistants, clinical nurse specialists, and nurse practitioners, who may, if state and local laws permit it, and when appropriate rules are followed, provide, certify or supervise therapy services.

PHYSICIAN with respect to outpatient rehabilitation therapy services means a doctor of medicine, osteopathy (including an osteopathic practitioner), podiatric medicine, or optometry (for low vision rehabilitation only). Chiropractors and doctors of dental surgery or dental medicine are not considered physicians for therapy services and may neither refer patients for rehabilitation therapy services nor establish therapy plans of care.

PATIENT client, resident, and beneficiary are terms used interchangeably to indicate enrolled recipients of Medicare covered services.

PROVIDERS of services are defined in §1861(u) of the Act, 42CFR400.202 and 42CFR485 Subpart H as participating hospitals, critical access hospitals (CAH), skilled nursing facilities (SNF), comprehensive outpatient rehabilitation facilities (CORF), home health agencies (HHA), hospices, participating clinics, rehabilitation agencies or outpatient rehabilitation facilities (ORF). Providers are also defined as public health agencies with agreements only to furnish outpatient therapy services, or community mental health centers with agreements only to furnish partial hospitalization services. To qualify as providers of services, these providers must meet certain conditions enumerated in the law and enter into an agreement with the Secretary in which they agree not to charge any beneficiary for covered services for which the program will pay and to refund any erroneous collections made. Note that the word PROVIDER in sections 220 and 230 is not used to mean a person who provides a service, but is used as in the statute to mean a facility or agency such as rehabilitation agency or home health agency.

QUALIFIED PROFESSIONAL means a physical therapist, occupational therapist, speech-language pathologist, physician, nurse practitioner, clinical nurse specialist, or physician's assistant, who is licensed or certified by the state to perform therapy services, and who also may appropriately perform therapy services under Medicare policies. Qualified professionals may also include physical therapist assistants (PTA) and occupational therapy assistants (OTA) when working under the supervision of a qualified therapist, within the scope of practice allowed by state law. Assistants are limited in the services they may provide (see section 230.1 and 230.2) and may not supervise others.

QUALIFIED PERSONNEL means staff (auxiliary personnel) who have been educated and trained as therapists and qualify to furnish therapy services only under direct supervision incident to a physician or NPP. See §230.5 of this manual. Qualified personnel may or may not be licensed as therapists but meet all of the requirements for therapists with the exception of licensure.

SIGNATURE means a legible identifier of any type acceptable according to policies in Pub. 100-08, Medicare Program Integrity Manual, Chapter 3, §3.4.1.1 (B) concerning signatures.

SUPPLIERS of therapy services include individual practitioners such as physicians, NPPs, physical therapists and occupational therapists who have Medicare provider numbers. Regulatory references on physical therapists in private practice (PTPPs) and occupational therapists in private practice (OTPPs) are at 42CFR410.60 (C)(1), 485.701-729, and 486.150-163. Speech-language pathologists are not suppliers because the Act does not provide coverage of any speech-language pathology services furnished by a speech-language pathologist as an independent practitioner. (See §230.3.)

THERAPIST refers only to qualified physical therapists, occupational therapists and speech-language pathologists, as defined in §230. Qualifications that define therapists are in §§230.1, 230.2, and 230.3. Skills of a therapist are defined by the scope of practice for therapists in the state.

THERAPY (or outpatient rehabilitation services) includes only outpatient physical therapy, occupational therapy and speech-language pathology services paid using the Medicare Physician Fee Schedule or the same services when provided in hospitals that are exempt from the hospital Outpatient Prospective Payment System and paid on a reasonable cost basis, including critical access hospitals.

Therapy services referred to in this manual are those skilled rehabilitative services provided according to the standards and conditions in CMS manuals, (e.g., in this chapter and in Pub. 100-04, Medicare Claims Processing Manual, Chapter 5), within their scope of practice by qualified professionals or qualified personnel, as defined in this section, represented by procedures found in the American Medical Association's "Current Procedural Terminology (CPT)." A list of CPT (HCPCS) codes is provided in Pub. 100-04, Chapter 5, §20, and in Local Coverage Determinations developed by contractors. Unless modified by the words "maintenance" or "not", the term therapy refers to rehabilitative therapy services as described in §220.2(C).

TREATMENT DAY means a single calendar day on which treatment, evaluation and/or reevaluation is provided. There could be multiple visits, treatment sessions/encounters on a treatment day.

VISITS OR TREATMENT SESSIONS begin at the time the patient enters the treatment area (of a building, office, or clinic) and continue until all services (e.g., activities, procedures, services) have been completed for that session and the patient leaves that area to participate in a non-therapy activity. It is likely that not all minutes in the visits/treatment sessions are billable (e.g., rest periods). There may be two treatment sessions in a day, for example, in the morning and afternoon. When there are two visits/treatment sessions in a day, plans of care indicate treatment amount of twice a day.

Specific policies may differ by setting. Other policies concerning therapy services are found in other manuals. When a therapy service policy is specific to a setting, it takes precedence over these general outpatient policies. For special rules on:

- CORFs - See Chapter 12 of this manual and also Pub. 100-04, Chapter 5;
- SNF - See Chapter 8 of this manual and also Pub. 100-04, Chapter 6, for SNF claims/billing;
- HHA - See Chapter 7 of this manual, and Pub. 100-04, Chapter 10;
- GROUP THERAPY AND STUDENTS - See Pub. 100-02, Chapter 15, §230;
- ARRANGEMENTS - Pub. 100-01, Chapter 5, §10.3;
- COVERAGE is described in the Medicare Program Integrity Manual, Pub. 100-08, Chapter 13, §13.5.1; and
- THERAPY CAPS - See Pub. 100-04, Chapter 5, §10.2, for a complete description of this financial limitation.

C. General

Therapy services are a covered benefit in §§1861(g), 1861(p), and 1861(ll) of the Act. Therapy services may also be provided incident to the services of a physician/NPP under §§1861(s)(2) and 1862(a)(20) of the Act.

Covered therapy services are furnished by providers, by others under arrangements with and under the supervision of providers, or furnished by suppliers (e.g., physicians, NPP, enrolled therapists), who meet the requirements in Medicare manuals for therapy services.

Where a prospective payment system (PPS) applies, therapy services are paid when services conform to the requirements of that PPS. For example, see Pub. 100-04 for a description of applicable Inpatient Hospital Part B and Outpatient PPS rules. Reimbursement for therapy provided to Part A inpatients of hospitals or residents of SNFs in covered stays is included in the respective PPS rates.

Payment for therapy provided by an HHA under a plan of treatment is included in the home health PPS rate. Therapy may be billed by an HHA on bill type 34x if there are no home health services billed under a home health plan of care at the same time (e.g., the patient is not home-bound), and there is a valid therapy plan of treatment.

In addition to the requirements described in this chapter, the services must be furnished in accordance with health and safety requirements set forth in regulations at 42CFR484, and 42CFR485.

▼ 220.1.2. PLANS OF CARE FOR OUTPATIENT PHYSICAL THERAPY, OCCUPATIONAL THERAPY, OR SPEECH-LANGUAGE PATHOLOGY SERVICES ▼

(Rev. 88, Issued: 05-07-08, Effective: 01-01-08, Implementation: 06-09-08)
Reference: 42CFR 410.61

A. Establishing the Plan (See §220.1.3 for certifying the plan.)

The services must relate directly and specifically to a written treatment plan as described in this chapter. The plan, (also known as a plan of care or plan of treatment) must be established before treatment is begun. The plan is established when it is developed (e.g., written or dictated).

The signature and professional identity (e.g., MD, OTR/L) of the person who established the plan, and the date it was established must be recorded with the plan. Establishing the plan, which is described below, is not the same as certifying the plan, which is described in §§220.1.1 and 220.1.3

Outpatient therapy services shall be furnished under a plan established by:

A physician/NPP (consultation with the treating physical therapist, occupational therapist, or speech-language pathologist is recommended. Only a physician may establish a plan of care in a CORF);

The physical therapist who will provide the physical therapy services;

The occupational therapist who will provide the occupational therapy services; or

The speech-language pathologist who will provide the speech-language pathology services.

The plan may be entered into the patient's therapy record either by the person who established the plan or by the provider's or supplier's staff when they make a written record of that person's oral orders before treatment is begun.

Treatment Under a Plan
The evaluation and treatment may occur and are both billable either on the same day or at subsequent visits. It is appropriate that treatment begins when a plan is established.

Therapy may be initiated by qualified professionals or qualified personnel based on a dictated plan. Treatment may begin before the plan is committed to writing only if the treatment is performed or supervised by the same clinician who establishes the plan. Payment for services provided before a plan is established may be denied.

Two Plans
It is acceptable to treat under two separate plans of care when different physician's/NPP's refer a patient for different conditions. It is also acceptable to combine the plans of care into one plan covering both conditions if one or the other referring physician/NPP is willing to certify the plan for both conditions. The Treatment Notes continue to require timed code treatment minutes and

total treatment time and need not be separated by plan. Progress Reports should be combined if it is possible to make clear that the goals for each plan are addressed. Separate Progress Reports referencing each plan of care may also be written, at the discretion of the treating clinician, or at the request of the certifying physician/NPP, but shall not be required by contractors.

B. Contents of Plan (See §220.1.3 for certifying the plan.)

The plan of care shall contain, at minimum, the following information as required by regulation (42CFR424.24 and 410.61) (See §220.3 for further documentation requirements):

Diagnoses;

Long term treatment goals; and

Type, amount, duration and frequency of therapy services.

The plan of care shall be consistent with the related evaluation, which may be attached and is considered incorporated into the plan. The plan should strive to provide treatment in the most efficient and effective manner, balancing the best achievable outcome with the appropriate resources.

Long term treatment goals should be developed for the entire episode of care in the current setting. When the episode is anticipated to be long enough to require more than one certification, the long term goals may be specific to the part of the episode that is being certified. Goals should be measurable and pertain to identified functional impairments. When episodes in the setting are short, measurable goals may not be achievable; documentation should state the clinical reasons progress cannot be shown.

The type of treatment may be PT, OT, or SLP, or, where appropriate, the type may be a description of a specific treatment or intervention. (For example, where there is a single evaluation service, but the type is not specified, the type is assumed to be consistent with the therapy discipline (PT, OT, SLP) ordered, or of the therapist who provided the evaluation.) Where a physician/NPP establishes a plan, the plan must specify the type (PT, OT, SLP) of therapy planned.

There shall be different plans of care for each type of therapy discipline. When more than one discipline is treating a patient, each must establish a diagnosis, goals, etc. independently. However, the form of the plan and the number of plans incorporated into one document are not limited as long as the required information is present and related to each discipline separately. For example, a physical therapist may not provide services under an occupational therapist plan of care. However, both may be treating the patient for the same condition at different times in the same day for goals consistent with their own scope of practice.

The amount of treatment refers to the number of times in a day the type of treatment will be provided. Where amount is not specified, one treatment session a day is assumed.

The frequency refers to the number of times in a week the type of treatment is provided. Where frequency is not specified, one treatment is assumed. If a scheduled holiday occurs on a treatment day that is part of the plan, it is appropriate to omit that treatment day unless the clinician who is responsible for writing Progress Reports determines that a brief, temporary pause in the delivery of therapy services would adversely affect the patient's condition.

The duration is the number of weeks, or the number of treatment sessions, for THIS PLAN of care. If the episode of care is anticipated to extend beyond the 90 calendar day limit for certification of a plan, it is desirable, although not required, that the clinician also estimate the duration of the entire episode of care in this setting.

The frequency or duration of the treatment may not be used alone to determine medical necessity, but they should be considered with other factors such as condition, progress, and treatment type to provide the most effective and efficient means to achieve the patients' goals. For example, it may be clinically appropriate, medically necessary, most efficient and effective to provide short term intensive treatment or longer term and less frequent treatment depending on the individuals' needs.

It may be appropriate for therapists to taper the frequency of visits as the patient progresses toward an independent or caregiver assisted self management program with the intent of improving outcomes and limiting treatment time. For example, treatment may be provided 3 times a week for 2 weeks, then 2 times a week for the next 2 weeks, then once a week for the last 2 weeks. Depending on the individual's condition, such treatment may result in better outcomes, or may result in earlier discharge than routine treatment 3 times a week for 4 weeks. When tapered frequency is planned, the exact number of treatments per frequency level is not required to be projected in the plan, because the changes should be made based on assessment of daily progress. Instead, the beginning and end frequencies shall be planned. For example, amount, frequency and duration may be documented as "once daily, 3 times a week tapered to once a week over 6 weeks." Changes to the frequency may be made based on the clinicians clinical judgment and do not require recertification of the plan unless requested by the physician/NPP. The clinician should consider any comorbidities, tissue healing, the ability of the patient and/or caregiver to do more independent self management as treatment progresses, and any other factors related to frequency and duration of treatment.

The above policy describes the minimum requirements for payment. It is anticipated that clinicians may choose to make their plans more specific, in accordance with good practice. For example, they may include these optional elements: short term goals, goals and duration for the current episode of care, specific treatment interventions, procedures, modalities or techniques and the amount of each. Also, notations in the medical record of beginning date for the plan are recommended but not required to assist Medicare contractors in determining the dates of services for which the plan was effective.

C. Changes to the Therapy Plan

Changes are made in writing in the patient's record and signed by one of the following professionals responsible for the patient's care:
The physician/NPP;

> The physical therapist (in the case of physical therapy);
> The speech-language pathologist (in the case of speech-language pathology services);
> The occupational therapist (in the case of occupational therapy services; or
> The registered professional nurse or physician/NPP on the staff of the facility
> pursuant to the oral orders of the physician/NPP or therapist.

While the physician/NPP may change a plan of treatment established by the therapist providing such services, the therapist may not significantly alter a plan of treatment established or certified by a physician/NPP without their documented written or verbal approval [See §220.1.3(C)]. A change in long-term goals, (for example if a new condition was to be treated) would be a significant change. Physician/NPP certification of the significantly modified plan of care shall be obtained within 30 days of the initial therapy treatment under the revised plan. An insignificant alteration in the plan would be a change in the frequency or duration due to the patient's illness, or a modification of short-term goals to adjust for improvements made toward the same long-term goals. If a patient has achieved a goal and/or has had no response to a treatment that is part of the plan, the therapist may delete a specific intervention from the plan of care prior to physician/NPP approval. This shall be reported to the physician/ NPP responsible for the patient's treatment prior to the next certification.

Procedures (e.g., neuromuscular reeducation) and modalities (e.g., ultrasound) are not goals, but are the means by which long and short term goals are obtained. Changes to procedures and modalities do not require physician signature when they represent adjustments to the plan that result from a normal progression in the patient's disease or condition *or adjustments to the plan due to lack of expected response to the planned intervention, when the goals remain unchanged*. Only when the patient's condition changes significantly, making revision of long term goals necessary, is a physician's/NPP's signature required on the change, (long term goal changes may be accompanied by changes to procedures and modalities).

▼ 220.1.3. CERTIFICATION AND RECERTIFICATION OF NEED FOR TREATMENT AND THERAPY PLANS OF CARE ▼

(Rev. 88, Issued: 05-07-08, Effective: 01-01-08, Implementation: 06-09-08)
Reference: 42CFR424.24(c)
See specific certification rules in Pub. 100-01, Chapter 4, §20 for hospital services.

A. Method and Disposition of Certifications

Certification requires a dated signature on the plan of care or some other document that indicates approval of the plan of care. It is not appropriate for a physician/NPP to certify a plan of care if the patient was not under the care of some physician/NPP at the time of the treatment or if the patient did not need the treatment. Since delayed certification is allowed, the date the certification is signed is important only to determine if it is timely or delayed. The certification must relate to treatment during the *interval* on the claim. Unless there is reason to believe the plan was not signed appropriately, or it is not timely, no further evidence that the patient was under the care of a physician/NPP and that the patient needed the care is required.

The format of all certifications and recertifications and the method by which they are obtained is determined by the individual facility and/or practitioner. Acceptable documentation of certification may be, for example, a physician's progress note, a physician/NPP order, or a plan of care that is signed and dated by a physician/NPP, and indicates the physician/NPP is aware that therapy service is or was in progress and the physician/NPP makes no record of disagreement with the plan when there is evidence the plan was sent (e.g., to the office) or is available in the record (e.g., of the institution that employs the physician/NPP) for the physician/NPP to review. For example, if during the course of treatment under a certified plan of care a physician sends an order for continued treatment for 2 more weeks, contractors shall accept the order as certification of continued treatment for 2 weeks under the same plan of care. If the new certification is for less treatment than previously planned and certified, this new certification takes the place of any previous certification. At the end of the 2 weeks of treatment (which might extend more than 2 calendar weeks from the date the order/certification was signed) another certification would be required if further treatment was documented as medically necessary.

The certification should be retained in the clinical record and available if requested by the contractor.

B. Initial Certification of Plan

The physician's/NPP's certification of the plan (with or without an order) satisfies all of the certification requirements noted above in §220.1 for the duration of the plan of care, or 90 calendar days from the date of the initial treatment, whichever is less. The initial treatment includes the evaluation that resulted in the plan.

Timing of Initial Certification

The provider or supplier (e.g., facility, physician/NPP, or therapist) should obtain certification as soon as possible after the plan of care is established, unless the requirements of delayed certification are met. "As soon as possible" means that the physician/NPP shall certify the *initial* plan as soon as it is obtained, or *within 30 days of* the initial therapy treatment. Since payment may be denied if a physician does not certify the plan, the therapist should forward the plan to the physician as soon as it is established. Evidence of diligence in providing the plan to the physician may be considered by the *Medicare* contractor during review in the event of a delayed certification.

Timely certification of the *initial plan* is met when physician/NPP certification of the plan is documented, by signature or verbal order, and dated *in the 30 days following the first day of treatment (including evaluation)*. If the order to certify is verbal, it must be followed within 14 days by a signature to be timely. A dated notation of the order to certify the plan should be made in the patient's medical record.

Recertification is not required if the duration of the initially certified plan of care is more than the duration (length) of the entire episode of treatment.

C. Review of Plan and Recertification

Reference: 42CFR424.24(c), 1861(r), 42CFR 410.61(e).

The timing of recertification changed on January 1, 2008. Certifications signed on or after January 1, 2008, follow the rules in this section. Certifications signed on or prior to December 31, 2007, follow the rule in effect at that time, which required recertification every 30 calendar days.

Payment and coverage conditions require that the plan must be reviewed, as often as necessary but at least whenever it is certified or recertified to complete the certification requirements. It is not required that the same physician/NPP who participated initially in recommending or planning the patient's care certify and/or recertify the plans.

Recertifications that document the need for continued or modified therapy should be signed whenever the need for a significant modification of the plan becomes evident, or at least every 90 days after initiation of treatment under that plan, unless they are delayed.

Physician/NPP Options for Certification

A physician/NPP may certify or recertify a plan for *whatever duration of treatment* the physician/NPP determines is appropriate, up to a maximum of 90 calendar days. Many episodes of therapy treatment last less than 30 calendar days. Therefore, it is expected that the physician/NPP should certify a plan that appropriately estimates the duration of care for the individual, even if it is less than 90 days. If the therapist writes a plan of care for a duration that is more or less than the duration approved by the physician/NPP, then the physician/NPP would document a change to the duration of the plan and certify it for the duration the physician/NPP finds appropriate (up to 90 days). Treatment beyond the duration certified by the physician/NPP requires that a plan be recertified for the extended duration of treatment. It is possible that patients will be discharged by the therapist before the end of the estimated treatment duration because some will improve faster than estimated and/or some were successfully progressed to an independent home program.

Physicians/NPPs may require that the patient make a physician/NPP visit for an examination if, in the professional's judgment, the visit is needed prior to certifying the plan, *or during the planned treatment*. Physicians/NPPs should indicate their requirement for visits, preferably on an order preceding the treatment, or on the plan of care that is certified. If the physician wishes to restrict the patient's treatment beyond a certain date when a visit is required, the physician should certify a plan only until the date of the visit. After that date, services will not be considered reasonable and necessary due to lack of a certified plan. Physicians/NPPs should not sign a certification if they require a visit and a visit was not made. However, Medicare does not require a visit unless the National Coverage Determination (NCD) for a particular treatment requires it (e.g., see Pub. 100-03, §270.1 - Electrical Stimulation (ES) and Electromagnetic Therapy for the Treatment of Wounds).

Restrictions on Certification

Certifications and recertifications by doctors of podiatric medicine must be consistent with the scope of the professional services provided by a doctor of podiatric medicine as authorized by applicable state law. Optometrists may order and certify only low vision services. Chiropractors may not certify or recertify plans of care for therapy services.

D. Delayed Certification

References: §1835(a)
of the Act 42CFR424.11(d)(3)

Certifications are required for each interval of treatment based on the patient's needs, not to exceed 90 calendar days from the initial therapy treatment. Certifications are timely when the initial certification (or certification of a significantly modified plan of care) is dated within 30 calendar days of the initial treatment under that plan. Recertification is timely when dated during the duration of the initial plan of care or within 90 calendar days of the initial treatment under that plan, whichever is less. *Delayed* certification and recertification requirements shall be deemed satisfied where, at any later date, a physician/NPP makes a certification accompanied by a reason for the delay. Certifications are acceptable without justification for 30 days after they are due. Delayed certification should include one or more certifications or recertifications on a single signed and dated document.

Delayed certifications should include any evidence the provider or supplier considers necessary to justify the delay. For example, a certification may be delayed because the physician did not sign it, or the original was lost. In the case of a long delayed certification (over 6 months), the provider or supplier may choose to submit with the delayed certification some other documentation (e.g., an order, progress notes, telephone contact, requests for certification or signed statement of a physician/NPP) indicating need for care and that the patient was under the care of a physician at the time of the treatment. Such documentation may be requested by the contractor for delayed certifications if it is required for review. It is not intended that needed therapy be stopped or denied when certification is delayed. The delayed certification of otherwise covered services should be accepted unless the contractor has reason to believe that there was no physician involved in the patient's care, or treatment did not meet the patient's need (and therefore, the certification was signed inappropriately).

EXAMPLE: Payment should be denied if there is a certification signed 2 years after treatment by a physician/NPP who has/had no knowledge of the patient when the medical record also shows *e.g.,* no order, note, physician/NPP attended meeting, correspondence with a physician/NPP, documentation of discussion of the plan with a physician/NPP, documentation of sending the plan to any physician/NPP, or other indication that there was a physician/NPP involved in the case.

EXAMPLE: Payment should not be denied, even when certified 2 years after treatment, when there is evidence that a physician approved needed treatment, such as an order, documentation of therapist/physician/NPP discussion of the plan, chart notes, meeting notes, requests for certification, certifications for intervals before or after the service in question, or physician/NPP services during which the medical record or the patient's history would, in good practice, be reviewed and would indicate therapy treatment is in progress.

EXAMPLE: Subsequent certifications of plans for continued treatment for the same condition in the same patient may indicate physician certification of treatment that occurred between certification dates, even if the signature for one of the plans in the episode is delayed. If a certified plan of care ends March 30th and a new plan of care for continued treatment after March 30th is developed or signed by a therapist on April 15th and that plan is subsequently certified, that certification may be considered delayed and acceptable effective from the first treatment date after March 30th for the frequency and duration as described in the plan. Of course, documentation should continue to indicate that therapy during the delay is medically necessary, as it would for any treatment. The certification of the physician/NPP is interpreted as involvement and approval of the ongoing episode of treatment, including the treatment that preceded the date of the certification unless the physician/NPP indicates otherwise.

E. Denials Due to Certification

Denial for payment that is based on absence of certification is a technical denial, which means a statutory requirement has not been met. Certification is a statutory requirement in SSA 1835(a)(2)- ("periodic review" of the plan).

For example, if a patient is treated and the provider/supplier cannot produce (on contractor request) a plan of care (timely or delayed) for the billed treatment dates certified by a physician/NPP, then that service might be denied for lack of the required certification. If an appropriate certification is later produced, the denial shall be overturned.

In the case of a service furnished under a provider agreement as described in 42CFR489.21, the provider is precluded from charging the beneficiary for services denied as a result of missing certification.

However, if the service is provided by a supplier (in the office of the physician/NPP, or therapist) a technical denial due to absence of a certification results in beneficiary liability. For that reason, it is recommended that the patient be made aware of the need for certification and the consequences of its absence.

A technical denial decision may be reopened by the contractor or reversed on appeal as appropriate, if delayed certification is later produced.

▼ 220.3. DOCUMENTATION REQUIREMENTS FOR THERAPY SERVICES ▼

(Rev. 88, Issued: 05-07-08, Effective: 01-01-08, Implementation: 06-09-08)

A. General

Therapy services shall be payable when the medical record and the information on the claim form consistently and accurately report covered therapy services. Documentation must be legible, relevant and sufficient to justify the services billed. In general, services must be covered therapy services provided according to the requirements in Medicare manuals. Medicare requires that the services billed be supported by documentation that justifies payment. Documentation must comply with all legal/regulatory requirements applicable to Medicare claims.

The documentation guidelines in sections 220 and 230 of this chapter identify the minimal expectations of documentation by providers or suppliers or beneficiaries submitting claims for payment of therapy services to the Medicare program. State or local laws and policies, or the policies of the profession, the practice, or the facility may be more stringent. Additional documentation not required by Medicare is encouraged when it conforms to state or local law or to professional guidelines of the American Physical Therapy Association, the American Occupational Therapy Association, or the American Speech-Language Hearing Association. It is encouraged but not required that narratives that specifically justify the medical necessity of services be included in order to support approval when those services are reviewed. (See also section 220.2- Reasonable and Necessary Outpatient Rehabilitation Therapy Services)

Contractors shall consider the entire record when reviewing claims for medical necessity so that the absence of an individual item of documentation does not negate the medical necessity of a service when the documentation as a whole indicates the service is necessary. Services are medically necessary if the documentation indicates they meet the requirements for medical necessity including that they are skilled, rehabilitative services, provided by clinicians (or qualified professionals when appropriate) with the approval of a physician/NPP, safe, and effective (i.e., progress indicates that the care is effective in rehabilitation of function).

B. Documentation Required

List of required documentation

These types of documentation of therapy services are expected to be submitted in response to any requests for documentation, unless the contractor requests otherwise. The timelines are minimum requirements for Medicare payment. Document as often as the clinician's judgment dictates but no less than the frequency required in Medicare policy:

- **Evaluation/and Plan of Care** (may be one or two documents). Include the initial evaluation and any re-evaluations relevant to the episode being reviewed;
- **Certification** (physician/NPP approval of the plan) and recertifications when records are requested after the certification/recertification is due. See definitions in section 220 and certification policy in section 220.1.3 of this chapter. Certification *(and recertification* of the plan *when applicable) are* required for payment *and must be submitted when records are requested after the certification or recertification is due.*
- **Progress Reports** *(including Discharge Notes, if applicable)* when records are requested after the reports are due. (See definitions in section 220 and descriptions in 220.3 D);
- **Treatment Notes** for each treatment day (may also serve as Progress Reports when required information is included in the notes); and
- A separate **justification statement** may be included either as a separate document or within the other documents if the provider/supplier wishes to assure the contractor understands their reasoning for services that are more extensive than is typical for the condition treated. A separate statement is not required if the record justifies treatment without further explanation.

Limits on Requirements

Contractors shall not require more specific documentation unless other Medicare manual policies require it. Contractors may request further information to be included in these documents concerning specific cases under review when that information is relevant, but not submitted with records.

Dictated Documentation

For Medicare purposes, dictated therapy documentation is considered completed on the day it was dictated. The qualified professional may edit and electronically sign the documentation at a later date.

Dates for Documentation

The date the documentation was made is important only to establish the date of the initial plan of care because therapy cannot begin until the plan is established unless treatment is performed or supervised by the same clinician who establishes the plan. However, contractors may require that treatment notes and progress reports be entered into the record within 1 week of the last date to which the Progress Report or Treatment Note refers. For example, if treatment began on the first of the month at a frequency of twice a week, a Progress Report would be required at the end of the month. Contractors may require that the Progress Report that describes that month of treatment be dated not more than 1 week after the end of the month described in the report.

Document Information to Meet Requirements

In documenting records, clinicians must be familiar with the requirements for covered and payable outpatient therapy services as described in the manuals. For example, the records should justify:

- The patient is under the care of a physician/NPP;
  - Physician/NPP care shall be documented by physician/NPP certification (approval) of the plan of care; and

- Although not required, other evidence of physician/NPP involvement in the patient's care may include, for example: order/referral, conference, team meeting notes, *and correspondence.*
- Services require the skills of a therapist.
  - Services must not only be provided by the qualified professional or qualified personnel, but they must require, for example, the expertise, knowledge, clinical judgment, decision making and abilities of a therapist that assistants, qualified personnel, caretakers or the patient cannot provide independently. A clinician may not merely supervise, but must apply the skills of a therapist by actively participating in the treatment of the patient during each Progress Report Period. In addition, a therapist's skills may be documented, for example, by the clinician's descriptions of their skilled treatment, the changes made to the treatment due to a clinician's assessment of the patient's needs on a particular treatment day or changes due to progress the clinician judged sufficient to modify the treatment toward the next more complex or difficult task.
  - A therapist's skill may also be required for safety reasons, if an unstable fracture requires the skill of a therapist to do an activity that might otherwise be done independently by the patient at home. Or the skill of a therapist might be required for a patient learning compensatory swallowing techniques to perform cervical auscultation and identify changes in voice and breathing that might signal aspiration. After the patient is judged safe for independent use of these compensatory techniques, the skill of a therapist is not required to feed the patient, or check what was consumed.
- Services are of appropriate type, frequency, intensity and duration for the individual needs of the patient.
  - Documentation should establish the variables that influence the patient's condition, especially those factors that influence the clinician's decision to provide more services than are typical for the individual's condition.
  - Clinicians and contractors shall determine typical services using published professional literature and professional guidelines. The fact that services are typically billed is not necessarily evidence that the services are typically appropriate. Services that exceed those typically billed should be carefully documented to justify their necessity, but are payable if the individual patient benefits from medically necessary services. Also, some services or episodes of treatment should be less than those typically billed, when the individual patient reaches goals sooner than is typical.
  - Documentation should establish through objective measurements that the patient is making progress toward goals. Note that regression and plateaus can happen during treatment. It is recommended that the reasons for lack of progress be noted and the justification for continued treatment be documented if treatment continues after regression or plateaus.
  - *Needs of the Patient.* When a service is reasonable and necessary, the patient also needs the services. Contractors determine the patient's needs through knowledge of the individual patient's condition, and any complexities that impact that condition, as described in documentation (usually in the evaluation, re-evaluation, and Progress Report). Factors that contribute to need vary, but in general they relate to such factors as the patient's diagnoses, complicating factors, age, severity, time since onset/acuity, self-efficacy/motivation, cognitive ability, prognosis, and/or medical, psychological and social stability. Patients who need therapy generally respond to therapy, so changes in objective and sometimes to subjective measures of improvement also help establish the need for services. The use of scientific evidence, obtained from professional literature, and sequential measurements of the patient's condition during treatment is encouraged to support the potential for continued improvement that may justify the patients need for therapy.

C. Evaluation/Re-Evaluation and Plan of Care

The initial evaluation, or the plan of care including an evaluation, should document the necessity for a course of therapy through objective findings and subjective patient self-reporting. Utilize the guidelines of the American Physical Therapy Association, the American Occupational Therapy Association, or the American Speech-Language and Hearing Association as guidelines, and not as policy. Only a clinician may perform an initial examination, evaluation, re-evaluation and assessment or establish a diagnosis or a plan of care. A clinician may include, as part of the evaluation or re-evaluation, objective measurements or observations made by a PTA or OTA within their scope of practice, but the clinician must actively and personally participate in the evaluation or re-evaluation. The clinician may not merely summarize the objective findings of others or make judgments drawn from the measurements and/or observations of others.

Documentation of the evaluation should list the conditions and complexities and, where it is not obvious, describe the impact of the conditions and complexities on the prognosis and/or the plan for treatment such that it is clear to the contractor who may review the record that the services planned are appropriate for the individual.

Evaluation shall include:

- A diagnosis (where allowed by state and local law) and description of the specific problem(s) to be evaluated and/or treated. The diagnosis should be specific and as relevant to the problem to be treated as possible. In many cases, both a medical diagnosis (obtained from a physician/NPP) and an impairment based treatment diagnosis related to treatment are relevant. The treatment diagnosis may or may not be identified by the therapist, depending on their scope of practice. Where a diagnosis is not allowed, use a condition description similar to the appropriate ICD-9 code. For example the medical diagnosis made by the physician is CVA; however, the treatment diagnosis or condition description for PT may be abnormality of gait, for OT, it may be hemiparesis, and for SLP, it may be dysphagia. For PT and OT, be sure to include the body part evaluated. Include all conditions and complexities that may impact the treatment. A description might include, for example, the pre-morbid function, date of onset, and current function;
- Results of one of the following four measurement instruments are recommended, but not required:

  > National Outcomes Measurement System (NOMS) by the American Speech-Language Hearing Association
  > Patient Inquiry by Focus On Therapeutic Outcomes, Inc. (FOTO)
  > Activity Measure – Post Acute Care (AM-PAC)
  > OPTIMAL by Cedaron through the American Physical Therapy Association

- If results of one of the four instruments above is not recorded, the record shall contain instead the following information indicated by asterisks (*) and should contain (but is not required to contain) all of the following, as applicable. Since published research supports its impact on the need for treatment, information in the following indented bullets may also be included with the results of the above four instruments in the evaluation report at the clinician's discretion. This information may be incorporated into a test instrument or separately reported within the required documentation. If it changes, update this information in the re-evaluation, and/or Treatment Notes, and/or Progress Reports, and/or in a separate record. When it is provided, contractors shall take this documented information into account to determine whether services are reasonable and necessary.

Documentation supporting illness severity or complexity including, e.g.,

- Identification of other health services concurrently being provided for this condition (e.g., physician, PT, OT, SLP, chiropractic, nurse, respiratory therapy, social services, psychology, nutritional/dietetic services, radiation therapy, chemotherapy, etc.), and/ or
- Identification of durable medical equipment needed for this condition, and/or

- Identification of the number of medications the beneficiary is talking (and type if known); and/or
- If complicating factors (complexities) affect treatment, describe why or how. For example: Cardiac dysrhythmia is not a condition for which a therapist would directly treat a patient, but in some patients such dysrhythmias may so directly and significantly affect the pace of progress in treatment for other conditions as to require an exception to caps for necessary services. Documentation should indicate how the progress was affected by the complexity. Or, the severity of the patient's condition as reported on a functional measurement tool may be so great as to suggest extended treatment is anticipated; and/or
- Generalized or multiple conditions. The beneficiary has, in addition to the primary condition being treated, another disease or condition being treated, or generalized musculoskeletal conditions, or conditions affecting multiple sites and these conditions will directly and significantly impact the rate of recovery; and/or.
- Mental or cognitive disorder. The beneficiary has a mental or cognitive disorder in addition to the condition being treated that will directly and significantly impact the rate of recovery; and/or.
- Identification of factors that impact severity including e.g., age, time since onset, cause of the condition, stability of symptoms, how typical/atypical are the symptoms of the diagnosed condition, availability of an intervention/treatment known to be effective, predictability of progress.

Documentation supporting medical care prior to the current episode, if any, (or document none) including, e.g.,

- Record of discharge from a Part A qualifying inpatient, SNF, or home health episode within 30 days of the onset of this outpatient therapy episode, or
- Identification of whether beneficiary was treated for this same condition previously by the same therapy discipline (regardless of where prior services were furnished); and
- Record of a previous episode of therapy treatment from the same or different therapy discipline in the past year.

Documentation required to indicate beneficiary health related to quality of life, specifically,

- The beneficiary's response to the following question of self-related health: "At the present time, would you say that your health is excellent, very good, fair, or poor?" If the beneficiary is unable to respond, indicate why; and

Documentation required to indicate beneficiary social support including, specifically,

- Where does the beneficiary live (or intend to live) at the conclusion of this outpatient therapy episode? (e.g., private home, private apartment, rented room, group home, board and care apartment, assisted living, SNF), and
- Who does beneficiary live with (or intend to live with) at the conclusion of this outpatient therapy episode? (e.g., lives alone, spouse/significant other, child/children, other relative, unrelated person(s), personal care attendant), and
- Does the beneficiary require this outpatient therapy plan of care in order to return to a premorbid (or reside in a new) living environment, and
- Does the beneficiary require this outpatient therapy plan of care in order to reduce Activities of Daily Living (ADL) or Instrumental Activities of Daily Living or (IADL) assistance to a premorbid level or to reside in a new level of living environment (document prior level of independence and current assistance needs); and

*Documentation required to indicate objective, measurable beneficiary physical function including, e.g.,

- Functional assessment individual item and summary scores (and comparisons to prior assessment scores) from commercially available therapy outcomes instruments other than those listed above; or

- Functional assessment scores (and comparisons to prior assessment scores) from tests and measurements validated in the professional literature that are appropriate for the condition/function being measured; or
- Other measurable progress towards identified goals for functioning in the home environment at the conclusion of this therapy episode of care.
- Clinician's clinical judgments or subjective impressions that describe the current functional status of the condition being evaluated, when they provide further information to supplement measurement tools; and
- A determination that treatment is not needed, or, if treatment is needed a prognosis for return to premorbid condition or maximum expected condition with expected time frame and a plan of care.

NOTE: When the Evaluation Serves as the Plan of Care. When an evaluation is the only service provided by a provider/supplier in an episode of treatment, the evaluation serves as the plan of care if it contains a diagnosis, or in states where a therapist may not diagnose, a description of the condition from which a diagnosis may be determined by the referring physician/NPP. The goal, frequency, and duration of treatment are implied in the diagnosis and one-time service. The referral/order of a physician/NPP is the certification that the evaluation is needed and the patient is under the care of a physician. Therefore, when evaluation is the only service, a referral/order and evaluation are the only required documentation. If the patient presented for evaluation without a referral or order and does not require treatment, a physician referral/order or certification of the evaluation is required for payment of the evaluation. A referral/order dated after the evaluation shall be interpreted as certification of the plan to evaluate the patient.

The time spent in evaluation shall not also be billed as treatment time. Evaluation minutes are untimed and are part of the total treatment minutes, but minutes of evaluation shall not be included in the minutes for timed codes reported in the treatment notes.

Re-evaluations shall be included in the documentation sent to contractors when a re-evaluation has been performed. See the definition in section 220. Re-evaluations are usually focused on the current treatment and might not be as extensive as initial evaluations. Continuous assessment of the patient's progress is a component of ongoing therapy services and is not payable as a re-evaluation. A re-evaluation is not a routine, recurring service but is focused on evaluation of progress toward current goals, making a professional judgment about continued care, modifying goals and/or treatment or terminating services. A formal re-evaluation is covered only if the documentation supports the need for further tests and measurements after the initial evaluation. Indications for a re-evaluation include new clinical findings, a significant change in the patient's condition, or failure to respond to the therapeutic interventions outlined in the plan of care.

A re-evaluation may be appropriate prior to planned discharge for the purposes of determining whether goals have been met, or for the use of the physician or the treatment setting at which treatment will be continued.

A re-evaluation is focused on evaluation of progress toward current goals and making a professional judgment about continued care, modifying goals and/or treatment or terminating services. Reevaluation requires the same professional skills as evaluation. The minutes for re-evaluation are documented in the same manner as the minutes for evaluation. Current Procedural Terminology does not define a re-evaluation code for speech-language pathology; use the evaluation code.

Plan of Care. See section 220.1.2 for requirements of the plan. The evaluation and plan may be reported in two separate documents or a single combined document.

D. Progress Report

The Progress Report provides justification for the medical necessity of treatment.

Contractors shall determine the necessity of services based on the delivery of services as directed in the plan and as documented in the Treatment Notes and Progress Report.

For Medicare payment purposes, information required in Progress Reports shall be written by a clinician that is, either the physician/NPP who provides or supervises the services, or by the therapist who provides the services and supervises an assistant. It is not required that the referring or supervising physician/NPP sign the Progress Reports written by a PT, OT or SLP.

Timing

The minimum Progress Report Period shall be at least once every 10 treatment days or at least once during each *30 calendar days*, whichever is less. The day beginning the first reporting period is the first day of the episode of treatment regardless of whether the service provided on that day is an evaluation, re-evaluation or treatment. Regardless of the date on which the report is actually written (and dated), the end of the Progress Report Period is either a date chosen by the clinician, the 10th treatment day, or *the 30th calendar day of the episode of treatment*, whichever is shorter. The next treatment day begins the next reporting period. The Progress Report Period requirements are complete when both the elements of the Progress Report and the clinician's active participation in treatment have been documented.

For example, for a patient evaluated on Monday, October 1 and being treated five times a week, on weekdays: On October 5, (before it is required), the clinician may choose to write a Progress Report for the last week's treatment (from October 1 to October 5). October 5 ends the reporting period and the next treatment on Monday, October 8 begins the next reporting period. If the clinician does not choose to write a report for the next week, the next report is required to cover October 8 through October 19, which would be 10 treatment days.

It should be emphasized that the dates for recertification of plans of care do not affect the dates for required Progress Reports. (Consideration of the case in preparation for a report may lead the therapist to request early recertification. However, each report does not require recertification of the plan, and there may be several reports between recertifications). In many settings, weekly Progress Reports are voluntarily prepared to review progress, describe the skilled treatment, update goals, and inform physician/NPPs or other staff. The clinical judgment demonstrated in frequent reports may help justify that the skills of a therapist are being applied, and that services are medically necessary. Particularly where the patient's medical status, or appropriate tapering of frequency due to expected progress towards goals, results in limited frequency e.g., (2-4 times a month), more frequent Progress Reports can differentiate rehabilitative from maintenance treatment, document progress and justify the continued necessity for skilled care.

Absences

Holidays, sick days or other patient absences may fall within the Progress Report Period. Days on which a patient does not encounter qualified professional or qualified personnel for treatment, evaluation or re-evaluation do not count as treatment days. However, absences do not affect the requirement for a Progress Report at least once during each *Progress Report Period*. If the patient is absent unexpectedly at the end of the reporting period, when the clinician has not yet provided the required active participation during that reporting period, a Progress Report is still required, but without the clinician's active participation in treatment, the requirements of the Progress Report Period are incomplete.

Delayed Reports

If the clinician has not written a Progress Report before the end of the Progress Reporting Period, it shall be written within 7calendar days *after* the end of the reporting period. If the clinician did not participate actively in treatment during the Progress Report Period, documentation of the delayed active participation shall be entered in the Treatment Note as soon as possible. The Treatment Note shall explain the reason for the clinician's missed active participation. Also, the Treatment Note shall document the clinician's guidance to the assistant or qualified personnel to justify that the skills of a therapist were required during the reporting period. It is not necessary to include in this Treatment Note any information already recorded in prior Treatment Notes or Progress Reports.

The contractor shall make a clinical judgment whether continued treatment by assistants or qualified personnel is reasonable and necessary when the clinician has not actively participated in treatment for longer than one reporting period. Judgment shall be based on the individual case and documentation of the application of the clinician's skills to guide the assistant or qualified personnel during and after the reporting period.

Early Reports

Often, Progress Reports are written weekly, or even daily, at the discretion of the clinician. Clinicians are encouraged, but not required to write Progress Reports more frequently than the minimum required in order to allow anyone who reviews the records to easily determine that the services provided are appropriate, covered and payable.

Elements of Progress Reports may be written in the Treatment Notes if the provider/supplier or clinician prefers. If each element required in a Progress Report is included in the Treatment Notes at least once during the Progress Report Period, then a separate Progress Report is not required. Also, elements of the Progress Report may be incorporated into a revised Plan of Care *when one is indicated*. Although the Progress Report written by a therapist does not require a physician/NPP signature when written as a stand-alone document, the *revised* Plan of Care accompanied by the Progress Report shall be re-certified by a physician/NPP. See the section 220.1.2C on Plan of Care for guidance on when a revised plan requires certification.

Progress Reports for Services Billed Incident to a Physician's Service. The policy for incident to services requires, for example, the physician's initial service, direct supervision of therapy services, and subsequent services of a frequency which reflect his/her active participation in and management of the course of treatment. (See section 60.1B of this chapter. Also, see the billing requirements for services incident to a physician in Pub. 100-04, Chapter 26, Items 17, 19, 24, and 31.) Therefore, supervision and reporting requirements for supervising physician/NPPs supervising staff are the same as those for PTs and OTs supervising PTAs and OTAs with certain exceptions noted below.

When a therapy service is provided by a therapist, supervised by a physician/NPP and billed incident to the services of the physician/NPP, the Progress Report shall be written and signed by the therapist who provides the services.

When the services incident to a physician are provided by qualified personnel who are not therapists, the ordering or supervising physician/NPP must personally provide at least one treatment session during each Progress Report Period and sign the Progress Report.

Documenting Clinician Participation in Treatment in the Progress Report

Verification of the clinician's required participation in treatment during the Progress Report Period shall be documented by the clinician's signature on the Treatment Note and/or on the Progress Report. When unexpected discontinuation of treatment occurs, contractors shall not require a clinician's participation in treatment for the incomplete reporting period.

The Discharge Note (or Discharge Summary) is required for each episode of outpatient treatment. In provider settings where the physician/NPP writes a discharge summary and the discharge documentation meets the requirements of the provider setting, a separate discharge note written by a therapist is not required. The Discharge Note shall be a Progress Report written by a clinician, and shall cover the reporting period from the last Progress Report to the date of discharge. In the case of a discharge unanticipated in the plan or previous Progress Report, the clinician may base any judgments required to write the report on the Treatment Notes and verbal reports of the assistant or qualified personnel.

In the case of a discharge anticipated within 3 treatment days of the Progress Report, the clinician may provide objective goals which, when met, will authorize the assistant or qualified personnel to discharge the patient. In that case, the clinician should verify that the services provided prior to discharge continued to require the skills of a therapist, and services were provided or supervised by a clinician. The Discharge Note shall include all treatment provided since the last Progress Report and indicate that the therapist reviewed the notes and agrees to the discharge.

At the discretion of the clinician, the discharge note may include additional information; for example, it may summarize the entire episode of treatment, or justify services that may have extended beyond those usually expected for the patient's condition. Clinicians should consider the discharge note the last opportunity to justify the medical necessity of the entire treatment episode in case the record is reviewed. The record should be reviewed and organized so that the required documentation is ready for presentation to the contractor if requested.

Assistant's Participation in the Progress Report Physical Therapist Assistants or Occupational Therapy Assistants may write elements of the Progress Report dated between clinician reports. Reports written by assistants are not complete Progress Reports. The clinician must write a Progress Report during each Progress Report Period regardless of whether the assistant writes other reports. However, reports written by assistants are part of the record and need not be copied into the clinicians report. Progress Reports written by assistants supplement the reports of clinicians and shall include:

- Date of the beginning and end of the reporting period that this report refers to;
- Date that the report was written (not required to be within the reporting period);
- Signature, and professional identification, or for dictated documentation, the identification of the qualified professional who wrote the report and the date on which it was dictated;
- Objective reports of the patient's subjective statements, if they are relevant. For example, "Patient reports pain after 20 repetitions." Or, "The patient was not feeling well on 11/05/06 and refused to complete the treatment session."; and
- Objective measurements (preferred) or description of changes in status relative to each goal currently being addressed in treatment, if they occur. Note that assistants may not make clinical judgments about why progress was or was not made, but may report the progress objectively. For example: "increasing strength" is not an objective measurement, but "patient ambulates 15 feet with maximum assistance" is objective.

Descriptions shall make identifiable reference to the goals in the current plan of care. Since only long term goals are required in the plan of care, the Progress Report may be used to add, change or delete short term goals. Assistants may change goals only under the direction of a clinician. When short-term goal changes are dictated to an assistant or to qualified personnel, report the change, clinician's name, and date. Clinicians verify these changes by cosignatures on the report or in the clinician's Progress Report. (See section 220.1.2(C) to modify the plan for changes in long term goals.)

The evaluation and plan of care are considered incorporated into the Progress Report, and information in them is not required to be repeated in the report. For example, if a time interval for the treatment is not specifically stated, it is assumed that the goals refer to the plan of care active for the current Progress Report Period. If a body part is not specifically noted, it is assumed the treatment is consistent with the evaluation and plan of care.

Any consistent method of identifying the goals may be used. Preferably, the long term goals may be numbered (1, 2, 3,) and the short term goals that relate to the long term goals may be numbered and lettered 1.A, 1.B, etc. The identifier of a goal on the plan of care may not be changed during the episode of care to which the plan refers. A clinician, an assistant on the order of a therapist or qualified personnel on the order of a physician/NPP shall add new goals with new identifiers or letters. Omit reference to a goal after a clinician has reported it to be met, and that clinician's signature verifies the change.

Content of Clinician (Therapist, Physician/NPP) Progress Reports
In addition to the requirements above for notes written by assistants, the Progress Report of a clinician shall also include:

- Assessment of improvement, extent of progress (or lack thereof) toward each goal;
- Plans for continuing treatment, reference to additional evaluation results, and/or treatment plan revisions should be documented in the clinician's Progress Report; and

- Changes to long or short term goals, discharge or an updated plan of care that is sent to the physician/NPP for certification of the next interval of treatment.

A re-evaluation should not be required before every Progress Report routinely, but may be appropriate when assessment suggests changes not anticipated in the original plan of care.

Care must be taken to assure that documentation justifies the necessity of the services provided during the reporting period, particularly when reports are written at the minimum frequency. Justification for treatment must include, for example, objective evidence or a clinically supportable statement of expectation that:

- The patient's condition has the potential to improve or is improving in response to therapy;
- Maximum improvement is yet to be attained; and
- There is an expectation that the anticipated improvement is attainable in a reasonable and generally predictable period of time.

Objective evidence consists of standardized patient assessment instruments, outcome measurements tools or measurable assessments of functional outcome. Use of objective measures at the beginning of treatment, during and/or after treatment is recommended to quantify progress and support justifications for continued treatment. Such tools are not required, but their use will enhance the justification for needed therapy.

EXAMPLE: The Plan states diagnosis is 787.2- Dysphagia secondary to other late effects of CVA. Patient is on a restricted diet and wants to drink thick liquids. Therapy is planned 3X week, 45 minute sessions for 6 weeks. Long term goal is to consume a mechanical soft diet with thin liquids without complications such as aspiration pneumonia. Short Term Goal 1: Patient will improve rate of laryngeal elevation/timing of closure by using the super-supraglottic swallow on saliva swallows without cues on 90% of trials. Goal 2: Patient will compensate for reduced laryngeal elevation by controlling bolus size to ½ teaspoon without cues 100%. The Progress Report for 1/3/06 to 1/29/06 states: 1. Improved to 80% of trials; 2. Achieved. Comments: Highly motivated; spouse assists with practicing, compliant with current restrictions. New Goal: "5. Patient will implement above strategies to swallow a sip of water without coughing for 5 consecutive trials. Mary Johns, CCC-SLP, 1/29/06." Note the provider is billing 92526 three times a week, consistent with the plan; progress is documented; skilled treatment is documented.

E. Treatment Note

The purpose of these notes is simply to create a record of all treatments and skilled interventions that are provided and to record the time of the services in order to justify the use of billing codes on the claim. Documentation is required for every treatment day, and every therapy service. The format shall not be dictated by contractors and may vary depending on the practice of the responsible clinician and/or the clinical setting.

The Treatment Note is not required to document the medical necessity or appropriateness of the ongoing therapy services. Descriptions of skilled interventions should be included in the plan or the Progress Reports and are allowed, but not required daily. Non-skilled interventions need not be recorded in the Treatment Notes as they are not billable. However, notation of non-skilled treatment or report of activities performed by the patient or non-skilled staff may be reported voluntarily as additional information if they are relevant and not billed. Specifics such as number of repetitions of an exercise and other details included in the plan of care need not be repeated in the Treatment Notes unless they are changed from the plan.

Documentation of each Treatment shall include the following required elements:

- Date of treatment; and
- Identification of each specific intervention/modality provided and billed, for both timed and untimed codes, in language that can be compared with the billing on the claim to verify correct coding. Record each service provided that is represented by a timed code, regardless of whether or not it is billed, because the unbilled timed services may impact the billing; and
- Total timed code treatment minutes and total treatment time in minutes. Total treatment time includes the minutes for timed code treatment and untimed code treatment. Total treatment time does not include time for services that are not billable (e.g., rest periods). For Medicare purposes, it is not required that unbilled services that are not part of the total treatment minutes be recorded, although they may be included voluntarily to provide an accurate description of the treatment, show consistency with the plan, or comply with state or local policies. The amount of time for each specific intervention/modality provided to the patient may also be recorded voluntarily, but contractors shall not require it, as it is indicated in the billing. The billing and the total timed code treatment minutes must be consistent. See Pub. 100-04, Chapter 5, section 20.2 for description of billing timed codes; and
- Signature and professional identification of the qualified professional who furnished or supervised the services and a list of each person who contributed to that treatment (i.e., the signature of Kathleen Smith, PTA, with notation of *phone consultation with* Judy Jones, PT, supervisor, when permitted by state and local law). The signature and identification of the supervisor need not be on each Treatment Note, unless the supervisor actively participated in the treatment. Since a clinician must be identified on the Plan of Care and the Progress Report, the name and professional identification of the supervisor responsible for the treatment is assumed to be the clinician who wrote the plan or report. When the treatment is supervised without active participation by the supervisor, the supervisor is not required to cosign the Treatment Note written by a qualified professional. When the responsible supervisor is absent, the presence of a similarly qualified supervisor on the clinic roster for that day is sufficient documentation and it is not required that the substitute supervisor sign or be identified in the documentation.

If a treatment is added or changed under the direction of a clinician during the treatment days between the Progress Reports, the change must be recorded and justified on the medical record, either in the Treatment Note or the Progress Report, as determined by the policies of the provider/supplier. New exercises added or changes made to the exercise program help justify that the services are skilled. For example: The original plan was for therapeutic activities, gait training and neuromuscular re-education. "On Feb. 1 clinician added electrical stim. to address shoulder pain."

Documentation of each treatment may also include the following optional elements to be mentioned only if the qualified professional recording the note determines they are appropriate and relevant. If these are not recorded daily, any relevant information should be included in the progress report.

- Patient self-report;
- Adverse reaction to intervention;
- Communication/consultation with other providers (e.g., supervising clinician, attending physician, nurse, another therapist, etc.);
- Significant, unusual or unexpected changes in clinical status;
- Equipment provided; and/or
- Any additional relevant information the qualified professional finds appropriate.

See Pub. 100-04, Chapter 5, section 20.2 for instructions on how to count minutes. It is important that the total number of timed treatment minutes support the billing of units on the claim, and that the total treatment time reflects services billed as untimed codes.

▼ 230.2. PRACTICE OF OCCUPATIONAL THERAPY ▼

(Rev. 88, Issued: 05-07-08, Effective: 01-01-08, Implementation: 06-09-08)

A. General

Occupational therapy services are those services provided within the scope of practice of occupational therapists and necessary for the diagnosis and treatment of impairments, functional disabilities or changes in physical function and health status. (See Pub. 100-03, the Medicare National Coverage Determinations Manual, for specific conditions or services.)

Occupational therapy is medically prescribed treatment concerned with improving or restoring functions which have been impaired by illness or injury or, where function has been permanently lost or reduced by illness or injury, to improve the individual's ability to perform those tasks required for independent functioning. Such therapy may involve:

The evaluation, and reevaluation as required, of a patient's level of function by administering diagnostic and prognostic tests;

The selection and teaching of task-oriented therapeutic activities designed to restore physical function; e.g., use of woodworking activities on an inclined table to restore shoulder, elbow, and wrist range of motion lost as a result of burns;

The planning, implementing, and supervising of individualized therapeutic activity programs as part of an overall "active treatment" program for a patient with a diagnosed psychiatric illness; e.g., the use of sewing activities which require following a pattern to reduce confusion and restore reality orientation in a schizophrenic patient;

The planning and implementing of therapeutic tasks and activities to restore sensory-integrative function; e.g., providing motor and tactile activities to increase sensory input and improve response for a stroke patient with functional loss resulting in a distorted body image;

The teaching of compensatory technique to improve the level of independence in the activities of daily living, for example:

- Teaching a patient who has lost the use of an arm how to pare potatoes and chop vegetables with one hand;
- Teaching an upper extremity amputee how to functionally utilize a prosthesis;
- Teaching a stroke patient new techniques to enable the patient to perform feeding, dressing, and other activities as independently as possible; or
- Teaching a patient with a hip fracture/hip replacement techniques of standing tolerance and balance to enable the patient to perform such functional activities as dressing and homemaking tasks.

The designing, fabricating, and fitting of orthotics and self-help devices; e.g., making a hand splint for a patient with rheumatoid arthritis to maintain the hand in a functional position or constructing a device which would enable an individual to hold a utensil and feed independently; or

Vocational and prevocational assessment and training, subject to the limitations specified in item B below.

Only a qualified occupational therapist has the knowledge, training, and experience required to evaluate and, as necessary, reevaluate a patient's level of function, determine whether an occupational therapy program could reasonably be expected to improve, restore, or compensate for lost function and, where appropriate, recommend to the physician/NPP a plan of treatment.

C. Services of Occupational Therapy Support Personnel

Services

The services of OTAs used when providing covered therapy benefits are included as part of the covered service. These services are billed by the supervising occupational therapist. OTAs may not provide evaluation services, make clinical judgments or decisions or take responsibility for the service. They act at the direction and under the supervision of the treating occupational therapist and in accordance with state laws.

An occupational therapist must supervise OTAs. The level and frequency of supervision differs by setting (and by state or local law). General supervision is required for OTAs in all settings except private practice (which requires direct supervision) unless state practice requirements are more stringent, in which case state or local requirements must be followed. See specific settings for details. For example, in clinics, rehabilitation agencies, and public health agencies, 42CFR485.713 indicates that when an OTA provides services, either on or off the organization's premises, those services are supervised by a qualified occupational therapist who makes an onsite supervisory visit at least once every 30 days or more frequently if required by state or local laws or regulation.

The services of an OTA shall not be billed as services incident to a physician/NPP's service, because they do not meet the qualifications of a therapist.

Services provided by aides, even if under the supervision of a therapist, are not therapy services in the outpatient setting and are not covered by Medicare. Although an aide may help the therapist by providing unskilled services, those services that are unskilled are not covered by Medicare and shall be denied as not reasonable and necessary if they are billed as therapy services.

D. Application of Medicare Guidelines to Occupational Therapy Services

Occupational therapy may be required for a patient with a specific diagnosed psychiatric illness. If such services are required, they are covered assuming the coverage criteria are met. However, where an individual's motivational needs are not related to a specific diagnosed psychiatric illness, the meeting of such needs does not usually require an individualized therapeutic program. Such needs can be met through general activity programs or the efforts of other professional personnel involved in the care of the patient. Patient motivation is an appropriate and inherent function of all health disciplines, which is interwoven with other functions performed by such personnel for the patient. Accordingly, since the special skills of an occupational therapist are not required, an occupational therapy program for individuals who do not have a specific diagnosed psychiatric illness is not to be considered reasonable and necessary for the treatment of an illness or injury. Services furnished under such a program are not covered.

Occupational therapy may include vocational and prevocational assessment and training. When services provided by an occupational therapist are related solely to specific employment opportunities, work skills, or work settings, they are not reasonable or necessary for the diagnosis or treatment of an illness or injury and are not covered. However, carriers and intermediaries exercise care in applying this exclusion, because the assessment of level of function and the teaching of compensatory techniques to improve the level of function, especially in activities of daily living, are services which occupational therapists provide for both vocational and nonvocational purposes. For example, an assessment of sitting and standing tolerance might be nonvocational for a mother of young children or a retired individual living alone, but could also be a vocational test for a sales clerk. Training an amputee in the use of prosthesis for telephoning is necessary for everyday activities as well as for employment purposes. Major changes in life style may be mandatory for an individual with a substantial disability. The techniques of adjustment cannot be considered exclusively vocational or nonvocational.

Model Forms: IEP, Prior Written Notice and Excerpts from Procedural Safeguards
Guidance on Required Content of Forms Under Part B of the IDEA

Part B of the Individuals with Disabilities Education Act (IDEA) sets forth requirements for States and local educational agencies (school districts) in providing special education and related services to children with disabilities, ages 3 through 21. Part B emphasizes the importance of including parents in decisions regarding the education of their children. Before a school district proposes or refuses to take action regarding the educational program of a child with a disability, the district must provide a "prior written notice" to the parents. The district must also, at specified times, provide parents with a "procedural safeguards notice" which explains their rights under Part B of the IDEA. Further, parents and school personnel must work together to develop an individualized education program (IEP) for each child which sets forth the services that the child will receive to meet his or her unique needs.

In the Individuals with Disabilities Education Improvement Act of 2004 (the 2004 reauthorization of the IDEA), the Congress required the U.S. Department of Education to publish and widely disseminate "model forms," that are "consistent with the requirements of [Part B of the IDEA]" and "sufficient to meet those requirements." Specifically, the reauthorization required the Department to develop forms for the: (1) IEP; (2) notice of procedural safeguards; and (3) prior written notice.

Attached to this introduction are the three forms that the Department has, consistent with the instructions from the Congress, developed to assist States and school districts in understanding the content that Part B requires for each of these three types of forms. The content of each of these forms is based upon the requirements set forth in the final Part B regulations. Although States must ensure that school districts include all of the content that Part B requires for each of the documents that they provide to parents, States are not required to use the format or specific language reflected in these forms. States may choose to add additional content to their forms, so long as any additional content is not inconsistent with Part B requirements.

These three forms closely track the language in the regulations. However, where appropriate, the Secretary has, in order to make the forms more user-friendly:

- Used "school district" or "district" in place of "public agency" and "local educational agency."
- Used "you" in place of "parent" (or the student, where parental rights have been transferred from the parent to the student at the age of majority).

In order to receive a copy of these model forms or the Part B regulations, please contact Mary Louise Dirrigl by either e-mail (mary.louise.dirrigl@ed.gov) or telephone (202 245 7324).

PART B

INDIVIDUALIZED EDUCATION PROGRAM

The Individualized Education Program (IEP) is a written document that is developed for each eligible child with a disability. The Part B regulations specify, at 34 CFR §§300.320-300.328, the procedures that school districts must follow to develop, review, and revise the IEP for each child. The document below sets out the IEP content that those regulations require.

A statement of the child's present levels of academic achievement and functional performance including:

- How the child's disability affects the child's involvement and progress in the general education curriculum (i.e., the same curriculum as for nondisabled children) or <u>for preschool children</u>, as appropriate, how the disability affects the child's participation in appropriate activities. [34 CFR §300.320(a)(1)]

```


```

A statement of measurable annual goals, including academic and functional goals designed to:

- Meet the child's needs that result from the child's disability to enable the child to be involved in and make progress in the general education curriculum. [34 CFR §300.320(a)(2)(i)(A)]
- Meet each of the child's other educational needs that result from the child's disability. [34 CFR §300.320(a)(2)(i)(B)]

```


```

For children with disabilities who take alternate assessments aligned to alternate achievement standards (in addition to the annual goals), a description of benchmarks or short-term objectives. [34 CFR §300.320(a)(2)(ii)]

```


```

A description of:

- How the child's progress toward meeting the annual goals will be measured. [34 CFR §300.320(a)(3)(i)]
- When periodic reports on the progress the child is making toward meeting the annual goals will be provided such as through the use of quarterly or other periodic reports, concurrent with the issuance of report cards. [34 CFR §300.320(a)(3)(ii)]

```


```

U.S. Department of Education
Office of Special Education and Rehabilitative Services,
Office of Special Education Program

Model From: Individualized Education Program

A statement of the <u>special education and related services</u> and <u>supplementary</u> aids and <u>services</u>, based on peer-reviewed research to the extent practicable, to be provided to the child, or on behalf of the child, and <u>a statement of the program modifications or supports</u> for school personnel that will be provided to enable the child:

- To advance appropriately toward attaining the annual goals. [34 CFR §300.320(a)(4)(i)]
- To be involved in and make progress in the general education curriculum and to participate in extracurricular and other nonacademic activities. [34 CFR §300.320(a)(4)(ii)]
- To be educated and participate with other children with disabilities and nondisabled children in extracurricular and other nonacademic activities. [34 CFR §300.320(a)(4)(iii)]

An explanation of the extent, if any, to which the child will not participate with nondisabled children in the regular classroom and in extracurricular and other nonacademic activities. [34 CFR §300.320(a)(5)]

A statement of any individual appropriate accommodations that are necessary to measure the academic achievement and functional performance of the child on State and districtwide assessments. [34 CFR §300.320(a)(6)(i)]

If the IEP Team determines that the child must take an alternate assessment instead of a particular regular State or districtwide assessment of student achievement, a statement of why:

- The child cannot participate in the regular assessment. [34 CFR §300.320(a)(6)(ii)(A)]
- The particular alternate assessment selected is appropriate for the child. [34 CFR §300.320(a)(6)(ii)(B)]

The projected date for the beginning of the services and modifications and the anticipated frequency, location, and duration of <u>special education and related services</u> and <u>supplementary aids and services</u> and <u>modifications and supports</u>. [34 CFR §300.320(a)(7)]

Service, Aid or Modification	Frequency	Location	Beginning Date	Duration

TRANSITION SERVICES

Beginning not later than the first IEP to be in effect when the child turns 16, or younger if determined appropriate by the IEP Team, and updated annually thereafter, the IEP must include:

- Appropriate measurable postsecondary goals based upon age-appropriate transition assessments related to training, education, employment, and where appropriate, independent living skills. [34 CFR §300.320(b)(1)]

        ```
        ```

- The transition services (including courses of study) needed to assist the child in reaching those goals. [34 CFR §300.320(b)(2)]

Transition Services (Including Courses of Study)

RIGHTS THAT TRANSFER AT AGE OF MAJORITY

- Beginning not later than one year before the child reaches the age of majority under State law, the IEP must include a statement that the child has been informed of the child's rights under Part B of the IDEA, if any, that will, consistent with 34 CFR §300.520, transfer to the child on reaching the age of majority. [34 CFR §300.320(c)]

PART B

PRIOR WRITTEN NOTICE

Under 34 CFR §300.503(a), the school district must give you a written notice (information received in writing), whenever the school district: (1) Proposes to begin or change the identification, evaluation, or educational placement of your child or the provision of a free appropriate public education (FAPE) to your child; or (2) Refuses to begin or change the identification, evaluation, or educational placement of your child or the provision of FAPE to your child. The required content under 34 CFR §300.503(b) is listed below in this model form. The school district must provide the notice in understandable language (34 CFR §300.503(c)). This model form provides a format that States and/or school districts may choose to adopt to construct the form that they will use to provide that notice. The school district will need to insert the required child- and situation-specific information, and must inform parents, as part of the notice, that they have protection under the procedural safeguards of Part B of the IDEA.

PRIOR WRITTEN NOTICE UNDER PART B OF THE IDEA

- Description of the action that the school district proposes or refuses to take:

        ```
        ```

U.S. Department of Education
Office of Special Education and Rehabilitative Services,
Office of Special Education Program

Model From: Prior Written Notice

- Explanation of why the school district is proposing or refusing to take that action:

- Description of each evaluation procedure, assessment, record, or report the school district used in deciding to propose or refuse the action:

- Description of any other choices that the Individualized Education Program (IEP) Team considered and the reasons why those choices were rejected:

- Description of other reasons why the school district proposed or refused the action:

- Resources for the parents to contact for help in understanding Part B of the IDEA:

- If this notice is not an initial referral for evaluation, how the parent can obtain a copy of a description of the procedural safeguards:

PART B

PROCEDURAL SAFEGUARDS NOTICE

The Individuals with Disabilities Education Act (IDEA), the Federal law concerning the education of students with disabilities, requires schools to provide parents of a child with a disability with a notice containing a full explanation of the procedural safeguards available under the IDEA and U.S. Department of Education regulations. A copy of this notice must be given to parents only one time a school year, except that a copy must be given to the parents: (1) upon initial referral or parent request for evaluation; (2) upon receipt of the first State complaint under 34 CFR §§300.151 through 300.153 and upon receipt of the first due process complaint under §300.507 in a school year; (3) when a decision is made to take a disciplinary action that constitutes a change of placement; and (4) upon parent request. [34 CFR §300.504(a)]

This procedural safeguards notice must include a full explanation of all of the procedural safeguards available under §300.148 (unilateral placement at private school at public expense), §§300.151 through 300.153 (State complaint procedures), §300.300 (consent), §§300.502 through 300.503, §§300.505 through 300.518, and §§300.530 through 300.536 (procedural safeguards in Subpart E of the Part B regulations), and §§300.610 through 300.625 (confidentiality of information provisions in Subpart F). This model form provides a format that States and/or school districts may choose to use to provide information about procedural safeguards to parents.

[NOTE TO STATES AND SCHOOL DISTRICTS: Where the Office of Special Education Programs (OSEP) has included bracketed NOTES in this document, these NOTES are intended as directions to States or school districts regarding content that they must include in the procedural safeguards notice provided to parents. The State or school district should insert the required State-specific language and delete the NOTES prior to providing the notice to parents.]

GENERAL INFORMATION

PRIOR WRITTEN NOTICE
34 CFR §300.503
Notice
Your school district must give you written notice (provide you certain information in writing), whenever it:

1. Proposes to initiate or to change the identification, evaluation, or educational placement of your child, or the provision of a free appropriate public education (FAPE) to your child; or
2. Refuses to initiate or to change the identification, evaluation, or educational placement of your child, or the provision of FAPE to your child.

Content of notice
The written notice must:

1. Describe the action that your school district proposes or refuses to take;
2. Explain why your school district is proposing or refusing to take the action;
3. Describe each evaluation procedure, assessment, record, or report your school district used in deciding to propose or refuse the action;
4. Include a statement that you have protections under the procedural safeguards provisions in Part B of the IDEA;
5. Tell you how you can obtain a description of the procedural safeguards if the action that your school district is proposing or refusing is not an initial referral for evaluation;
6. Include resources for you to contact for help in understanding Part B of the IDEA;
7. Describe any other choices that your child's individualized education program (IEP) Team considered and the reasons why those choices were rejected; and
8. Provide a description of other reasons why your school district proposed or refused the action.

Notice in understandable language
The notice must be:

1. Written in language understandable to the general public; and
2. Provided in your native language or other mode of communication you use, unless it is clearly not feasible to do so.

If your native language or other mode of communication is not a written language, your school district must ensure that:

1. The notice is translated for you orally by other means in your native language or other mode of communication;
2. You understand the content of the notice; and
3. There is written evidence that 1 and 2 have been met.

NATIVE LANGUAGE
34 CFR §300.29
Native language, when used with an individual who has limited English proficiency, means the following:

1. The language normally used by that person, or, in the case of a child, the language normally used by the child's parents;
2. In all direct contact with a child (including evaluation of the child), the language normally used by the child in the home or learning environment.

For a person with deafness or blindness, or for a person with no written language, the mode of communication is what the person normally uses (such as sign language, Braille, or oral communication).

ELECTRONIC MAIL
34 CFR §300.505
If your school district offers parents the choice of receiving documents by e-mail, you may choose to receive the following by e-mail:

1. Prior written notice;
2. Procedural safeguards notice; and
3. Notices related to a due process complaint.

PARENTAL CONSENTDEFINITION
34 CFR §300.9
Consent
Consent means:

1. You have been fully informed in your native language or other mode of communication (such as sign language, Braille, or oral communication) of all information about the action for which you are giving consent.
2. You understand and agree in writing to that action, and the consent describes that action and lists the records (if any) that will be released and to whom; and
3. You understand that the consent is voluntary on your part and you may withdraw your consent at anytime.

Your withdrawal of consent does not negate (undo) an action that has occurred after you gave your consent and before you withdrew it.

PARENTAL CONSENT
34 CFR §300.300
Consent for initial evaluation
Your school district cannot conduct an initial evaluation of your child to determine whether your child is eligible under Part B of the IDEA to receive special education and related services without first providing you with prior written notice of the proposed action and without obtaining your consent as described under the heading Parental Consent.

Your school district must make reasonable efforts to obtain your informed consent for an initial evaluation to decide whether your child is a child with a disability.

Your consent for initial evaluation does not mean that you have also given your consent for the school district to start providing special education and related services to your child.

If your child is enrolled in public school or you are seeking to enroll your child in a public school and you have refused to provide consent or failed to respond to a request to provide consent for an initial evaluation, your school district may, but is not required to, seek to conduct an initial evaluation of your child by utilizing the Act's mediation or due process complaint, resolution meeting, and impartial due process hearing procedures (unless required to do so or prohibited from doing so under State law). Your school district will not violate its obligations to locate, identify and evaluate your child if it does not pursue an evaluation of your child in these circumstances, unless State law requires it to pursue the evaluation.

Special rules for initial evaluation of wards of the State

If a child is a ward of the State and is not living with his/her parent—

The school district does not need consent from the parent for an initial evaluation to determine if the child is a child with a disability if:

1. Despite reasonable efforts to do so, the school district cannot find the child's parent;
2. The rights of the parents have been terminated in accordance with State law; or
3. A judge has assigned the right to make educational decisions and to consent for an initial evaluation to an individual other than the parent.

Ward of the State, as used in the IDEA, means a child who, as determined by the State where the child lives, is:

1. A foster child;
2. Considered a ward of the State under State law; or
3. In the custody of a public child welfare agency.

Ward of the State does not include a foster child who has a foster parent.

Parental consent for services

Your school district must obtain your informed consent before providing special education and related services to your child for the first time.

The school district must make reasonable efforts to obtain your informed consent before providing special education and related services to your child for the first time.

If you do not respond to a request to provide your consent for your child to receive special education and related services for the first time, or if you refuse to give such consent, your school district may not use the procedural safeguards (i.e., mediation, due process complaint, resolution meeting, or an impartial due process hearing) in order to obtain agreement or a ruling that the special education and related services (recommended by your child's IEP Team) may be provided to your child without your consent.

If you refuse to give your consent for your child to receive special education and related services for the first time, or if you do not respond to a request to provide such consent and the school district does not provide your child with the special education and related services for which it sought your consent, your school district:

1. Is not in violation of the requirement to make a free appropriate public education (FAPE) available to your child for its failure to provide those services to your child; and
2. Is not required to have an individualized education program (IEP) meeting or develop an IEP for your child for the special education and related services for which your consent was requested.

Parental consent for reevaluations

Your school district must obtain your informed consent before it reevaluates your child, unless your school district can demonstrate that:

1. It took reasonable steps to obtain your consent for your child's reevaluation; and
2. You did not respond.

If you refuse to consent to your child's reevaluation, the school district may, but is not required to, pursue your child's reevaluation by using the mediation, due process complaint, resolution meeting, and impartial due process hearing procedures to seek to override your refusal to consent to your child's reevaluation. As with initial evaluations, your school district does not violate its obligations under Part B of the IDEA if it declines to pursue the reevaluation in this manner.

Documentation of reasonable efforts to obtain parental consent

Your school must maintain documentation of reasonable efforts to obtain parental consent for initial evaluations, to provide special education and related services for the first time, to reevaluation and to locate parents of wards of the State for initial evaluations. The documentation must include a record of the school district's attempts in these areas, such as:

1. Detailed records of telephone calls made or attempted and the results of those calls;
2. Copies of correspondence sent to the parents and any responses received; and
3. Detailed records of visits made to the parent's home or place of employment and the results of those visits.

Other consent requirements

Your consent is not required before your school district may:

1. Review existing data as part of your child's evaluation or a reevaluation; or
2. Give your child a test or other evaluation that is given to all children unless, before that test or evaluation, consent is required from all parents of all children.

[NOTE: If the State requires consent for other services and activities (in addition to those listed above), the notice must specify what those other services and activities are, and then also state: "The school district must develop and implement procedures to ensure that your refusal to consent to any of these other services and activities does not result in a failure to provide your child with a free appropriate public education (FAPE)."]

Your school district may not use your refusal to consent to one service or activity to deny you or your child any other service, benefit, or activity.

If you have enrolled your child in a private school at your own expense or if you are home schooling your child, and you do not provide your consent for your child's initial evaluation or your child's reevaluation, or you fail to respond to a request to provide your consent, the school district may not use its consent override procedures (i.e., mediation, due process complaint, resolution meeting, or an impartial due process hearing) and is not required to consider your child as eligible to receive equitable services (services made available to parentally-placed private school children with disabilities).

INDEPENDENT EDUCATIONAL EVALUATIONS
34 CFR §300.502
General
As described below, you have the right to obtain an independent educational evaluation (IEE) of your child if you disagree with the evaluation of your child that was obtained by your school district.

If you request an independent educational evaluation, the school district must provide you with information about where you may obtain an independent educational evaluation and about the school district's criteria that apply to independent educational evaluations.

Definitions
Independent educational evaluation means an evaluation conducted by a qualified examiner who is not employed by the school district responsible for the education of your child.

Public expense means that the school district either pays for the full cost of the evaluation or ensures that the evaluation is otherwise provided at no cost to you, consistent with the provisions of Part B of the IDEA, which allow each State to use whatever State, local, Federal and private sources of support are available in the State to meet the requirements of Part B of the Act.

Parent right to evaluation at public expense
You have the right to an independent educational evaluation of your child at public expense if you disagree with an evaluation of your child obtained by your school district, subject to the following conditions:

1. If you request an independent educational evaluation of your child at public expense, your school district must, without unnecessary delay, either: (a) File a due process complaint to request a hearing to show that its evaluation of your child is appropriate; or (b) Provide an independent educational evaluation at public expense, unless the school district demonstrates in a hearing that the evaluation of your child that you obtained did not meet the school district's criteria.
2. If your school district requests a hearing and the final decision is that your school district's evaluation of your child is appropriate, you still have the right to an independent educational evaluation, but not at public expense.
3. If you request an independent educational evaluation of your child, the school district may ask why you object to the evaluation of your child obtained by your school district. However, your school district may not require an explanation and may not unreasonably delay either providing the independent educational evaluation of your child at public expense or filing a due process complaint to request a due process hearing to defend the school district's evaluation of your child.

You are entitled to only one independent educational evaluation of your child at public expense each time your school district conducts an evaluation of your child with which you disagree.

Parent-initiated evaluations
If you obtain an independent educational evaluation of your child at public expense or you share with the school district an evaluation of your child that you obtained at private expense:

1. Your school district must consider the results of the evaluation of your child, if it meets the school district's criteria for independent educational evaluations, in any decision made with respect to the provision of a free appropriate public education (FAPE) to your child; and
2. You or your school district may present the evaluation as evidence at a due process hearing regarding your child.

Requests for evaluations by hearing officers
If a hearing officer requests an independent educational evaluation of your child as part of a due process hearing, the cost of the evaluation must be at public expense.

School district criteria

If an independent educational evaluation is at public expense, the criteria under which the evaluation is obtained, including the location of the evaluation and the qualifications of the examiner, must be the same as the criteria that the school district uses when it initiates an evaluation (to the extent those criteria are consistent with your right to an independent educational evaluation).

Except for the criteria described above, a school district may not impose conditions or timelines related to obtaining an independent educational evaluation at public expense.

CONFIDENTIALITY OF INFORMATION

DEFINITIONS
34 CFR §300.611

As used under the heading Confidentiality of Information:

- *Destruction means* physical destruction or removal of personal identifiers from information so that the information is no longer personally identifiable.
- *Education records* means the type of records covered under the definition of "education records" in 34 CFR Part 99 (the regulations implementing the Family Educational Rights and Privacy Act of 1974, 20 U.S.C. 1232g (FERPA)).
- *Participating agency* means any school district, agency or institution that collects, maintains, or uses personally identifiable information, or from which information is obtained, under Part B of the IDEA.

PERSONALLY IDENTIFIABLE
34 CFR §300.32

Personally identifiable means information that has:

A. Your child's name, your name as the parent, or the name of another family member;
B. Your child's address;
C. A personal identifier, such as your child's social security number or student number; or
D. A list of personal characteristics or other information that would make it possible to identify your child with reasonable certainty.

NOTICE TO PARENTS
34 CFR §300.612

The State Educational Agency must give notice that is adequate to fully inform parents about confidentiality of personally identifiable information, including:

1. A description of the extent to which the notice is given in the native languages of the various population groups in the State;
2. A description of the children on whom personally identifiable information is maintained, the types of information sought, the methods the State intends to use in gathering the information (including the sources from whom information is gathered), and the uses to be made of the information;
3. A summary of the policies and procedures that participating agencies must follow regarding storage, disclosure to third parties, retention, and destruction of personally identifiable information; and
4. A description of all of the rights of parents and children regarding this information, including the rights under the Family Educational Rights and Privacy Act (FERPA) and its implementing regulations in 34 CFR Part 99.

Before any major identification, location, or evaluation activity (also known as "child find"), the notice must be published or announced in newspapers or other media, or both, with circulation adequate to notify parents throughout the State of the activity to locate, identify, and evaluate children in need of special education and related services.

ACCESS RIGHTS
34 CFR §300.613

The participating agency must permit you to inspect and review any education records relating to your child that are collected, maintained, or used by your school district under Part B of the IDEA. The participating agency must comply with your request to inspect and review any education records on your child without unnecessary delay and before any meeting regarding an individualized education program (IEP), or any impartial due process hearing (including a resolution meeting or a hearing regarding discipline), and in no case more than

45 calendar days after you have made a request.

Your right to inspect and review education records includes:

1. Your right to a response from the participating agency to your reasonable requests for explanations and interpretations of the records;
2. Your right to request that the participating agency provide copies of the records if you cannot effectively inspect and review the records unless you receive those copies; and
3. Your right to have your representative inspect and review the records.

The participating agency may presume that you have authority to inspect and review records relating to your child unless advised that you do not have the authority under applicable State law governing such matters as guardianship, or separation and divorce.

RECORD OF ACCESS
34 CFR §300.614

Each participating agency must keep a record of parties obtaining access to education records collected, maintained, or used under Part B of the IDEA (except access by parents and authorized employees of the participating agency), including the name of the party, the date access was given, and the purpose for which the party is authorized to use the records.

RECORDS ON MORE THAN ONE CHILD
34 CFR §300.615

If any education record includes information on more than one child, the parents of those children have the right to inspect and review only the information relating to their child or to be informed of that specific information.

LIST OF TYPES AND LOCATIONS OF INFORMATION
34 CFR §300.616

On request, each participating agency must provide you with a list of the types and locations of education records collected, maintained, or used by the agency.

FEES
34 CFR §300.617

Each participating agency may charge a fee for copies of records that are made for you under Part B of the IDEA, if the fee does not effectively prevent you from exercising your right to inspect and review those records. A participating agency may not charge a fee to search for or to retrieve information under Part B of the IDEA.

AMENDMENT OF RECORDS AT PARENT'S REQUEST
34 CFR §300.618

If you believe that information in the education records regarding your child collected, maintained, or used under Part B of the IDEA is inaccurate, misleading, or violates the privacy or other rights of your child, you may request the participating agency that maintains the information to change the information.

The participating agency must decide whether to change the information in accordance with your request within a reasonable period of time of receipt of your request.

If the participating agency refuses to change the information in accordance with your request, it must inform you of the refusal and advise you of the right to a hearing for this purpose as described under the heading Opportunity For a Hearing.

OPPORTUNITY FOR A HEARING
34 CFR §300.619

The participating agency must, on request, provide you an opportunity for a hearing to challenge information in education records regarding your child to ensure that it is not inaccurate, misleading, or otherwise in violation of the privacy or other rights of your child.

HEARING PROCEDURES
34 CFR §300.621

A hearing to challenge information in education records must be conducted according to the procedures for such hearings under the Family Educational Rights and Privacy Act (FERPA).

CONSENT FOR DISCLOSURE OF PERSONALLY IDENTIFIABLE INFORMATION
34 CFR §300.622

Unless the information is contained in education records, and the disclosure is authorized without parental consent under the Family Educational Rights and Privacy Act (FERPA), your consent must be obtained before personally identifiable information is disclosed to parties other than officials of participating agencies. Except under the circumstances specified below, your consent is not required before personally identifiable information is released to officials of participating agencies for purposes of meeting a requirement of Part B of the IDEA.

Your consent, or consent of an eligible child who has reached the age of majority under State law, must be obtained before personally identifiable information is released to officials of participating agencies providing or paying for transition services.

If your child is in, or is going to go to, a private school that is not located in the same school district you reside in, your consent must be obtained before any personally identifiable information about your child is released between officials in the school district where the private school is located and officials in the school district where you reside.

SAFEGUARDS
34 CFR §300.623

Each participating agency must protect the confidentiality of personally identifiable information at collection, storage, disclosure, and destruction stages.

One official at each participating agency must assume responsibility for ensuring the confidentiality of any personally identifiable information.

All persons collecting or using personally identifiable information must receive training or instruction regarding your State's policies and procedures regarding confidentiality under Part B of the IDEA and the Family Educational Rights and Privacy Act (FERPA).

Each participating agency must maintain, for public inspection, a current listing of the names and positions of those employees within the agency who may have access to personally identifiable information.

DESTRUCTION OF INFORMATION
34 CFR §300.624

Your school district must inform you when personally identifiable information collected, maintained, or used is no longer needed to provide educational services to your child.

The information must be destroyed at your request. However, a permanent record of your child's name, address, and phone number, his or her grades, attendance record, classes attended, grade level completed, and year completed may be maintained without time limitation.

Reproducible Sample Forms

OCCUPATIONAL THERAPY PEDIATRIC EVALUATION REPORT

BACKGROUND INFORMATION
Date of report: __/__/20__

Date of birth &/or age: _____

Primary intervention diagnosis/concern:

Secondary diagnosis/concern:

Precautions/contraindications:

Reason for referral to OT: *(or questions to be answered)*

Therapist: *(Print or type your name, sign and date the report at the end.)*

Client's name or initials:

Date of referral: __/__/20__

Assessments performed:

❑ Play Observation

❑ Self-care Observation

❑ Parent Interview

❑ Pediatric Evaluation of Disability Inventory (PEDI)

❑ Sensory Profile

❑ Peabody Developmental Motor Scales 2nd ed. (PDMS-2)

❑ Bruininks-Oseretsky Test of Motor Proficiency, 2nd ed. (BOT-2)

❑ Beery Visual Motor Integration (VMI)

❑ Sensory Integration and Praxis Test (SIPT)

❑ Sensorimotor Performance Analysis (SPA)

❑ Evaluation Tool of Children's Handwriting (ETCH)

❑ Other: _____

FINDINGS
Occupational Profile: *(Describe the client's occupational history and experience, patterns of living, interests, values, and needs that are relevant to the current situation.)*

Occupational Analysis:

Areas of Occupation:	Not Tested	Dependent	Max Assist	Mod Assist	Min Assist	Equipment	Independent
Bathing	❑	❑	❑	❑	❑	❑	❑
Toileting	❑	❑	❑	❑	❑	❑	❑
Eating	❑	❑	❑	❑	❑	❑	❑
Feeding	❑	❑	❑	❑	❑	❑	❑
Dressing	❑	❑	❑	❑	❑	❑	❑
Functional Mobility	❑	❑	❑	❑	❑	❑	❑
Grooming	❑	❑	❑	❑	❑	❑	❑
Safety	❑	❑	❑	❑	❑	❑	❑
Handwriting	❑	❑	❑	❑	❑	❑	❑
Meal prep	❑	❑	❑	❑	❑	❑	❑
Play	❑	❑	❑	❑	❑	❑	❑
Other (describe)		❑	❑	❑	❑	❑	❑

Performance Skills:	Not Tested	Absent	Developing	Proficient	Comments:
Posture	❑	❑	❑	❑	
Balance	❑	❑	❑	❑	
Fine motor coordination	❑	❑	❑	❑	
Gross motor coordination	❑	❑	❑	❑	
Visual motor integration	❑	❑	❑	❑	
Following directions	❑	❑	❑	❑	
Sensory processing	❑	❑	❑	❑	
Emotional regulation	❑	❑	❑	❑	
Cognitive skills	❑	❑	❑	❑	
Communication and social skills	❑	❑	❑	❑	
Other (describe)		❑	❑	❑	

Performance patterns: Describe the client's

Habits:

Routines:

Roles:

Rituals:

Client factors:

Body Functions:	Not Tested	Absent	Impaired	Adequate	Comments:
Attention	❑	❑	❑	❑	
Distractability	❑	❑	❑	❑	
Memory	❑	❑	❑	❑	
Sequencing	❑	❑	❑	❑	
Initiative	❑	❑	❑	❑	
Sight	❑	❑	❑	❑	
Hearing	❑	❑	❑	❑	
Smell	❑	❑	❑	❑	
Taste	❑	❑	❑	❑	
Touch	❑	❑	❑	❑	
Vestibular	❑	❑	❑	❑	
Kinesthetic	❑	❑	❑	❑	
Proprioception	❑	❑	❑	❑	
Temperature	❑	❑	❑	❑	
Pain	❑	❑	❑	❑	
Muscle tone	❑	❑	❑	❑	
Reflexes	❑	❑	❑	❑	
Endurance	❑	❑	❑	❑	
Joint stability	❑	❑	❑	❑	
Bilateral integration	❑	❑	❑	❑	
Praxis	❑	❑	❑	❑	
Other (describe)		❑	❑	❑	

OCCUPATIONAL THERAPY PEDIATRIC EVALUATION REPORT (PAGE 3)

Body Structure:	Deformity	Movement Limitation	Normal	Comments:
Head	❏	❏	❏	
Neck	❏	❏	❏	
Shoulders	❏	❏	❏	❏ R ❏ L ❏ B
Elbows	❏	❏	❏	❏ R ❏ L ❏ B
Forearms	❏	❏	❏	❏ R ❏ L ❏ B
Wrists	❏	❏	❏	❏ R ❏ L ❏ B
Hands	❏	❏	❏	❏ R ❏ L ❏ B
Trunk	❏	❏	❏	
Hips	❏	❏	❏	❏ R ❏ L ❏ B
Knees	❏	❏	❏	❏ R ❏ L ❏ B
Legs	❏	❏	❏	❏ R ❏ L ❏ B
Ankles	❏	❏	❏	❏ R ❏ L ❏ B
Feet	❏	❏	❏	❏ R ❏ L ❏ B
Other (describe)	❏	❏	❏	

Activity demands and contexts: *(describe)*

Specific test results:

Name of Test (subtest)	Raw Score	Standard Score	Percentile Rank	Age Equivalent	Comments

INTERPRETATION
Strengths and areas in need of intervention:
Supports and hindrances to occupational performance:
Prioritization of need areas:

1.

2.

3.

PLAN

Mutually Agreed-On Long-Term Goals	Mutually Agreed-On Short-Term Goals	Recommended Intervention Methods and Approaches

OCCUPATIONAL THERAPY PEDIATRIC EVALUATION REPORT (PAGE 4)

**Plans for coordination/
communication with school-based team**   ❑ Phone   **Frequency:**

❑ Email   **At least __x/mo**

❑ Conferences   **More often as
needed**

**Plans for coordination/
communication with family**   ❑ Phone   **Frequency:**

❑ Email   **At least __x/wk**

❑ Conferences   **More often as
needed**

Intervention will be provided ___ x/ week, ____ min sessions, for ___ weeks at
❑ clinic   ❑ home   ❑ other _____

Anticipated D/C environment: ❑ school   ❑ home   ❑ other _____

_____
Signature   **Date**

OCCUPATIONAL THERAPY EVALUATION REPORT

BACKGROUND INFORMATION

Date of report:	Client's name or initials:
Date of birth &/or age:	Date of referral: M F
Primary intervention diagnosis/concern:	
Secondary diagnosis/concern:	

Reason for referral to OT: *(or questions to be answered)*

Therapist: *(Print or type your name, sign and date the report at the end.)*

Assessments performed: *(Give a brief description of the method(s) used to gather evaluation data; i.e. interview, informal observation, name of formal assessments, etc.)*

FINDINGS

Occupational Profile: *(Describe the client's occupational history and experience, patterns of living, interests, values and needs that are relevant to the current situation.)*

Occupational Analysis:

    Areas of occupation:

    Performance skills:

    Performance patterns:

    Client factors:

    Activity demands:

    Contexts:

INTERPRETATION
Supports and hindrances to occupational performance

Prioritization of need areas:

PLAN

Mutually Agreed-On Long-Term Goals	Mutually Agreed-On Short-Term Goals	Intervention Methods and Approaches

Expected frequency, duration and intensity:

Location of intervention:

Anticipated D/C environment:

_____

Signature   **Date**

OCCUPATIONAL THERAPY INTERVENTION PLAN

BACKGROUND INFORMATION:

Date of report:

Date of birth &/or age:

Primary intervention diagnosis/concern:

Secondary diagnosis/concern:

Client's name or initials:

Date of referral: M   F

Reason for referral to OT: *(or questions to be answered)*

Therapist: *(Print or type your name and credential, you will sign and date the report at the end.)*

FINDINGS

Occupational profile: *(Describe the client's occupational history and experience, patterns of living, interests, values and needs that are relevant to the current situation.)*

Progress Toward Goals So Far; Reasons for Progress or Lack Thereof in:

    Areas of occupation:

    Performance skills:

    Performance patterns:

    Activity demands:

    Client factors:

    Contexts:

Equipment/Orthotics issued:

Home programs/training:

OCCUPATIONAL THERAPY INTERVENTION PLAN (PAGE 2)

INTERPRETATION

Analysis of occupational performance: *(Describe the barriers and challenges, supports and strengths.)*

PLAN

Long-Term Goals	Short-Term Goals	Methods/Approaches

Expected frequency, duration and intensity:

Location of intervention:

Anticipated discontinuation environment:

Signature   *Date*

OCCUPATIONAL THERAPY NARRATIVE NOTES

DATE: **NOTE:**

Client name:
Record number:
Physician name:
Diagnosis/condition:

OCCUPATIONAL THERAPY SOAP NOTES

SOAP NOTES

S:

O:

A:

P:

> **Client name:**
> **Record number:**
> **Physician name:**
> **Diagnosis/condition:**

S:

O:

A:

P:

> **Client name:**
> **Record number:**
> **Physician name:**
> **Diagnosis/condition:**

SAMPLE DISCONTINUATION SUMMARY REPORT

Date of report: **Name:**
Date of birth &/or age: **Date of initial referral:**   M   F
Primary intervention diagnosis/concern:
Secondary diagnosis/concern:
Precautions/contraindications:
Reason for referral to OT:
Reason for OT discontinuation:

Therapist: *(Print or type your name and credential, you will sign and date the report at the end.)*

Description of OT intervention: *(Include service delivery model, duration/frequency of interventions, # of intervention sessions or beginning and end dates of interventions, location of interventions and types of interventions provided.)*

Brief summary of progress toward goals: *(Statements of progress toward or achievement of long-term goals or reasons why goals were not met.)*

Occupational therapy outcomes:
    Initial performance in areas of occupation:
    (Concise summary of changes in the client's performance in the areas of activities of daily living, instrumental activities of daily living, education, work, play, leisure, and social participation.)

    Current level of performance in areas of occupation:
    (Concise summary of current performance and expectations for performance within the contexts of the client's anticipated environments following discontinuation.)

Contextual aspects related to discontinuation:
    (Concise summary of the cultural, physical, social, personal, spiritual, temporal and/or virtual contexts.)

Discontinuation recommendations:
    (Concise description of discontinuation plans other referrals, follow-up, home program suggestions, support systems, and caregiver suggestions.)

_____

Signature   **Date**

SAMPLE IEP GOAL PAGE

Individualized Education Program for:

IEP Dates: from _____ **to** _____   **DOB:** _____

Current Level of Performance/Measurable Annual Goals/Benchmarks

Goal # _____
Educational need area: _____ Academic/cognitive   _____ Behavior   _____ Communication
_____ Motor   _____ Self-help   _____ Social   _____ Vocational

Current Level of Performance:

Measurable Annual Goal:

Benchmark/Objectives:

PLAN OF TREATMENT FOR OUTPATIENT REHABILITATION
(COMPLETE FOR INITIAL CLAIMS ONLY)

1. PATIENT'S LAST NAME	FIRST NAME	M.I.	2. PROVIDER NO.	3. HICN

4. PROVIDER NAME	5. MEDICAL RECORD NO. *(Optional)*	6. ONSET DATE	7. SOC. DATE

8. TYPE ☐ PT ☐ OT ☐ SLP ☐ CR ☐ RT ☐ PS ☐ SN ☐ SW	9. PRIMARY DIAGNOSIS *(Pertinent Medical D.X.)*	10. TREATMENT DIAGNOSIS	11. VISITS FROM SOC.

12. PLAN OF TREATMENT FUNCTIONAL GOALS

GOALS *(Short Term)*

OUTCOME *(Long Term)*

PLAN

13. SIGNATURE *(professional establishing POC including prof. designation)*

14. FREQ/DURATION *(e.g., 3/Wk. x 4 Wk.)*

I CERTIFY THE NEED FOR THESE SERVICES FURNISHED UNDER THIS PLAN OF TREATMENT AND WHILE UNDER MY CARE   ☐ N/A

15. PHYSICIAN SIGNATURE

16. DATE

17. CERTIFICATION

FROM   THROUGH   N/A

18. ON FILE *(Print/type physician's name)*
☐

20. INITIAL ASSESSMENT *(History, medical complications, level of function at start of care. Reason for referral.)*

19. PRIOR HOSPITALIZATION

FROM   TO   N/A

21. FUNCTIONAL LEVEL *(End of billing period)* PROGRESS REPORT   ☐ CONTINUE SERVICES **OR**   ☐ DC SERVICES

22. SERVICE DATES
FROM   THROUGH

Form CMS-700-(11-91)

INSTRUCTIONS FOR COMPLETION OF FORM CMS-700

(Enter dates as 6 digits, month, day, year)

1. **Patient s Name** - Enter the patient's last name, first name and middle initial as shown on the health insurance Medicare card.

2. **Provider Number** - Enter the number issued by Medicare to the billing provider *(i.e., 00–7000)*.

3. **HICN** - Enter the patient's health insurance number as shown on the health insurance Medicare card, certification award, utilization notice, temporary eligibility notice, or as reported by SSO.

4. **Provider Name** - Enter the name of the Medicare billing provider.

5. **Medical Record No.** - *(optional)* Enter the patient's medical/clinical record number used by the billing provider.

6. **Onset Date** - Enter the date of onset for the patient's primary medical diagnosis, if it is a new diagnosis, or the date of the most recent exacerbation of a previous diagnosis. If the exact date is not known enter 01 for the day *(i.e., 120191)*. The date matches occurrence code 11 on the UB-92.

7. **SOC** *(start of care)* **Date** - Enter the date services began at the billing provider (the date of the first Medicare billable visit which **remains the same on subsequent claims** until discharge or denial corresponds to occurrence code 35 for PT, 44 for OT, 45 for SLP and 46 for CR on the UB-92).

8. **Type** - Check the type therapy billed; i.e., physical therapy (PT), occupational therapy (OT), speech-language pathology (SLP), cardiac rehabilitation (CR), respiratory therapy (RT), psychological services (PS), skilled nursing services (SN), or social services (SW).

9. **Primary Diagnosis** - Enter the pertinent written medical diagnosis resulting in the therapy disorder and relating to 50% or more of effort in the plan of treatment.

10. **Treatment Diagnosis** - Enter the written treatment diagnosis for which services are rendered. For example, for PT the primary medical diagnosis might be Degeneration of Cervical Intervertebral Disc while the PT treatment DX might be Frozen R Shoulder or, for SLP, while CVA might be the primary medical DX, the treatment DX might be Aphasia. If the same as the primary DX enter SAME.

11. **Visits From Start of Care** - Enter the **cumulative total** visits *(sessions)* completed since services were started at the billing provider for the diagnosis treated, through the last visit on this bill. *(Corresponds to UB-92 value code 50 for PT, 51 for OT, 52 for SLP, or 53 for cardiac rehab.)*

12. **Plan of Treatment/Functional Goals** - Enter brief current plan of treatment goals for the patient for this billing period. Enter the major short-term goals to reach overall long-term outcome. Enter the major plan of treatment to reach stated goals and outcome. Estimate time-frames to reach goals, when possible.

13. **Signature** - Enter the signature *(or name)* and the professional designation of the professional establishing the plan of treatment.

14. **Frequency/Duration** - Enter the current frequency and duration of your treatment; e.g., 3 times per week for 4 weeks is entered 3/Wk x 4Wk.

15. **Physician's Signature** - If the form CMS-700 is used for certification, the physician enters his/her signature. **If certification is required and the form is not being used for certification, check the ON FILE box in item 18.** If the certification is not required for the type service rendered, check the N/A box.

16. **Date** - Enter the date of the physician's signature only if the form is used for certification.

17. **Certification** - Enter the inclusive dates of the certification, **even if the ON FILE box is checked in item 18.** Check the N/A box if certification is not required.

18. **ON FILE** (Means certification signature and date) - Enter the **typed/printed name of the physician** who certified the plan of treatment that is on file at the billing provider. If certification is not required for the type of service checked in item 8, type/print the name of the physician who referred or ordered the service, **but do not check the ON FILE box.**

19. **Prior Hospitalization** - Enter the inclusive dates of recent hospitalization *(1st to DC day)* **pertinent** to the patient's current plan of treatment. Enter N/A if the hospital stay does not relate to the rehabilitation being rendered.

20. **Initial Assessment** - Enter only **current relevant history** from records or patient interview. Enter the major functional limitations stated, if possible, in objective measurable terms. Include only relevant surgical procedures, prior hospitalization and/or therapy for the same condition. Include only pertinent baseline tests and measurements from which to judge future progress or lack of progress.

21. **Functional Level** (end of billing period) - Enter the pertinent progress made and functional levels obtained at the end of the billing period compared to levels shown on initial assessment. Use objective terminology. Date progress when function can be consistently performed. When only a few visits have been made, enter a note indicating the training/treatment rendered and the patient's response if there is no change in function.

22. **Service Dates** - Enter the From and Through dates which represent this billing period *(should be monthly)*. Match the From and Through dates in field 6 on the UB-92. DO NOT use 00 in the date. Example: 01 08 91 for January 8, 1991.

UPDATED PLAN OF PROGRESS FOR OUTPATIENT REHABILITATION

(Complete for Interim to Discharge Claims. Photocopy of CMS-700 or 701 is required.)

1. PATIENT'S LAST NAME	FIRST NAME	M.I.	2. PROVIDER NO.	3. HICN

4. PROVIDER NAME	5. MEDICAL RECORD NO. *(Optional)*	6. ONSET DATE	7. SOC. DATE

8. TYPE ☐PT ☐OT ☐SLP ☐CR ☐RT ☐PS ☐SN ☐SW	9. PRIMARY DIAGNOSIS *(Pertinent Medical D.X.)* 12. FREQ/DURATION *(e.g., 3/Wk. x 4 Wk.)*	10.TREATMENT DIAGNOSIS	11. VISITS FROM SOC.

13. CURRENT PLAN UPDATE, FUNCTIONAL GOALS *(Specify changes to goals and plan.)*

GOALS *(Short Term)*

OUTCOME *(Long Term)*

PLAN

I HAVE REVIEWED THIS PLAN OF TREATMENT AND RECERTIFY A CONTINUING NEED FOR SERVICES. ☐ N/A ☐ DC	14. RECERTIFICATION FROM THROUGH N/A
15. PHYSICIAN'S SIGNATURE	16. DATE	17. ON FILE *(Print/type physician's name)* ☐

18. REASON(S) FOR CONTINUING TREATMENT THIS BILLING PERIOD *(Clarify goals and necessity for continued skilled care.)*

19. SIGNATURE *(or name of professional, including prof. designation)*	20. DATE	21. ☐ CONTINUE SERVICES **OR** ☐ DC SERVICES

22. FUNCTIONAL LEVEL *(At end of billing period — Relate your documentation to functional outcomes and list problems still present.)*

22. SERVICE DATES
FROM   THROUGH

Form CMS-701(11-91)

INSTRUCTIONS FOR COMPLETION OF FORM CMS-701

(Enter dates as 6 digits, month, day, year)

1. **Patient's Name** - Enter the patient's last name, first name and middle initial as shown on the health insurance Medicare card.

2. **Provider Number** - Enter the number issued by Medicare to the billing provider *(i.e., 00–7000)*.

3. **HICN** - Enter the patient's health insurance number as shown on the health insurance Medicare card, certification award, utilization notice, temporary eligibility notice, or as reported by SSO.

4. **Provider Name** - Enter the name of the Medicare billing provider.

5. **Medical Record No.** - *(optional)* Enter the patient's medical/ clinical record number used by the billing provider. *(This is an item which you may enter for your own records.)*

6. **Onset Date** - Enter the date of onset for the patient's primary medical diagnosis, if it is a new diagnosis, or the date of the most recent exacerbation of a previous diagnosis. If the exact date is not known enter 01 for the day *(i.e., 120191)*. The date matches occurrence code 11 on the UB-92.

7. **SOC** *(start of care)* **Date** - Enter the date services began at the billing provider (the date of the first Medicare billable visit which **remains the same on subsequent claims** until discharge or denial corresponds to occurrence code 35 for PT, 44 for OT, 45 for SLP and 46 for CR on the UB-92).

8. **Type** - Check the type therapy billed; i.e., physical therapy (PT), occupational therapy (OT), speech-language pathology (SLP), cardiac rehabilitation (CR), respiratory therapy (RT), psychological services (PS), skilled nursing services (SN), or social services (SW).

9. **Primary Diagnosis** - Enter the pertinent written medical diagnosis resulting in the therapy disorder and relating to 50% or more of effort in the plan of treatment.

10. **Treatment Diagnosis** - Enter the written treatment diagnosis for which services are rendered. For example, for PT the primary medical diagnosis might be Degeneration of Cervical Intervertebral Disc while the PT treatment DX might be Frozen R Shoulder or, for SLP, while CVA might be the primary medical DX, the treatment DX might be Aphasia. If the same as the primary DX enter SAMPLE.

11. **Visits From Start of Care** - Enter the **cumulative total** visits *(sessions)* completed since services were started at the billing provider for the diagnosis treated, through the last visit on this bill. *(Corresponds to UB-92 value code 50 for PT, 51 for OT, 52 for SLP, or 53 for cardiac rehab.)*

12. **Current Frequency/Duration** - Enter the current frequency and duration of your treatment; e.g., 3 times per week for 4 weeks is entered 3/Wk x 4Wk.

13. **Current Plan Update, Functional Goals** - Enter the current plan of treatment goals for the patient for this billing period. *(If the same as shown on the CMS-700 or previous 701 enter "same".)* Enter the short-term goals to reach overall long-term outcome. Justify intensity if appropriate. Estimate time-frames to meet goals, when possible.

14. **Recertification** - Enter the inclusive dates when recertification is required, **even if the ON FILE box is checked in item 17.** Check the N/A box if recertification is not required for the type of service rendered.

15. **Physician's Signature** - If the form CMS-701 is used for recertification, the physician enters his/her signature. If recertification is not required for the type of service rendered, check N/A box. **If the form CMS-701 is not being used for recertification, check the ON FILE box - item 17.** If discharge is ordered, check DC box.

16. **Date** - Enter the date of the physician's signature only if the form is used for recertification.

17. **On File** *(Means certification signature and date)* - Enter the **typed/printed name of the physician** who certified the plan of treatment that is on file at the billing provider. If recertification is not required for the type of service checked in item 8, type/print the name of the physician who referred or ordered the service, **but do not check the ON FILE box.**

18. **Reason(s) For Continuing Treatment This Billing Period** - Enter the **major reasons** why the patient needs to continue skilled rehabilitation **for this billing period** (e.g., briefly state the patient's need for specific functional improvement, skilled training, reduction in complication or improvement in safety and how long you believe this will take, if possible or state your reasons for recommending discontinuance). Complete by the rehab specialist prior to physician's recertification.

19. **Signature** - Enter the signature *(or name)* and the professional designation of the individual justifying or recommending need for care *(or discontinuance)* for this billing period.

20. **Date** - Enter the date of the rehabilitation professional's signature.

21. Check the box if services are continuing or discontinuing at end of this billing period.

22. **Functional Level** *(end of billing period)* - Enter the pertinent progress made through the end of this billing period. Use objective terminology. Compare progress made to that shown on the previous CMS-701, item 22, or the CMS-700, items 20 and 21. Date progress when function can be consistently performed or when meaningful functional improvement is made or when significant regression in function occurs. Your intermediary reviews this progress compared to that on the prior CMS-701 or 700 to determine coverage for this billing period. Send a photocopy of the form covering the previous billing period.

23. **Service Dates** - Enter the From and Through dates which represent this billing period *(should be monthly)*. Match the From and Through dates in field 6 on the UB-92. DO NOT use 00 in the date. Example: 01 08 91 for January 8, 1991.

MEDICARE REDETERMINATION REQUEST FORM

1. Beneficiary's Name: _____

2. Medicare Number: _____

3. Description of Item or Service in Question: _____

4. Date the Service or Item was Received: _____

5. I do not agree with the determination of my claim. MY REASONS ARE:

_____

_____

_____

6. Date of the initial determination notice _____
    (If you received your initial determination notice more than 120 days ago, include your reason for not making this request earlier.)

_____

_____

_____

7. Additional Information Medicare Should Consider: _____

_____

_____

_____

8. Requester's Name: _____

9. Requester's Relationship to the Beneficiary: _____

10. Requester's Address: _____

_____

11. Requester's Telephone Number: _____

12. Requester's Signature: _____

13. Date Signed: _____

14. ❑ I have evidence to submit. (Attach such evidence to this form.)
    ❑ I do not have evidence to submit.

NOTICE: Anyone who misrepresents or falsifies essential information requested by this form may upon conviction be subject to fine or imprisonment under Federal Law.

Form CMS-20027 (05/05) EF 05/2005

TRANSFER OF APPEAL RIGHTS

Important: This form allows you to transfer your appeal rights to your health care provider for an item or service. If your provider accepts your appeal rights, he or she cannot charge you for this item or service (except for applicable coinsurance and deductible amounts) even if Medicare will not pay the claim. **Please see the back for more information before you complete this form.**

Section I must be completed and signed by the beneficiary.

SECTION I: TRANSFER OF APPEAL RIGHTS

1. Name of Patient *(Please Print)*

2. Medicare Number *(9 digits followed by an alpha/numeric suffix)*
☐☐☐ ☐☐ ☐☐☐☐ ☐

4. Phone Number *(Include area code)*

3. Address *(Street)*

City

State

ZIP

5. Item or Service

6. I, _____, voluntarily transfer my appeal rights to _____. I understand that I will have no right to appeal a denied claim for this item or service unless I cancel the transfer in writing. I also understand that I cannot be charged for this item or service (except for applicable coinsurance and deductible amounts) unless I cancel the transfer.

7. Signature

Date

Section II must be completed and signed by the health care provider or supplier.

SECTION II: ACCEPTANCE OF APPEAL RIGHTS

8. I, _____, accept the appeal rights for the item or service listed Line 5. I will not collect payment from the patient for this item or service, except for any applicable deductible or coinsurance.

9. Signature

Date

11. Phone Number

10. Address *(Street)*

City

State

ZIP

Form CMS-20031 (05/05) EF 05/2005   **See the back of this form for more information.**

Appendix H   **333**

1. Why am I receiving this form?

A provider or supplier may not have the right to appeal in some situations, so they may ask you to transfer your appeal rights to them. This allows them to appeal on their own to Medicare.

2. What are my appeal rights?

You have the right to appeal if Medicare decides that they will not pay for an item or service. Your "appeal rights" are your rights to ask Medicare to reconsider their decision to not pay for the item or service.

3. What does it mean to transfer my appeal rights?

You have the right to transfer your appeal rights to your health care provider or supplier for an item or service. If Medicare decides not to pay for the item or service, your provider or supplier will be allowed to appeal the decision. You will not be able to appeal the decision; your provider must do it for you.

4. Who can I transfer my appeal rights to?

You may transfer your appeal rights only to the individual who provided the item or service that you listed in Section I of this form.

5. What financial risks do I take when I transfer my appeal rights?

If a provider or supplier accepts your appeals rights, they cannot bill you for the item or service, unless you cancel the transfer or you already signed an Advance Beneficiary Notice. Whether or not you choose to transfer your appeal rights, you will be responsible for paying the appropriate deductible or coinsurance amounts.

6. Am I transferring my appeal rights for all of my claims?

No, you are only transferring your appeal rights for the item or service that you listed in Section I of this form.

7. How long does the transfer last?

This transfer is permanent, unless you decide to cancel it. However, if you cancel the transfer, you may be responsible for payment if Medicare decides that they will not pay for the item or service.

8. How can I cancel the transfer?

You can cancel the transfer by indicating in writing that you no longer wish to transfer your appeal rights for this item or service. You can do this at any time. For information about canceling the transfer, call 1-800-MEDICARE (1-800-633-4227).

9. Who can I contact if I need help completing this form?

State Health Insurance Assistance Programs (SHIPs) are located in every State. These programs have volunteer counselors who can give you free assistance with Medicare questions. Please check your **Medicare and You handbook** to locate a program in your State. Or, for more information, visit *www.medicare.gov*.

Summary of the Occupational Therapy Practice Framework (2nd ed.)

Domain	Categories	Examples
Area of Occupation	Activities of Daily Living	• Bathing, showering • Bowel and bladder management • Dressing • Eating • Feeding • Functional mobility • Personal device care • Personal hygiene and grooming • Sexual activity • Toilet hygiene
	Instrumental Activities of Daily Living	• Care of others • Care of pets • Child rearing • Communication management • Community mobility • Financial management • Health management and maintenance • Home establishment and management • Meal preparation and cleanup • Religious observance • Safety and emergency maintenance • Shopping
	Rest and Sleep	• Rest • Sleep • Sleep preparation • Sleep participation
	Education	• Formal educational participation • Informal personal education needs or interests exploration • Informal personal education participation
	Work	• Employment interests and pursuits • Employment seeking and acquisition • Job performance • Retirement preparation and adjustment

(Continued)

Domain	Categories	Examples
		• Volunteer exploration • Volunteer participation
	Play	• Play exploration • Play participation
	Leisure	• Leisure exploration • Leisure participation
	Social Participation	• Community • Family • Peer, friend
Client Factors	Values, Beliefs, and Spirituality	• Honesty • Fairness • Work before play • Religious beliefs

	Body Functions	• Specific mental functions
		  ° Higher level cognitive
		  ° Attention
		  ° Memory
		  ° Perception
		  ° Thought
		  ° Mental functions of sequencing complex movement
		  ° Emotional
		  ° Experience of self and time
		• Global mental functions
		  ° Consciousness
		  ° Orientation
		  ° Temperament and personality
		  ° Energy and drive
		  ° Sleep (physiological process)
		• Sensory functions and pain
		  ° Seeing and related functions
		  ° Hearing functions
		  ° Vestibular functions
		  ° Taste functions
		  ° Smell functions
		  ° Proprioceptive functions
		  ° Touch functions
		  ° Pain (sharp, dull, diffuse, phantom)
		  ° Temperature
		  ° Pressure
		• Neuromusculoskeletal and movement-related functions
		  ° Joint mobility
		  ° Joint stability
		  ° Muscle power
		  ° Muscle tone
		  ° Muscle endurance
		  ° Motor reflexes
		  ° Involuntary movement reactions
		  ° Control of voluntary movement
		  ° Gait patterns

Domain	Categories	Examples

		• Cardiovascular, hematological, immunological, and respiratory functions
		  ◦ Endurance
		  ◦ Depth of respiration
		  ◦ Fatigability
		• Voice and speech functions
		  ◦ Voice functions
		  ◦ Fluency and rhythm
		  ◦ Alternative vocalization functions
		• Digestive, metabolic, and endocrine system functions
		• Genitourinary and reproductive functions
		  ◦ Urinary functions
		  ◦ Genital and reproductive functions
		• Skin and related-structure functions
		  ◦ Wound care/wound healing
		  ◦ Skin integrity

	Body Structures	• Structures of the nervous system • Eye, ear, and related structures • Structures involved in voice and speech • Structures of the cardiovascular, immunological, and respiratory systems • Structures related to the digestive, metabolic, and endocrine systems • Structures related to the genitourinary and reproductive systems • Structures related to movement • Skin and related structures
Performance Skills	Motor and Praxis Skills	• Bending • Reaching • Pacing and tempo • Coordination • Balance • Posture • Manipulative skills
	Sensory Perceptual Skills	• Ability to locate sound • Stereognosis • Kinesthesia • Depth perception • Figure/ground discrimination • Visual motor integration
	Emotional Regulation Skills	• Responding to feelings of others • Persistence • Controlling emotions • Recovering from emotional events • Displaying situationally appropriate emotions • Coping strategies

(Continued)

Domain	Categories	Examples
	Cognitive Skills	• Judgment • Sequencing • Organizing • Prioritizing • Creating • Multitasking
	Communication and Social Skills	• Eye contact • Verbal communication • Nonverbal communication • Turn taking • Initiating • Terminating • Personal space
Performance Patterns	Habits	• Automatic behaviors
	Routines	• Following sequence of steps • Following schedules • Following policies and procedures
	Roles	• Parent • Student • Employee • Teacher • Coach • Sick person • Victim • Humanitarian
	Rituals	• Religious observance • Cultural events • Personally meaningful events
Context and Environment	Cultural	• Customs • Beliefs • Activity patterns • Behavioral standards • Expectations
	Personal	• Age • Gender • Socioeconomic status • Educational status • Diagnosis/condition • Ethnicity
	Physical	• Natural environment (e.g., geographic terrain, plants, animals) • Man-made environment (e.g., buildings, furniture, tools, devices)
	Social	• Relationships • Expectations of others • Systems (e.g., political, legal, economic, institutional)

Domain	Categories	Examples
	Temporal	• Stages of life • Time of year • Time of day • Time since diagnosis • Rhythm of activity
	Virtual	• E-mail • Chat rooms • Social networking websites • Videoconferencing
Activity Demands	Objects Used and Their Properties	• Tools • Materials • Equipment
	Space Demands	• Arrangement • Lighting • Temperature • Noise • Ventilation • Humidity • Size
	Social Demands	• Rules • Expectations • Language
	Sequencing and Timing	• Steps of the task • Sequence of steps/tasks • Timing of steps
	Required Actions and Performance Skills	• Sensory • Perceptual • Motor • Praxis • Emotional • Cognitive • Communication • Social performance skills
	Required Body Functions	• Mobility of joints • Level of consciousness • Strength • Endurance
	Required Body Structures	• Hands • Eyes • Ears • Arms • Hips • Lungs • Brain

Adapted from American Occupational Therapy Association (2008). Occupational therapy practice framework: Domain and process, 2nd ed., *American Journal of Occupational Therapy* 62, 625–683. Additional examples provided by K. M. Sames, MBA, OTR/L, FAOTA.

Index

'b' indicates boxed material; 'e' indicate an exercise; 'f' indicates a figure; 't' indicates a table

▼ A ▼

Abbreviated notes, translation, 23e
Abbreviations, 12
  body parts and diagnoses, 14b–17b
  clinical procedures, 18b–21b
  educationally related, 23b
  frequency, 14b
  payment and administration,
    21b–22b
  professional credentials and job
    titles, 12b–13b
  range of motion, 18b
  "x" abbreviations, 17b
ABCD (Audience, Behavior, Condition,
    Degree) goal format, 114–115,
    115e, 121e, 122e
Academic integrity exercise, 72e
Accuracy, CARE documentation system,
    47–48, 50b
Achievable
  RHUMBA goal format, 117, 118e
  SMART goal format, 119, 120e–121e
Action, FEAST goal format, 115, 116e
Action format meeting minute-taking,
    221f
Action verbs, goal writing, 111b–112b
Active voice, 4
Activities of daily living, 28
Activity demands, 28f, 30
Activity Measure-Post Acute Care
    (AM-PAC), 106
Acute care settings, short-term goals,
    111
Additional functions, job description,
    245
Administration, abbreviations, 21b–22b
Administrative documentation, 201–202
  appeal letters, 208
  grants, 222–229
  incident reports, 204
  job descriptions, 237–246
  meetings, 215–221
  policies and procedures, 231–236
Administrative law judge (ALJ), appeals
    process, 211
"Adverse events," 203
Ages 3–21, 178, 182
All capitals, as shouting, 4
American Academy of Pediatrics, 66
American Health Information
    Management Association
    (AHIMA), 63
*American Journal of Occupational
    Therapy* (AJOT), 27
American Occupational Therapy
    Association (AOTA), 25, 66
  appeals, 210
  discontinuation of services, 167

documentation guidelines, 1, 54
documentation standards, 78–80
ethical standards, 58
evaluation process, 91
insurance company denials support,
    214
intervention planning, 126–130
progress reporting, 141
screening standards, 86
American Occupational Therapy
    Association (AOTA) Code of
    ethics
on fraud, 67
on plagiarism, 71
on progress, 129
American Physical Therapy
    Association, 66
American Psychological Association
    (APA)
  professional writing, 4
  standards for writing, 4, 69
American Speech-Language-Hearing
    Association, 66
Americans with Disabilities Act (ADA),
    job descriptions, 237, 244–245
Angier, M., 119
Annual goals
  IEP, 197, 199f, 200
  IFSP, 184, 184f, 189
Appeal letters, 208–213
  Medicare, 213–214
  private insurers, 211–214,
    212e–213e
  sample, 210f
Areas of occupation, 28b, 28–29,
    33e–34e
Assessment
  Medicare definition, 87
  notice and consent, educational
    services, 179e
  occupational therapy definition, 34
  SOAP note, 148–149
  tools bias, 94
Assistance, change measurement, 113b
Asterisk, emphasis, 4
Attendance logs, 160–162, 161f
Audience, ABCD goal format, 114, 115e

▼ B ▼

Background information (Bi)
  evaluation report, 99, 99f, 200f
  intervention plan, 126, 135f
Baum, C., 36
Behavior, ABCD goal format, 114, 115e
Behavioral model/framework,
    documentation influence, 37t
Behavioral, RHUMBA goal format, 117,
    118e

BiFIP format
  evaluation report, 99, 103, 107
  intervention plan, 126
Billable time, 66
Billing code fraud, 66
Billing information protection, 61
Biomechanical model/framework,
    documentation influence, 38t
Birth through age 2, 174, 178,
    182
Body functions and structures, activity
    demands, 30
Body parts, abbreviations, 14b–17b
Bottom-up approach, 44, 44e–45e
  evaluation, 91
Braille, notice and consent forms, 175
Brennan, C., 125
Broad categorizations, 4
Business letter, forms, 6
Buzzwords, 9–10

▼ C ▼

Canadian Model of Occupational
    Performance, documentation
    influence, 38t
Cap exceptions, Medicare
    B therapy, 66
Care plan. *See* Intervention plan
CARE documentation system, 47,
    51e–52e
  accuracy, 47–48, 50b
  clarity, 47, 50b
  exceptions, 49, 50b
  relevance, 48–49, 50b
Career Onestop, Minnesota, 239
"Catchall" sentences, job
    description, 245
Center for Academic Integrity, Duke
    University, 70
Centers for Medicare and Medicaid
    Services (CMS), 66, 87, 105
Certification and re-certification,
    Medicare, 83
Change
  description and measurement, 112,
    113b–114b
  words describing, 129b–130b, 132
Cheating, attitudes toward, 70–71
Children with special needs,
    documentation of services, 1
Christiansen, C., 36
Clarification orders, 83
Clarity, CARE documentation system,
    47, 50b
Client
  occupational therapy definition, 34
  *Occupational Therapy Practice
    Framework* definition, 28